Contents

Diseases of the Goat

Second Edition

John G. Matthews
BSc, BVMS, MRCVS

Clarendon House Veterinary Centre,
Chelmsford, UK

Blackwell
Science

> **To my wife Hilary who understands goats**
> **and my mother Lesley who never will**

© 1999
Blackwell Science Ltd
Editorial Offices:
Osney Mead, Oxford OX2 0EL
25 John Street, London WC1N 2BL
23 Ainslie Place, Edinburgh EH3 6AJ
350 Main Street, Malden
  MA 02148 5018, USA
54 University Street, Carlton
  Victoria 3053, Australia
10, rue Casimir Delavigne
  75006 Paris, France

Other Editorial Offices:

Blackwell Wissenschafts-Verlag GmbH
Kurfürstendamm 57
10707 Berlin, Germany

Blackwell Science KK
MG Kodenmacho Building
7-10 Kodenmacho Nihombashi
Chuo-ku, Tokyo 104, Japan

The right of the Author to be identified as the
Author of this Work has been asserted in
accordance with the Copyright, Designs and
Patents Act 1988.

First edition published as Outline of Clinical
Diagnosis in the Goat by Butterworth-
Heinemann Ltd, 1991
Second edition published by Blackwell Science,
1999
Reprinted 2001

Set in 10/12pt Palatino
by DP Photosetting, Aylesbury, Bucks
Printed and bound in Great Britain by
Biddles Ltd, *www.biddles.co.uk*

DISTRIBUTORS

Marston Book Services Ltd
PO Box 269
Abingdon
Oxon OX14 4YN
(*Orders:* Tel: 01235 465500
          Fax: 01235 465555)

USA
Blackwell Science, Inc.
Commerce Place
350 Main Street
Malden, MA 02148 5018
(*Orders:* Tel: 800 759 6102
          781 388 8250
          Fax: 781 388 8255)

Canada
Login Brothers Book Company
324 Saulteaux Crescent
Winnipeg, Manitoba R3J 3T2
(*Orders:* Tel: 204-837-2987
          Fax: 204-837-3116)

Australia
Blackwell Science Pty Ltd.
54 University Street
Carlton, Victoria 3053
(*Orders:* Tel: 3 9347 0300
          Fax: 3 9347 5001)

A catalogue record for this title
is available from the British Library

Library of Congress
Cataloging-in-Publication Data

For further information on
Blackwell Science, visit our website:
www.blackwell-science.com

Matthews, John G.
    Diseases of the goat/John G. Matthews. — 2nd 3d.
        p. cm.
    Rev. ed. of : Outline of clinical diagnosis in the goat.
    1991.
    Includes bibliographical references (p.   ).
    ISBN 0–632–05167–1 (pbk.)
    1. Goats—Diseases—Diagnosis. 2. Veterinary clinical
    pathology.
    I. Matthews, John D. Outline of clinical diagnosis in the
goat/
    II. Title.
    SF968.M37   1999
    636.3′90896—dc21   99–34208
                                            CIP

The Blackwell Science logo is a trade mark of Blackwell
Science Ltd, registered at the United Kingdom Trade Marks
Registry

Preface to First Edition

The increasing interest in goats in the UK, both for milk and fibre production, has been matched by a corresponding awareness in the veterinary profession that the species merits consideration as an animal in its own right. The formation of the Goat Veterinary Society in 1979 provided a means of collating and disseminating information on goat management and disease control, but until now there has been no readily available text covering goat diseases. Hopefully this book will, at least in part, fill that gap.

The book gives an outline of the more common clinical problems likely to be met by the general practitioner involved with goat medicine, with each chapter covering a major presenting sign. Each chapter starts with the initial assessment and clinical examination of the patient, together with further investigations which may aid diagnosis, before considering specific diseases, their diagnosis, clinical signs and treatment. At the end of each chapter there is a short list of references – these are generally review articles which the clinician will find of interest. A list of general references is included at the end of the book. In addition there is a chapter on plant poisoning.

It has been said that the goat is 'mostly sheep and partly cow' and, undoubtedly, any veterinary surgeon with a working knowledge of other ruminants should be able satisfactorily to diagnose and treat most medical conditions in the goat. There are, however, important behavioural and physiological differences between the species, resulting, in many instances, in important differences in their response to disease, so that it is not always safe to extrapolate from one species to another. In addition, drug metabolism shows species variation, with the result that dose rates and excretion times for goats are not simply obtained from cow or sheep data. I hope that having read this book, the clinician will feel confident in treating not a small cow or a large milking sheep but the animal in its own right – the goat.

Preface to Second Edition

In the 8 years since the publication of the first edition of this book in 1991, the population of goats in the UK and hence the veterinary surgeon's involvement with them has changed. The hype surrounding Angora goats has subsided and their numbers have stabilised. There are fewer small herds of dairy goats being kept for milk and showing, but truly commercial dairy goat farming is well established, with herds of 1000, or even 2000, milkers becoming a reality and British goat products featured on the supermarket shelves. The veterinary surgeon is as likely to be presented with a Pygmy goat as one of its larger cousins. I hope this book will continue to provide the veterinary surgeons with a readily accessible source of information on the diagnosis and treatment of the diseases of the goat, which they will find useful, however great or small their professional involvement with the species.

Drugs in the text marked 'G' are licensed for use in goats in the UK.

John Matthews
May 1999

Acknowledgements

I acknowledge with grateful thanks the forbearance of my colleagues at Clarendon House Veterinary Centre during the writing of this book.

My wife Hilary has provided encouragement and support and given valuable advice on goat husbandry.

Author's Note

For many medical conditions, there are no drugs available which are specifically licensed for goats. Dose rates are quoted in the book for many unlicensed drugs. These dose rates have been obtained from published reports, data held on file by the drug manufacturers and from personal experience. Wherever possible, the clinician should use drugs which carry a full product licence for caprine treatment. If in doubt about the use or dosage of any drug, consult the manufacturer. In all cases where unlicensed drugs are used, milk should not be used for human consumption for 7 days and meat for 28 days following the administration of the drug.

Wherever possible drugs are matched with licensed products currently available in the UK, but these change monthly, and not all drugs quoted have a current licence for food-producing animals in the UK. It is the reader's responsibility to ensure that he/she is legally entitled to use any drug mentioned.

1 Female Infertility

The normal female goat

In temperate regions, female goats are seasonally polyoestrus. Most goats are totally anoestrus in the northern hemisphere between March and August, although fertile matings have been recorded in all months of the year. Anglo-Nubian and Pygmy goats in particular have extremely long breeding seasons. Recently imported goats from the southern hemisphere may take time to adjust to a new seasonality. The breeding season is initiated largely in response to decreasing day length, but is also dependent on temperature, the environment (particularly nutrition) and the presence of a male. Decreasing day length also stimulates reproductive activity in the buck. Table 1.1 details the reproductive aspects of the goat.

Table 1.1 Reproduction in the goat.

Breeding season	September to March (northern hemisphere)
Puberty	5 months
Age at first service	4 to 6 months (male) 7 to 18 months (female)
Oestrus cycle	19 to 21 days (dairy goats) 18 to 24 days (Pygmy goats)
Duration of oestrus	24 to 96 hours (usually 36 to 40 hours)
Ovulation	24 to 48 hours after start of oestrus
Gestation length	150 days (145 to 156 days)

Investigation of female infertility

Because of the seasonal pattern of breeding, infertility must be investigated as early as possible in the breeding season.

The investigation of female infertility in the goat presents major difficulties when compared with that in the cow because of the inability to palpate the ovaries and because of the seasonal pattern of breeding – does are often presented towards the end of the season, limiting the time available for remedial measures (Figure 1.1).

Initial assessment

The preliminary history should consider:

- ❏ Individual or herd/flock problem.
- ❏ Feeding, including mineral supplementation.
- ❏ Management practices – handmating, artificial insemination (AI), buck running with does.
- ❏ Disease status of herd/flock.

If there is a *herd problem* (Figure 1.1), investigate:

- ❏ Male infertility (qv).
- ❏ Intercurrent disease – parasitism, footrot, etc.
- ❏ Nutritional status – energy or protein deficit, mineral deficiency (phosphorus, copper, iodine, manganese).
- ❏ Stress – overcrowding, recent grouping of goats.
- ❏ Poor heat detection.
- ❏ Services at incorrect time.

Assessment of individual doe

General assessment

- ❏ Conformation.
- ❏ Body condition.
- ❏ Dentition.
- ❏ Clinical examination.

Any obvious clinical signs such as debility, anaemia or lameness should be investigated and corrected where possible before commencing specific therapy aimed at correcting a reproductive disorder.

In the UK overfeeding is probably a greater cause of infertility than poor condition.

Specific examination

- ❏ Specific examination of the reproductive and mammary systems. Include, where necessary, examination of the vagina and cervix with a speculum to identify anatomical abnormalities.

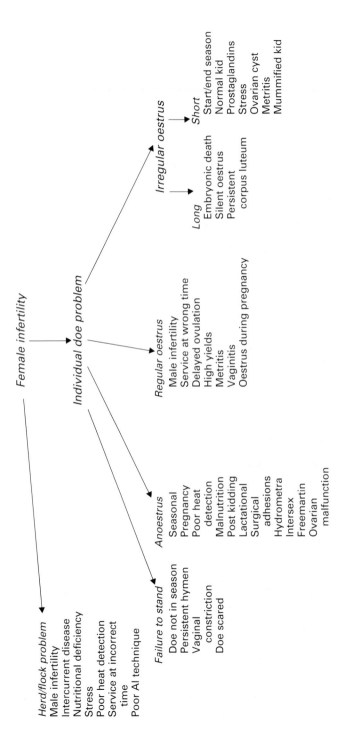

Figure 1.1 Causes of female infertility

Specific history

- ❏ Date of last kidding/stage of lactation.
- ❏ Daily milk yield.
- ❏ Presence or absence of obvious oestrus signs.
- ❏ Length of oestrus cycles.
- ❏ Date of last service.
- ❏ Willingness to stand for male.
- ❏ Kidding difficulties last time – malpresentation/manipulation, metritis, retained placenta, abortion, mummified fetus, stillbirths.

Further investigations

- ❏ Specific laboratory tests:
  - ■ progesterone assay
  - ■ oestrone sulphate assay
  - ■ bacteriological examination of vaginal or uterine samples
  - ■ feed analysis
- ❏ Laparoscopy or laparotomy.
- ❏ Realtime ultrasound scanning.

The four main individual infertility problems

Individual infertility problems will generally fall into one of four categories:

(1) Difficulty at service.
(2) Anoestrus.
(3) Irregular oestrus cycles.
(4) Regular oestrus cycles.

Difficulty at service

- ❏ Doe not in season.
- ❏ Doe scared – common with maiden animals, particularly if a large buck is used on a small doe.
- ❏ Persistent hymen or vaginal constriction.

Anoestrus

> Always consider the possibility of an undetected pregnancy (even if the owner insists that no mating has occurred) before attempting treatment, particularly with prostaglandins.

The causes of anoestrus are listed in Table 1.2 and discussed below.

❑ *Seasonal* – most goats are totally anoestrus between March and August.
❑ *Pregnancy.*
❑ *Poor heat detection.*

Table 1.2   Causes of anoestrus.

Seasonal
Pregnancy
Poor heat detection
Malnutrition
Post-kidding anoestrus
Lactational anoestrus
Adhesions following surgery
Hydrometra
Intersex
Freemartin
Ovarian malfunction

Although some dairy goats show only minor behavioural changes during oestrus, oestrus detection is generally easier than in Angora goats, with most does showing obvious signs of tail wagging, frequent bleating, urination near the buck, swelling of the vulva and a mucous vaginal discharge. The signs are generally accentuated in the presence of a male or even a 'billy rag', i.e. a cloth which has been rubbed on the head of a buck and stored in a sealed jar.

Oestrus can be determined visually by means of a speculum. At the onset of heat, the cervix changes from its normal white colour, becoming hyperaemic, and the cervical secretions are thin and clear. The secretions rapidly thicken, becoming grey/white and collecting on the floor of the vagina. Unlike cows, most does will not stand to be ridden by other females even when in oestrus. Riding behaviour is sometimes seen as an expression of dominance in the herd or as part of the nymphomaniac behaviour of goats with cystic ovaries. Many young bucks will mount and serve females which are not in true standing oestrus if the female is restrained, although older bucks are more discriminating. The doe will stand to be mated only when she is in oestrus.

In the milking doe, a rise in milk production may occur 8 to 12 hours before the start of oestrus and milk production may fall below normal during oestrus.

When the buck is running with the flock or herd, sire harnesses with raddles or marker paste will aid oestrus detection. A marked vasectomised ('teaser') buck can be used to detect (and help initiate) the start of oestrus in a group of does.

❏ *Malnutrition* – an energy or protein deficit due either to poor nutrition or intercurrent disease may cause anoestrus.
  Deficiencies of minerals such as cobalt, selenium, manganese, zinc, phosphorus, iodine and copper and deficiencies of vitamins B_{12} and D are all reported to cause infertility.

❏ *Post-kidding anoestrus* – many does will not show signs of oestrus for 3 months or more after kidding even if kidding takes place during the normal breeding season.

❏ *Lactational anoestrus* – some high yielding does do not exhibit marked signs of oestrus. These animals may respond to prostaglandin injections with careful observation for oestrus 24 to 48 hours later. Animals which do not respond may need a further injection 11 days later.

❏ *Adhesions following surgery* – the goat's reproductive tract is sensitive to handling and adhesions will occur unless very high standards of surgery are maintained during embryo transplant or other surgical procedures. Talc from surgical gloves will produce a marked tissue reaction.

❏ *False pregnancy (hydrometra, cloudburst)*
  False pregnancy occurs when aseptic fluid accumulates in the uterus in the absence of pregnancy but in the presence of a persistent corpus luteum which continues to secrete progesterone. The incidence of false pregnancies is fairly high, particularly in some strains of dairy goats.

Aetiology

❏ A persistent corpus luteum following an oestrus cycle in which pregnancy did not occur. This may occur in any sexually mature female but is particularly common in goats in their second year of a lactation ('running through') without being mated. Certain families seem prone to develop the condition.

❏ A persistent corpus luteum following embryonic death with resorption of the embryo.

Clinical signs

The doe acts as if pregnant, with enlargement of the abdomen and a degree of udder development if not milking. Milking does may show a sharp drop in yield and this may result in a significant economic loss if the condition is not corrected. Fetal fluids collect in the abdomen (*hydrometra*) and the doe may become enormously distended, although the amount of fluid varies from 1 to 7 l or more. When the hydrometra occurs following embryonic death, the false pregnancy generally persists for the full gestational length or longer before luteolysis occurs, progesterone secretion ceases and the fetal fluids are released (*cloudburst*). Some does milk adequately following a natural cloudburst.

When the false pregnancy occurs in a doe which has not been mated, the release of fluid often occurs in less than the normal gestation period, the doe may cycle again and a further false pregnancy may occur if she is not mated. Subsequent pregnancies are not generally affected, but the doe is likely to develop the condition again the following year. The expelled fluid is generally clear and mucoid so that the tail becomes sticky. Some goats that spontaneously cloudburst early, before a large amount of fluid has accumulated, have a bloody discharge.

If the false pregnancy follows fetal death, fetal membranes and possibly a decomposed fetus are present; otherwise no fetal membranes are formed.

Diagnosis

❑ Realtime ultrasound scanning of the right ventrolateral abdominal wall in early false pregnancy, or of either flank later, shows large fluid-filled compartments with the absence of fetuses or caruncles. Scanning should take place at least 40 days after mating to avoid confusion with early pregnancy.
❑ Elevated milk or plasma progesterone levels consistent with pregnancy, but low milk or plasma oestrone sulphate levels.
❑ X-ray fails to show fetal skeletons in an anoestrus doe with a distended abdomen.

Treatment

❑ Prostaglandin injection:
   Dinaprost, 2 ml i.m. or **s.c. (Lutalyse**, Pharmacia & Upjohn)
   Clorprostenol, 0.5 ml i.m. or **s.c. (Estrumate**, Schering-Plough).
   Lutalyse has a direct effect on uterine muscle and may be preferable to Estrumate.
❑ An oxytocin injection a few days after treatment with prostaglandin stimulates uterine contractions and aids involution:
   Oxytocin, 2–10 units, 0.2–1.0 ml i.m. or **s.c. (Oxytocin-S**, Intervet) (G)
   Pituitary extract (posterior lobe), 20–50 units, 2–5 ml i.m. or **s.c. (Hyposton**, Pharmacia & Uphohn) (G) or **2–10 units, 0.2–1.0 ml i.m.** (preferred) or **s.c. [Pituitary Extract (Synthetic)**, Animalcare] (G)

A false pregnancy may need to be distinguished from *hydrops uteri*. Hydrops uteri is an unusual condition of pregnant goats caused by an abnormal accumulation of fluid in either the amniotic (hydamnios) or allantoic (hydrallantois) sacs. Distension of the uterus is caused by accumulation of fluid which may be greater than 10 litres, leading to bilateral, rapidly progressive abdominal distension. Other clinical signs, similar to those of pregnancy toxaemia, are a result of compression of other organs by the fluid – lethargy, inappetence, decreased defaecation, recumbency, tachycardia and dyspnoea.

Ultrasonography can be used to distinguish between false pregnancy (hydrometra), where the uterus is distended with fluid but no fetuses, membranes or cotyledons are present, and hydrops uteri, where fluid, fetuses, membranes and cotyledons are present. Most fetuses of animals with hydrops uteri have congenital defects and are underdeveloped, but may appear normal although not viable.

Treatment is by caesarian section or by induction of parturition with prostaglandins, but cardiovascular support with intravenous fluids should be provided because of the danger of hypotension from the sudden loss of large volumes of fluid.

❏ *Intersex (pseudohermaphrodite)* – an animal which shows both male and female characteristics. In goats the dominant gene for absence of horns (polled condition) is associated with a recessive gene for intersex. Thus an intersex is normally polled with two polled parents. Intersex is a recessive sex-linked incompletely penetrant trait resulting from the breeding of two polled goats.

A mating between a homozygous (PP) polled male and a heterozygous (Pp) polled female will produce 50% intersexes; a mating between a heterozygous (Pp) polled male and a heterozygous (Pp) polled female will produce 25% intersexes.

Affected animals are genetically female with a normal female chromosome complement (60 XX), but phenotypically show great variation from phenotypic male to phenotypic female. Some animals are obviously abnormal at birth with a normal vulva but enlarged clitoris or a penile clitoris. The gonads are generally testes or ovotestes which may be abdominal or scrotal and phenotypic males may have a shortened penis (hypospadias), hypoplastic testes, or sperm granuloma in the head of the epididymis. Other animals may reach maturity before being detected and may present as being anoestrus. A phenotypically female animal may have male characteristics due to internal testes.

❏ *Freemartins* – a freemartin is a female rendered sterile in utero when her placenta and that of her twin male fuses in early gestation, allowing vascular anastomosis and exchange of cells and hormones between the two fetuses and resulting in hypoplasia of the female gonads and XX/XY chimaerism. A freemartin may be polled or horned. Most females born cotwin to males are normal females, i.e. placental fusion is unusual. There is some evidence that the condition is slightly more common when the female shares the uterus with two or more male fetuses.

❑ *Ovarian malfunction* – ovarian inactivity is poorly understood in the goat, but some anoestrus goats will respond to treatment with gonadotrophin releasing hormone:

> **Buserelin, 5 ml i.m., s.c.** or **i.v. (Receptal**, Hoechst Roussel)
> **Gonadorellin, 5 ml i.m. (Fertagyl**, Intervet).

Other goats will respond to treatment with prostaglandins, suggesting a *persistent corpus luteum* or *luteinised cystic ovaries.* Increased use of laparoscopic techniques may aid the diagnosis of these conditions.

Irregular oestrus cycles (Table 1.3)

Long oestrus cycles

❑ *Embryonic death* – early embryonic death with loss of the corpus luteum will produce a subsequent return to oestrus following resorption of the embryonic material. Following embryonic death, a percentage of does will not return to oestrus but develop hydrometra.

❑ *Silent oestrus* – some does will exhibit oestrus early in the season and then show no further oestrus signs for some months. These goats may be cycling silently and will respond to treatment with prostaglandins.

❑ *Persistent corpus luteum* – failure of the corpus luteum to undergo luteolysis at the correct time will delay the return to oestrus. Treat with prostaglandins.

Table 1.3   Irregular oestrus cycles.

Long	Short
Embryonic death	Start/end of season
Silent oestrus	Normal kid behaviour
Persistent corpus luteum	Prostaglandins
	Stress
	Ovarian follicular cyst
	Metritis
	Mummified kid

Short oestrus cycles (less than 18 to 21 days)

❏ Short anovulatory cycles of about 7 days are common at the start of the breeding season and occasionally occur at the end of the breeding season.

❏ Kids commonly show short cycles during their first breeding season.

❏ Very short oestrus cycles have been recorded following administration of prostaglandins to abort does. A normal oestrus pattern returns after 3 to 4 weeks.

❏ Premature regression of the corpus luteum is recognised as a problem in goats undergoing oestrus synchronisation for embryo transplant. In some cases this will be a result of stress (see below). In other cases, the cause is unknown.

❏ Groups of goats which are stressed will often show short cycles of around 7 days presumably because of premature regression of the corpus luteum. For this reason goats being brought together for a breeding programme, e.g. for embryo transplant, should be grouped at least 3 months before the start of the programme.

❏ Ovarian follicular cysts produce oestrogens which result in a shortened oestrus cycle of between 3 and 7 days or continuous heat. Eventually the oestrogenic effects produce relaxed pelvic ligaments and the goat displays male-like mounting behaviour. The diagnosis can be confirmed by laparoscopy or laparotomy.

Medical treatment with

Chorionic gonadotrophin 1000 U, i.m. or i.v. (Chorulon, Intervet) or with

Gonadotrophin releasing hormone:

Buserelin, 5 ml i.m., s.c. or i.v. (Receptal, Hoechst Roussel) or

Gonadorellin, 5 ml i.m. (Fertagyl, Intervet)

is only successful if commenced early. Surgical treatment to exteriorise and rupture the thick wall of the cyst should be considered in valuable animals. Treatment is exceptionally difficult in goats because the relatively short breeding season means that by the time treatment is completed the doe has already entered seasonal anoestrus.

❏ Endometritis may cause short cycling or return to oestrus at the normal time.

❏ Vaginitis – see 'Regular oestrus cycles'.

❏ The presence of fetal bone remaining from a mummified kid which is not expelled at parturition will act as a constant source of stimulation and result in short oestrus cycles. There may be a history of bones and fetal material being expelled at kidding or subsequently.

Regular oestrus cycles (Table 1.4)

❏ *Male infertility* (qv).
❏ *Service at the wrong time.*
❏ *Delayed ovulation/follicular atresia* – there is little scientific evidence describing these conditions in goats, but in practice a 'holding' injection given at the time of service or AI will aid fertility in some animals by stimulating ovulation on the day of service:
   Chorionic gonadotrophin, 500 U (Chorulon, Intervet) or
   Gonadotrophin releasing hormones, 2.5 ml i.m. (Receptal, Hoechst Roussel).
❏ *High yielding females* – some high yielding females may have sub-optimum fertility possibly due to a pituitary dysfunction resulting from the heavy lactation.
   Chorionic gonadotrophin, 500 U, i.m. or i.v. (Chorulon, Intervet)
   may promote maturation of follicles, ovulation and formation of the corpus luteum.
❏ *Metritis* – a low-grade metritis may result in the failure of the embryo to implant and subsequent return to service at the normal time.
❏ *Vaginitis* – this occasionally occurs, particularly after the removal of vaginal sponges. Vaginitis may result in short oestrus cycles or repeated return to service at a normal cycle length.
   In New Zealand and Australia, caprine herpes virus type 1 causes vulvovaginitis with short oestrus cycles.
❏ *Oestrus during pregnancy* – a few goats exhibit regular oestrus signs during pregnancy although this is less common than in cattle. Ovulation does not occur and the signs of oestrus are usually rather weak. Accurate pregnancy diagnosis is important before attempting treatment, particularly with prostaglandins.

Table 1.4 Regular oestrus cycles.

Male infertility
Service at the wrong time
Delayed ovulation
High yielders
Metritis
Vaginitis
Oestrus during pregnancy

Pregnancy diagnosis

> Non-return to service is not a reliable method of pregnancy diagnosis. Many does do not outwardly cycle throughout the breeding season and the non-return may be due to seasonal anoestrus or false pregnancy.
>
> Neither is mammary development in primarous goats a reliable method of pregnancy diagnosis as maiden milkers are common.
>
> Nor is abdominal distension.

Accurate pregnancy diagnosis is essential to distinguish between pregnant goats, those with false pregnancies and those which are not cycling.

Oestrone sulphate assay

Oestrone sulphate concentrations in milk and plasma increase steadily during pregnancy and can be used to diagnose pregnancy 50 days post service. Milk samples can be submitted to Genus Veterinary Laboratory, Cleeve House, Lower Wick, Worcester WR2 4NS and milk or blood to other commercial laboratories.

This test will distinguish between true pregnancy and hydrometra, but occasional false negatives do occur, particularly if the sampling is close to 50 days, and repeat sampling may be indicated before the induction of oestrus with prostaglandins to avoid the possibility of aborting a pregnant doe.

Ultrasonic scanning

Realtime ultrasonic scanning has the added advantage of giving *some* indication of the number of kids being carried, thus enabling a better estimate of the nutritional requirements of the doe during pregnancy. The technique is virtually 100% accurate in determining pregnancy and 96 to 97% accurate in determining twins and triplets. Good operators can distinguish hydrometra and resorbed fetuses as well as live kids.

Scanning can be used from 28 days post service when a fluid-filled uterus can be identified, but is best used between 50 and 100 days of pregnancy. Cotyledons can be distinguished from about 40 days and individual fetuses by 45 to 50 days. By 100 days individual fetuses more than fill the entire screen, making accurate determination of numbers difficult.

Transabdominal scanning is usually carried out with the goat standing. Early in pregnancy (30 to 45 days), the uterus lies towards the pelvis inlet, but later is usually against the right abdominal wall. A 5-MHz transducer is suitable for most of the pregnancy, but may not penetrate as far as the fetus in late gestation, although caruncles will be visible. Between 40 and 100 days, the length of the fetuses and the fetal head width or biparietal diameter (BPD) correlate closely with gestational age (see Figure 1.2). Later in pregnancy, the variation in size of fetuses is too great to permit accurate age determination.

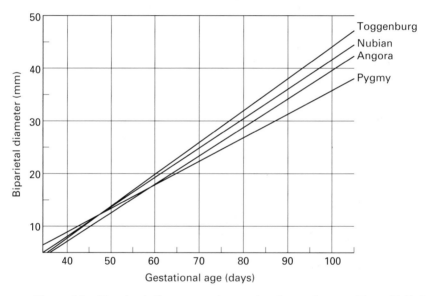

Figure 1.2 Biparietal diameter and gestational age of goats. (From Haibel *et al.*, 1989)

Doppler ultrasound techniques

Doppler ultrasound techniques can detect the fetal pulse after about 2 months' gestation, using either an intrapelvic probe or an external probe placed on a clipped site immediately in from the right udder or lateral to the left udder using vegetable oil to improve contact.

Between 60 and 120 days' gestation the accuracy in detecting non-pregnancy is more than 90%, but the method is unreliable in detecting multiple fetuses.

Other methods are sometimes useful:

Progesterone assay

Progesterone secreted by the corpus luteum of a pregnant goat can be detected by radioimmunoassay or by ELISA methods in milk or in plasma. Progesterone levels remain high throughout pregnancy.

Random sampling will not lead to accurate pregnancy diagnosis because the corpus luteum of the normal oestrus cycle and that of hydrometra also produce progesterone. A sample taken 24 days after mating will give nearly 100% accuracy in determining non-pregnancy but only about 85 to 90% accuracy in determining pregnancy because of factors such as early embryonic death and hydrometra. A low progesterone level always indicates non-pregnancy.

X-ray

Fetal skeletons are detectable by X-ray between 70 and 80 days, although the technique is more useful after 90 days. An enlarged uterus may be detected at 38 days and over.

Rectoabdominal palpation

In the non-pregnant goat a plastic rod inserted in the rectum can be palpated at the body wall. Between 70 and 100 days post service, the pregnant uterus prevents palpation of the rod. However, the technique produces unacceptably high levels of fetal mortality and risk of rectal perforation.

Ballotment

Ballotment of the right flank or ventrally is a time-honoured goat-keepers' technique for pregnancy diagnosis, but in the author's experience it is extremely unreliable. Fetal movements can often be observed in the right flank of the doe during the last 30 days of gestation.

Use of prostaglandins

Unlike other ruminants where placenta-derived progesterone becomes significant, the goat depends on corpus-luteum-derived progesterone throughout pregnancy, and is thus susceptible to luteolytic agents, including prostaglandins, throughout the whole of the pregnancy.

Prostaglandins can be used for:

❏   Timing of oestrus.
❏   Synchronisation of oestrus.

❏ Misalliance.
❏ Abortion.
❏ Timing and synchronisation of parturition.
❏ Treatment of hydrometra.
❏ Treatment of persistent corpus luteum.

> Prostaglandins can be used to terminate pregnancy throughout the whole gestation period.

Suggested doses of prostaglandins in dairy goats are:
  Clorprostenol, 0.5 ml i.m. or **s.c.** (**Estrumate**, Schering-Plough);
  Dinaprost, 5 ml i.m. or **s.c.** (**Lutalyse**, Pharmacia & Upjohn).
Smaller doses will produce luteolysis in Angora goats. The effect of prostaglandin administration is seen between 24 and 48 hours (generally around 36 hours) post-injection, provided the animal being injected has an active corpus luteum, i.e. between days 4 and 17 of the normal oestrus cycle or during pregnancy.

For induction of parturition where live kids are required, prostaglandins should not be used before day 144 of gestation, because prostaglandins bypass the steps involved in producing fetal lung surfactant. Before day 144, dexamethasone should be used and will produce parturition in about 48 to 96 hours (Figure 1.3).

Where rapid termination is required and the viability of the kids is not critical, e.g. collapsed doe, prostaglandins can be used at any stage of gestation.

There is generally no problem with retained fetal membranes following induction with prostaglandins or dexamethasone.

Control of the breeding season

Out-of-season breeding is being increasingly used to enable milk producers to maintain regular supplies of fresh milk and to produce three kid crops in 2 years from fibre goats. Best results are obtained when the techniques are used to extend the breeding season, i.e. by early or late season breeding, rather than in deep anoestrus.

Introduction of a buck or teaser male

Introduction of a buck or teaser male produces oestrus before the start of the breeding season, with loose synchronisation of oestrus. The introduction of a teaser or entire male into a group of does, which have been deprived of the sound, sight and smell of a male

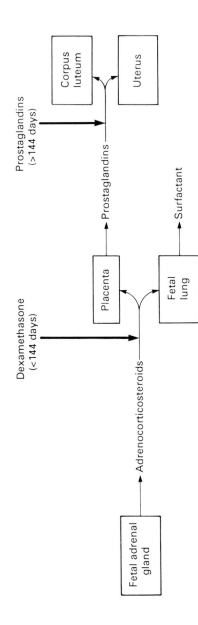

Figure 1.3 Induction of parturition.

for at least 4 to 6 weeks during the transitional period before the start of the normal breeding season, will produce oestrus cycles within 3 to 10 days, but the first one or two oestruses may be silent, without any sign of behavioural oestrus. A silent oestrus may be followed by a fertile oestrus 21 days later or the first silent oestrus may be followed by a short cycle and a second silent oestrus or fertile oestrus after about 5 days, following premature regression of the corpus luteum.

The fertility of the females after exposure is variable – the closer to the breeding season, the higher the fertility.

Lighting regimes

Lighting extends the breeding season into the spring, with synchronisation of oestrus. Does respond to a shortening daylength by ovulation and oestrus. Keeping goats under an artificially long daylight regime during the winter months, followed by a sudden change to normal daylength in the spring, enables out-of-season breeding to be achieved from April to June during the normal anoestrus period.

From 1 January, give 20 hours of artificial light for 60 days. After 60 days, return the goats to normal lighting. Oestrus occurs 7 to 10 weeks later. The oestrus period may be shorter than normal and the signs of oestrus not very obvious, so best results are obtained if the males are run with the females. Sudden introduction of the male to the females after their return to normal daylength increases the percentage of successful matings.

The lights must be of sufficient number and intensity to simulate daylight and the males should undergo light treatment at the same time as females. With this regime, kidding rates of 50 to 60% can be expected, although up to 90% has been obtained.

Theoretically, it is not necessary to provide continuous lighting for the extended long day period. In sheep, a long day effect can be obtained by providing one extra hour of light during the night, provided it is given 7 to 8 hours before dawn. However, equivocal results have been obtained with goats, so the practical application of short light pulses remains to be established.

Progestagen-impregnated intravaginal sponges

Progestagen-impregnated intravaginal sponges enable:

❑ Oestrus synchronisation within the breeding season.
❑ Extension of the breeding season.
❑ Out-of-season breeding.

Two types of intravaginal sponge are currently available in the UK:

Medroxyprogesterone, 60 mg (Veramix Sheep Sponge, Pharmacia & Upjohn)

Flugestone acetate, 30 mg (Chronogest, Intervet).

Applicators are available for insertion of the sponges, but because the goat's vagina is more delicate than that of sheep, it is generally better to insert the sponges manually with a gloved hand using a small amount of antiseptic cream. If the animals are handled gently, the incidence of vaginitis or vaginal adhesions is low, but antibiotic powder may be used at insertion:

Oxytetracycline powder (Oxytetracycline, Bimeda; **Terramycin**, Pfizer).

Chronogest sponges are removed after 11 to 14 days. Veramix sponges are removed after 11 to 17 days. Short progesterone treatments seem to give the best results but should be used in combination with a prostaglandin injection (qv) given 2 days before withdrawal, during the breeding season. Removal of the sponges promotes oestrus in 95 to 100% of animals in the transitionary and normal breeding periods, but in only about 70% of animals outside these periods. Two days before sponge removal, or at sponge removal if during the breeding season, a dose of follicle stimulating hormone is administered to ensure optimum ovulation:

Serum gonadotrophin, s.c. or **i.m. (Folligon**, Intervet; **Fostim**, Pharmacia & Upjohn) (G).

The dose depends on the size of the goat, its yield and the season when the sponges are being used (Table 1.5). If high doses of serum gonadotrophin are used, superovulation may occur, with resultant multiple births. There are usually very strong signs of oestrus following sponging. Oestrus occurs 24 to 72 hours after sponge removal

Table 1.5 Serum gonadotrophin treatments for sponged goats.

	Time of injection of serum gonadotrophin	Dose of serum gonadotrophin (U)	
		Production of milk/day	
		<3.5 kg	>3.5 kg
Out of season (March–June)	48 hours before sponge removal	600	700
Transitory period	48 hours before sponge removal	500	600
Breeding season (Sept–Feb)	At sponge removal	400	500

(generally 30 to 36 hours). The optimum time for fixed time AI is probably 36 to 40 hours after sponge removal.

Breeding season
Day 0: sponge inserted
Day 9: prostaglandin injection
Day 11: sponge removed + serum gonadotrophin injection
Day 12–13: onset of oestrus

Out of breeding season
Day 0: sponge inserted
Day 9: serum gonadotrophin injection
Day 11: sponge removed
Day 12–13: onset of oestrus

Transitory period
Day 0: sponge inserted
Day 9: prostaglandin injection + serum gonadotrophin injection
Day 11: sponge removed
Day 12–13: onset of oestrus

CIDR (controlled internal drug release)

A CIDR, a silicon rubber elasomer moulded over a nylon spine, is inserted into the vagina like a sponge and similarly releases a controlled amount of progesterone into the bloodstream. However, there is no CIDR suitable for goats available in the UK at present.

Melatonin

Animals measure daylength using melatonin secreted during the hours of darkness by the pineal gland. In sheep, treatment with melatonin provides a short day/long night signal that will advance the breeding season. Goats appear to need exposure to long days, provided by artificial light, before they will respond to melatonin. Twenty hours of artificial light from 1 January for 60 days followed by a return to natural light, combined with melatonin treatment by subcutaneous implant, will advance the breeding season by 2 to 3 months. Males should be light-treated under the same regime as the females and their fertility may be further increased by melatonin treatment. The males should be removed from the herd at the start of the melatonin treatment and kept apart (out of sight, sound and smell) until they are reintroduced 35 to 40 days later. Fertile oestrus will occur from 2 to 6 weeks after the introduction of the males (i.e. from late April to June), with peak mating activity occurring 3 to 4 weeks after introduction (during May) and peak kidding during November.

Melatonin can also be used in cashmere goats to delay the shedding of fleece, so obviating the need for winter shearing when weather conditions require goats to be housed and there is increased risk of post-shearing deaths.

Melatonin, 18 mg implant, **s.c.** behind ear (**Regulin**, Sanoffi).

Further reading

General

Evans, G. and Maxwell, W.M.C. (1987) *Salamon's Artificial Insemination of Sheep and Goats.* Butterworths, London.

Howe, P.A. (1984) Breeding problems in goats. *Proc. Univ. Sydney Post Grad. Comm. Vet Sci.,* **73**, 511–14.

Mews, A. (1981) Breeding and fertility in goats. *Goat Vet. Soc. J.,* **2** (2), 2–11.

Peaker, M. (1978) Gestation period and litter size in the goat. *Br. Vet. J.,* **134**, 379–83.

Skelton, M. (1978) Reproduction and breeding of goats. *J. Dairy Sci.,* **61**, 994–1010.

Ward, W.R. (1980) Some aspects of infertility in the goat. *Goat Vet. Soc. J.,* **1** (2), 2–5.

Control of the breeding season

Corteel, J.M., *et al.* (1982) Research and development in the control of reproduction. In: *Proc. III Int. Conf. Goat Prod. and Dis.,* Arizona, 1982, 584–91.

Evans, G., Holt, N., Pedrana, R.G. and Pemberton, D.H. (1987) Artificial breeding in sheep and goats. *Proc. Univ. Sydney Post Grad. Comm. Vet. Sci.,* **96**.

Geary, M.R. (1982) Use of Chronogest sponges and PMSG. *Goat Vet. Soc. J.,* **3** (2), 5–6.

Haibel, G.K. (1990) Out-of-season breeding in goats. *Vet. Clin. North Am.: Food Animal Practice,* **6** (3) November, 577–83.

Henderson, D.C. (1985) Control of the breeding season in sheep and goats. In *Practice,* July 1985, 118–23.

Henderson, D.C. (1987) Manipulation of the breeding season in goats – a review. *Goat Vet. Soc. J.,* **8** (1), 7–16.

False pregnancy

Hesslink, J.W. (1993) Incidence of hydrometra in dairy goats. *Vet. Rec.,* **132**, 110–112.

Pieterse, M.C. and Taverne, M.A.M. (1986) Hydrometra in goats: diagnosis with realtime ultrasound and treatment with prostaglandins or oxytocin. *Theriogenology,* **26**, 813–21.

Fetal age determination

Haibel, G.K., Perkins, N.R. and Lidi, G.M. (1989) Breed differences in biparietal diameters of second trimester Toggenburg, Nubian and Angora goat fetuses. *Theriogenology*, **32** (5), 827–34.

Hydrops uteri

Jones, S.L. and Fecteau, G. (1995) Hydrops uteri in a caprine doe pregnant with goat–sheep hybrid fetuses. *JAVMA*, **206** (12), 1920–22.
Morin, D.E., Hornbuckle II, T., Rowan, L.L. and Whiteley, H.E. (1994) Hydrallantois in a caprine doe. *JAVMA*, **204** (1), 108–111.

Intersexes

Hamerton, J.L., Dickson, J.M., Pollard, C.E., Grieves, S.A. and Short, R.V. (1969) Genetic intersexuality in goats. *J. Reprod. Fert. Suppl.*, **7**, 25–51.

Laparoscopy

Van Reven, G. (1988) Laparoscopy in goats. *Goat Vet. Soc. J.*, **9** (1/2), 24–32.

2 Abortion

The most common cause of abortion is 'unknown'. A list of causes of abortion is provided in Table 2.1.

Initial advice to owners

- ❏ Instruct the owner to save all the products of abortion for further examination – fetus/fetuses, fetal membranes. *The diagnosis will probably depend on laboratory investigation of aborted material.*
- ❏ Advise isolation of the aborted doe until a diagnosis is reached and/or uterine discharges have ceased.
- ❏ Warn of possible zoonoses, particularly during pregnancy. Care should be taken when handling aborted products – wear gloves. Any aborted material not required for laboratory examination should be burned or buried. Dogs and cats should be kept away from the aborted material.

Initial assessment

The preliminary history should consider:

- ❏ Individual or flock/herd problem.

Table 2.1 Causes of abortion.

Luteolysis	*Infection*
Trauma	Enzootic abortion
Stress	Toxoplasmosis
Iatrogenic	Listeriosis
Prostaglandins	Campylobacter
Corticosteroids	Q-fever
Poisoning	Leptospirosis
Plant	Salmonellosis
Wormers	Tickborne fever
Nutrition	Border disease
Starvation	Brucellosis
Vitamin A deficiency	Sarcocystosis
Manganese deficiency	*Fetal developmental abnormalities*

❏ Possible exposure to infected animals – bought-in stock, etc.
❏ Feeding, e.g. silage.
❏ Vaccination.
❏ Known disease status.

Specific enquiries should cover:

❏ The length of gestation/timing of abortion (see Table 2.2).
❏ The general breeding history – return to service, etc.
❏ The incidence of abortion, still births, weak kids.
❏ Signs of illness in the aborted doe.
❏ Drugs used on herd, e.g. prostaglandins.
❏ Access to possible poisons.
❏ The possibility of stress on the doe.

Table 2.2 Timing of abortion.

Abortion throughout gestation	Abortion in late gestation
Toxoplasmosis	Listeriosis
Chlamydia	Campylobacter
Leptospirosis	Q-fever
Prostaglandins	Salmonellosis
Stress	Border disease
Tickborne fever	Corticosteroids
	Multiple fetuses
	Energy deficit
	Mineral deficiency

Clinical examination

The doe should be fully examined for signs of disease. Aborting does may be ill and the clinical signs may aid diagnosis, but because abortion may occur some time after infection, many aborting does will show few additional clinical signs. Abortion may follow acute septicaemia and pyrexia caused by conditions not normally associated with abortion, e.g. enterotoxaemia. A blood sample should be taken for laboratory investigation.

The aborted fetuses and placentae should be examined grossly before submitting to the laboratory. If a number of does have aborted, samples from several animals should be submitted because of the possibility of more than one infectious agent being involved.

Laboratory investigation

Submission of correct specimens is essential for accurate diagnosis.

❏ Gross appearance of placentae and fetuses. Submit:
  (1) Placenta including cotyledons – fresh or fixed in formol-saline.
  (2) Fresh fetuses or
    ■ fetal lung and liver – fresh and fixed
    ■ fetal abomasal contents – fresh
    ■ fetal heart blood or exudate from serous cavities – fresh
    ■ fetal brain – fixed.
❏ Demonstration of a pathogen, e.g. microscopy, direct culture, virus isolation.
❏ Serological examination of the dam.
❏ Serological examination of the fetus.

Infectious causes

> There are important differences between sheep and goats in the behaviour of some infectious organisms which cause abortion. Because the epidemiology of these conditions is different in the two species, the control measures taken to limit the spread of disease in sheep will not necessarily be applicable to goats.
>
> More than one infective agent may be involved in an 'abortion storm'.

Enzootic abortion (chlamydia)

❏ Abortion occurs at any stage of pregnancy (unlike sheep where abortion is restricted to the last 2 to 4 weeks) because of the luteolytic effect from endometrial inflammation. The incubation period is as short as 2 weeks, so infection and abortion may occur within one pregnancy, even if infection occurs late in pregnancy.

Aetiology

❏ *Chlamydia psittaci*, an intracellular organism containing both RNA and DNA.

Transmission

❏ Ingestion of the organism shed in faeces but more generally from aborted material as *Chlamydia* is not very resistant in the environment. Shedding in vaginal secretions may begin as early as 9 days before abortion and last as long as 12 days after abortion.

❏ Carrier does or males in endemic herds and bought-in does continue the spread of infection. Kids born live will also carry the infection, although they remain negative serologically, and may shed organisms when they kid themselves.

Clinical signs

❏ Often abortion is the only clinical sign and the doe rapidly recovers, but severe illness with metritis, keratoconjunctivitis and pneumonia has been reported.

Postmortem findings

❏ Placenta – intercotyledonary placentitis often with a covering of yellow purulent material, giving a leathery appearance. Advanced autolysis occurs.

❏ Fetus – no specific gross lesions occur; the fetus may be autolysed or fresh.

Diagnosis

❏ Examination of smears from the placenta, the mouth or nostrils of the fetus or the vagina of the doe using modified Ziehl-Neelsen stain.

❏ Serological diagnosis of the disease using the complement fixation test, but males and young infected kids remain negative.

❏ Isolation of the organism in tissue culture or in embryonic eggs.

Treatment and control

❏ Segregate aborting animals for 2 weeks until the excretion of chlamydia has ceased.

❏ Dispose of aborted material and disinfect the area.

❏ Cull any live kids born to infected does.

❏ Treat all pregnant goats in the herd with tetracyclines for 10 days and move them to uncontaminated pasture halfway through treatment:

> Dairy goats: **20 mg long-acting oxytetracycline/kg i.m. every 3 days**
>
> Fibre goats: as dairy goats, or **400–450 mg oxytetracycline/head/ day orally.**

❏ Consider a vaccination programme, but only where infection is already present in the herd. **Enzovax** (Intervet) is a live vaccine licensed in the UK for use in sheep but not goats. Vaccination of

healthy females should prevent infection but may not prevent abortion in goats already infected. Annual vaccination should continue indefinitely as vaccination does not eliminate infection. **Mydiavac** (C-Vet) is an inactivated vaccine, licensed in sheep. As an inactivated vaccine, it does not pose a zoonotic risk and can be safely handled by women of childbearing age.
❑ Fertility is usually normal in pregnancies subsequent to the abortion, but immunity may wane after about 3 years.

Public health considerations

The organism is excreted in body fluids including milk. Pregnant women are particularly at risk from contact with aborted material and from drinking unpasteurised milk.

Toxoplasmosis

Aetiology

❑ *Toxoplasma gondii*, a protozoan parasite of endothelial cells.

Transmission

❑ Direct contact with the products of abortion.
❑ Infective oocysts passed in the faeces of cats which act as the intermediate host, multiplying and disseminating infection and contaminating stored foodstuffs or pastures. A reservoir of infection for susceptible cats exists in birds and wild rodents, which may pass the infection vertically between generations. Cats then amplify and spread the infection.
❑ Transplacental infection of kids. Very low levels of infection may result in abortion.

Clinical signs

❑ Pyrexia and lethargy may occur in the doe about 2 weeks after infection, but the doe will be clinically normal at the time of abortion. Occasional fatalities occur in adult goats – postmortem findings include nephritis, cystitis, encephalitis, hepatitis, enteritis and abomasitis.
❑ Resorption, fetal death and mummification occur if infection is during the first third of pregnancy.
❑ Abortions, stillbirths and weak kids are produced if infection occurs later in pregnancy.
❑ Normal but infected kids may be produced to does affected in late pregnancy.
❑ Up to 80% of females may be infected and abort.

Postmortem findings

❑ Placenta – yellow or white focal lesions, 1 to 3 mm in diameter on the cotyledons, with the intercotyledonary areas not affected.

❑ Fetus – there are usually no specific gross lesions on the fetus.

Diagnosis

❑ Fluorescent antibody examination of cotyledonary material.

❑ Examination of fetal fluid using latex agglutination test (available for practice laboratory use).

❑ Serological examination of dam may be confusing due to high serological levels in the normal population, but rising titre between paired samples is indicative of infection and a low titre means that the abortion was not due to *Toxoplasma.*

❑ Serological examination of live kids before suckling will demonstrate high specific antibodies.

❑ Histological examination of fetal tissues – brain, lung, liver, heart, kidney and spleen – shows necrotic foci surrounded by inflammatory cells and focal leucomalocia in the brain.

Treatment and control

❑ Animals remain infected for life.

❑ Unlike sheep, infected goats may abort in subsequent pregnancies, so it may be advisable to cull infected does.

❑ Chemoprophylaxis is likely to be of limited value in goats because of the risk of abortion during subsequent pregnancies.

❑ Infection can be prevented by stopping the access of cats to grain stores, feeding troughs and hay barns.

❑ Destroy the products of abortion as soon as possible.

❑ Oocysts may persist on pasture or in soil for over a year and are very resistant to most disinfectants.

❑ Cats acquire immunity to reinfection and do not subsequently present a threat to livestock unless they become immunosuppressed. Preventing cats breeding on the premises will prevent the spread of the disease via the intermediate host – younger cats generally pose the greatest threat.

❑ Rodent and bird control will reduce the reservoir of infection which exists for susceptible cats.

❑ Vaccination – a single injection 3 to 4 weeks prior to mating – gives a minimum of two seasons' protection. Vaccination will not introduce infection into the herd. **Toxovac** (Intervet) contains living tachyzoites of *Toxoplasma gondii* and is licensed in the UK for use in sheep but not goats.

Public health considerations

Toxoplasma tachyzoites are passed in the milk of infected does, so there is a risk to children and pregnant women from drinking infected milk as well as from handling aborted material. Aborted material should never be handled with bare hands.

Neosporosis

Aetiology

❏ *Neospora caninum*, a protozoan parasite that naturally infects dogs, cattle, sheep, goats, horses and deer and until 1988 was misdiagnosed as *Toxoplasma gondii*. The full life cycle is not known.

Transmission

❏ No definitive host, i.e. in which *Neospora* has a sexual replication cycle producing oocysts, has been identified.
❏ Vertical (transplacental) transmission is the only proven route of transmission and can occur repeatedly in the same animal.

Clinical signs

❏ Abortion, stillbirth and weak kids. Dams generally show no other clinical signs.

Diagnosis

❏ Serological examination by immunofluorescent antibody test (IFAT) and ELISA.
❏ Histological examination of brain and heart, parasites found in tissues by specific staining [immunoperoxidase (IFX) test]; characteristic non-suppurative encephalitis.

Treatment

❏ No drugs have been shown to prevent transplacental transmission.

Listeriosis

See Chapter 11.

❏ Abortion occurs from the 12th week but generally in late pregnancy.
❏ Retained placentae and metritis are common after abortion.
❏ Some kids are born alive but die soon afterwards.

Postmortem findings

❏ Placenta – placentitis with cotyledons and intercotyledonary areas affected.
❏ Fetus – necrotic grey yellow foci 1 to 2 mm diameter in the liver and sometimes the lung.

Diagnosis

❏ The organism is easily grown and identified in the laboratory as a gram-positive beta-haemolytic bacillus and can be isolated from the fetal stomach, uterine discharges, milk and the placenta.
❏ Fluorescent antibody examination of aborted material.

Treatment and control

❏ Clinically ill animals can be treated with ampicillin or potentiated sulphonamide.
❏ Aborted does are considered immune and should be retained in the herd.

Campylobacter (vibriosis)

Aetiology

❏ Comma-shaped bacteria. *Campylobacter fetus* (formerly *Vibrio fetus*). *Campylobacter jejuni* is also implicated in the USA.

Transmission

❏ Ingestion of organisms from aborted material.
❏ Some does remain permanent carriers.
❏ Wildlife can act as vectors.

Clinical signs

❏ Abortion in the last 4 to 6 weeks of gestation; some infected goats do not abort but produce weak kids at full term. These kids usually die within a few days.
❏ Does may be pyrexic and lethargic with diarrhoea for a few days either side of the abortion, but often the goat appears clinically normal.
❏ A post abortion vaginal discharge is usual.
❏ Males are infected but do not show clinical signs.

Postmortem findings

❏ Placenta – changes minimal.
❏ Fetus – may have doughnut-shaped foci of 10 to 20 mm diameter in the liver; the fetus is usually autolysed.

Diagnosis

❏ Direct smear of fetal abomasal contents.
❏ Culture of fetal abomasal contents.

Treatment and control

❏ Segregate aborting animals immediately and then cull them because of the possibility of a carrier state.
❏ Cull any live kids born.
❏ Treat the remainder of the herd with penicillin/dihydrostreptomycin or tetracyclines.

Public health considerations

Campylobacter causes acute gastroenteritis in humans, usually by faecal contamination from diarrhoeic or apparently healthy goats. Faecal contamination of raw goats milk produced human disease in an outbreak in the UK.

Q-fever

Aetiology

❏ Very small intracellular parasite *Coxiella burnettii*, a member of the Rickettsia family.

Transmission

❏ By ingestion after direct contamination with abortion material or the urine, faeces and milk of an infected animal.
❏ By inhalation or through injured skin after contact with the organism.
❏ By infected ticks (unconfirmed in the UK).
❏ Healthy carrier goats spread the infection.

Clinical signs

❏ Most infected goats are healthy carriers, but some aborting animals will be clinically ill with a retained placenta.
❏ Abortion occurs in the last month of pregnancy and weak infected kids may be born.

Postmortem findings

❏ Placenta – placentitis with clay-coloured cotyledons and inter-cotyledonary thickening.
❏ Fetus – autolysed with no specific lesions.

Diagnosis

❏ Smears from the placenta or fetal organs stained with a modified Ziehl-Neelsen stain show acid fast pleomorphic cocci and rods.
❏ By fluorescent antibody examination of cotyledonary material.
❏ A complement fixation test on the dam's serum shows the antibody level rising about a week after infections and persisting for a month.

Treatment and control

❏ Tetracyclines will probably control an outbreak.

Public health considerations
The disease is most important as a human infection which occurs via contact or inhalation of the organism from the fetus, placenta and uterine fluids and possibly by drinking infected milk.

Leptospirosis

See Chapter 17.

Salmonellosis

Three *Salmonella* serotypes have been reported to cause abortion in sheep and goats: *S. abortus ovis*, *S. typhimurium* and *S. dublin.* The latter two cause systemic illness with diarrhoea in addition to abortion, stillbirths or very weak live kids which die shortly afterwards.

Tickborne fever

Aetiology

❏ *Cytoecetes phagocytophilia,* an intracellular parasite of the Rickettsia family, transmitted by the tick vector *Ixodes ricinus.*

Epidemiology

❏ In endemic areas most ticks are infected and thus virtually all ruminants and deer exposed to ticks also become infected, generally very early in life.

Clinical signs

- ❏ Pyrexia, lethargy, weight loss (often not recognised).
- ❏ Abortion and metritis.
- ❏ Temporary infertility in male goats.

In addition, infection may increase the pathogenicity of other diseases such as tick pyaemia, louping ill, listeriosis and pasteurellosis.

Anglo-Nubian goats react more severely than other breeds of British goats.

Diagnosis

- ❏ Detection of the organism in polymorphonuclear leucocytes in Giemsa-stained blood smears.

Control

- ❏ Susceptible pregnant animals should not be exposed to tick infected pastures.

Border disease (hypomyelinogenesis congenita, hairy shaker disease)

Aetiology

- ❏ Pestivirus, serologically related to bovine virus diarrhoea and swine fever virus.

Epidemiology

- ❏ The incidence of the disease in the goat population is not known, but experimentally goats have been affected as well as sheep, and the virus should be considered as a possible cause of abortion. Direct animal contact by ingestion or aerosol is the main source of infection – sheep, goats, deer and possibly pigs are potential sources of infection. Surviving infected kids will remain carriers.

Clinical signs

- ❏ Abortion, stillbirths, barren does, fetal death and maceration from 70th day.
- ❏ Small weak kids with varying degrees of tremor and abnormal conformation, although hairy coat abnormalities as seen in lambs rarely, if ever, occur.

Postmortem findings

❏ Kids – affected kids show hydrocephalus and cerebellar hypoplasia.
❏ Placenta – severe necrotising caruncular placentitis.

Diagnosis

❏ Live animal: virus isolation and serology from kid or doe blood (clotted or heparinised).
❏ Postmortem: antigen can be detected in fresh samples of thyroid, kidney, brain, spleen, intestine, lymph nodes or placenta; virus can be isolated from postmortem material sent in virus transport medium; heart blood can be used for serology; histopathology of brain and spinal cord shows hypomyelinogenesis.

Brucellosis

Brucella abortus

Goats can be infected with *Brucella abortus* and hence are included in dairy cow testing programmes, but the incidence of infection is minute in all parts of the world. In infected goats abortion is rare and mastitis common. Serological testing of goats for brucellosis is reported to have severe limitations.

Brucella melitensis

Goats are most susceptible to *Brucella melitensis* which occurs mainly in southern Europe and is important as a major zoonosis producing Malta fever in humans who drink infected milk.

Abortion is the main clinical sign and usually occurs during the last months of gestation. The organism is excreted in uterine and vaginal secretions, urine, faeces and milk after parturition or abortion.

Sarcocystosis

Aetiology

❏ *Sarcocystis capracanis*, a protozoan parasite using the goat as an intermediate, with a carnivore as the definitive host. The incidence of the organism in the UK is unknown.

Clinical signs

❏ Clinical signs depend on the number of sporocysts ingested.
❏ They are non-specific and include pyrexia, anorexia, lethargy,

haemolytic anaemia, jaundice, nervous signs and abortion due to maternal failure – placenta and fetus are not infected; weak kids may be born alive.

Diagnosis

❑ No antemortem diagnostic test is available.

Postmortem findings

❑ Non-specific findings; petechial haemorrhages in many organs.
❑ Haemorrhages in heart and skeletal muscle.
❑ Immunofluorescent and immunoperoxidase techniques used to identify meronts in endothelial cells including the maternal caruncle.

Other organisms

Other organisms which have been implicated in abortion are:

❑ *Corynebacterium pyogenes.*
❑ *Yersinia pseudotuberculosis.*
❑ *Pasteurella haemolytica.*
❑ *Bacillus* spp.
❑ *Mycoplasma* spp.
❑ Caprine herpes virus.

Non-infectious causes

Medication

Prostaglandin administration will produce abortion at any stage of the gestation. Phenothiazine used as a worm drench is reported to cause abortion in late pregnancy as will corticosteroids given in late pregnancy.

Trauma and stress

> As the doe is dependent on corpus-luteum-derived progesterone throughout pregnancy, anything which causes luteolysis will produce abortion.

This means goats may be more susceptible than other species to abortion from trauma or stress. Any condition which causes release of prostaglandins, and thus luteolysis, will cause abortion.

Developmental abnormalities

Very few deformed fetuses are produced, but a fetus with developmental abnormalities may be aborted. An hereditary defect of Angora does in South Africa led to chronic hyperadrenocorticism, death of the fetus and then its expulsion.

Multiple fetuses

Abortions or early parturition appear more common in Anglo-Nubian goats which commonly carry three, four or more fetuses. In these cases placental insufficiency probably leads to fetal expulsion.

Poisons

Plant poisonings are occasionally implicated in abortion, e.g. *Astragulus* spp. and *Lathyrus* spp., but are unlikely to be of significance in the UK. Poisonings from non-plant sources also occasionally occur, generally causing abortion by producing a systemic illness.

Malnutrition

❏ *Energy deficit* – frank starvation will cause abortion particularly if the energy input is insufficient during the last third of pregnancy.
❏ *Mineral deficiencies* – mineral deficiencies, e.g. selenium, copper and iodine, generally cause the birth of dead or weak kids at full term, rather than abortion, but manganese deficiency has been shown to cause abortion at 80 to 105 days of gestation.
❏ *Vitamin deficiencies* – prolonged vitamin A deficiency has been shown to cause abortion, stillbirth, illthrift, retained placenta and night blindness due to the absence of visual purple in the retina. However, deficiency is extremely unlikely even in severe drought.

Further reading

General

East, N. (1983) Pregnancy toxaemia, abortions and periparturient diseases. *Vet. Clin. North. Am.: Large Anim. Pract.*, **5** (3), November, Sheep and Goat Medicine, 601–618.
Harwood, D.G. (1987) Abortion in the goat, an investigative approach. *Goat Vet. Soc. J.*, **8** (1), 25–8.

Merrall, M. (1985) The aborting goat. *Proc. of a Course in Goat Husbandry and Medicine*, Massey University, November 1985, **106**, 181–98.

Campylobacter

Anderson, K.L., Hammond, M.M., Urbane, J.W., Rhoades, H.E. and Bryner, J.H. (1983) Isolation of *Campylobacter jejuni* from an aborted caprine fetus. *JAVMA*, **183**, 90–92.

Chlamydial abortion

Appleyard, W.T. (1986) Chlamydial abortion in goats. *Goat Vet. Soc. J.*, **7** (2), 45–7.

Q-fever

Waldhalm, D.G., Stoenner, H.G., Simmons, E.E. and Thomas, A.L. (1978) Abortion associated with *Coxiella burnetii* infection in dairy goats. *JAVMA*, **173**, 1580–81.

Toxoplasmosis

Buxton, D. (1989) Toxoplasmosis in sheep and other farm animals. *In Practice*, January 1989, 9–12.

Dubey, J.P., Miller, S. and Desmonts, G. (1986) *Toxoplasma gondii* induced abortion in dairy goats. *JAVMA*, **188**, 159–62.

Herbert, I.V. (1986) Sarcocystosis and toxoplasmosis in goats. *Goat Vet. Soc. J.*, **7** (2), 25–31.

3 Male Infertility

Investigation of male infertility

See Figure 3.1 for the causes of male infertility.

Initial assessment

The preliminary history should consider:

- ❏ Individual or flock/herd problem.
- ❏ Management practices – handmating/buck running with does.
- ❏ Feeding, including mineral supplementation.
- ❏ Workload of the bucks.
- ❏ Age of bucks.

If more than one buck is involved consider:

- ❏ Overuse of bucks – particularly if used out of season or on synchronised groups of does. One buck can mate over 100 does over a season, but a ratio of one mature buck to about 70 does or two bucklings (two toothbucks) to 70 does is more satisfactory. A well-grown kid could serve up to 30 does in a season.
- ❏ Low sexual drive – if bucks used out of season on light-treated or sponged does.
- ❏ Disease status – parasitism, footrot, etc.
- ❏ Nutritional status.
- ❏ Poor heat detection.

If there is a problem with an individual goat, the specific history should determine whether the problem is:

- ❏ Return to service of females.
- ❏ Failure to serve at all.
- ❏ Failure to serve properly.

Assessment of individual buck

General assessment

- ❏ Body condition.
- ❏ Arthritis.

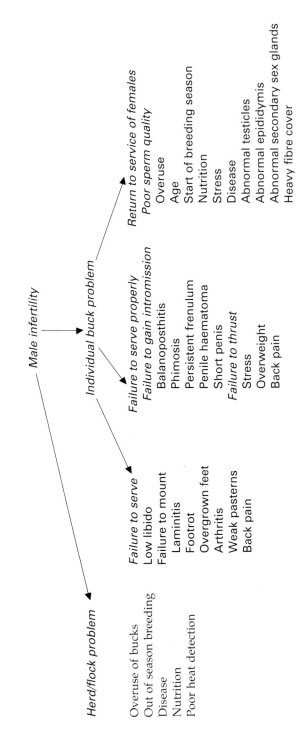

Figure 3.1 Causes of male infertility

❏ Weak pasterns.
❏ Poorly trimmed feet.

Specific examination

❏ Observe sexual activity using a doe in season as a teaser (prostaglandin treatment of doe during breeding season can be used to induce oestrus at a time suitable for examination).
❏ Libido.
❏ Failure to mate.
❏ Examine and palpate the external genitalia – check the scrotum and contents; note the size, shape, consistency and symmetry of the testes, epididymis and spermatic cord; the testes should move freely in the scrotum; measure the scrotal circumference and the epididymal diameter.

Scrotum

Scrotal dermatitis, abscesses, fly strike and trauma can all lead to temporary or permanent testicular degeneration and reduced fertility.

Testes

The testes should be symmetrical, large, oval and firm during the breeding season. Asymmetry suggests injury, disease or anatomical abnormality.

Cryptorchidism

Cryptorchidism may be unilateral or bilateral. Unilateral cryptorchids are generally fertile, but semen quality may be affected; bilateral cryptorchids are sterile. A genetically female intersex may be a cryptorchid. In Angora goats cryptorchidism has been shown to be inherited as a recessive trait.

Enlarged testes

❏ An inguinal hernia causing distension of the scrotum may be confused with enlarged testicles.
❏ *Orchitis* – inflammation of the testes may be unilateral or bilateral, acute or chronic. In the acute condition, the testes will be swollen and painful and the buck will be pyrexic, lethargic and unwilling to move. In chronic orchitis, fibrous adhesions may limit movement within the scrotum and the testicles become atrophied and fibrous.

❏ *Neoplasia* is an uncommon cause of infertility in bucks, but seminomas, adenomas and carcinomas have been reported.
❏ *Haematoma* – intratesticular haemorrhage may cause enlargement of a testis.

Small testes

❏ *Testicular hypoplasia* – underdeveloped testes occur particularly in polled males as part of the intersex condition (qv). The condition is generally bilateral, occasionally unilateral.
❏ *Testicular atrophy* occurs as a sequel to scrotal trauma, orchitis, sperm granuloma or systemic disease, if the goat is debilitated and as part of the ageing process in some bucks. With fibrosis the testicle feels very firm on palpation.
❏ *Testicular degeneration* – the testes feel soft and doughy due to tubular degeneration.

Conditions of the spermatic cord

❏ *Varicocoele* presents as a hard swelling in the dorsal part of the pampiniform plexus; caused by dilation and thrombosis in the internal spermatic vein.

Abnormal epididymis

❏ *Sperm granulomas* are palpable as hard knots at the head of the epididymis although the testes are normal in consistency. The condition occurs particularly in polled males as part of the intersex condition (qv) but can also arise from an infection causing epididymitis. If the condition is bilateral the buck is sterile.
❏ *Epididymitis* uncommonly occurs in goats as a result of infection with a variety of pathogens or following trauma.

Penis/prepuce

Balanoposthitis

❏ Inflammation of the penis and prepuce often leads to scar tissue and adhesions. The acute inflammation and the resulting fibrosis both cause infertility.
❏ *Caprine herpes virus type 1* causes balanoposthitis in goats in New Zealand and Australia with hyperaemia of the penis and ulceration of the prepuce.
❏ *Orf* (qv) occasionally infects the prepuce.
❏ Mycoplasmas and ureaplasms *may* be involved.

Persistent frenulum

The adhesions between the penis and prepuce which are present in the prepubertal male kid normally disappear by about 4 months of age, but occasionally persist.

Phimosis

Phimosis is seen as an inability to extrude the penis at service. It may result from trauma but is occasionally congenital.

Paraphimosis

Paraphimosis is the inability to withdraw the penis into the prepuce, resulting in the penis becoming swollen and oedematous.

Short penis

A short penis results in inability to protrude the penis beyond the prepuce. The condition is not treatable.

Haematoma of the penis

Haematoma of the penis follows trauma, such as caused by head-butting.

Examination of semen

❏ Collection of semen:
  ■ using an artificial vagina gives better quality semen than electroejaculation; if possible use a doe in oestrus as a teaser.
  ■ electroejaculation should only be used on an anaesthetised animal.
  ■ best semen samples are obtained during the breeding season.
  ■ some idea of sperm motility can be gained from a vaginal semen sample examined on a warmed slide.
❏ Examination of semen – volume, motility, numbers, morphology, absence of inflammatory cells/debris, live:dead ratio (see 'Reproductive data', Appendix 1).

Individual buck problems

Failure to serve at all

Low libido

❏ Season – the normal breeding season is September to March, but many bucks are now expected to work out of season following light or sponge treatment of does. If possible, bucks should be stimulated, e.g. by light, at the same time as the does. Most bucks will mate at any time of the year, but some reduction in libido must be expected out of season.
❏ Poor condition – intercurrent disease such as parasitism; energy or protein deficit.
❏ Hereditary – sexual drive is hereditable.
❏ Presence of other males – competition may increase libido, or a dominant male may suppress libido in subordinates.

Note: many (particularly older) bucks will only serve a female that is definitely in season. Some bucks will only serve each female once within a short period of time, rather than twice as expected by dairy goatkeepers.

Failure to mount

❏ Skeletal or muscular lesions:
  ■ foot problems: laminitis, footrot, overgrown feet
  ■ arthritis
  ■ weak pasterns
  ■ back pain.

Failure to serve properly

Failure to gain intromission

❏ Conditions of prepuce – phimosis due to trauma or infection, persistent frenulum (rare), adhesions/scarring.

Note: a very young male kid (<4 months) may have difficulty protruding the penis because of adhesions between penis and prepuce.
❏ Conditions of penis – adhesions/scarring, haematoma, short penis.

Failure to thrust

❏ Stress:
  ■ too many people 'assisting'

- ■ tiredness
- ■ strange surroundings.
- ❏ Overweight.
- ❏ Back pain.

Return to service

Return to service is generally caused by poor sperm quality.

- ❏ Overuse – particularly out of season and if large numbers of does are synchronised; reduced sperm density may take 6 weeks or more to recover.
- ❏ Age – old or young animals may have reduced sperm density and/ or poor quality semen.
- ❏ Start of breeding season – maximum sperm production occurs several weeks after onset of the breeding season.
- ❏ Nutrition – young males are particularly sensitive to poor nutrition including protein and energy deficits and vitamin deficiency (particularly vitamin A). The role of trace elements is not well documented, but copper, manganese, cobalt, zinc and phosphorus deficiencies may affect sperm production.
- ❏ Stress.
- ❏ Intercurrent disease – pyrexia will reduce sperm density through damage to epididymis and testes, causing permanent damage in some cases and a minimum of 6 weeks to recover. The spermatogenic cycle is about 22 days in the goat and normal fertility is not restored until a full spermatogenic cycle is completed.
- ❏ Abnormal testicles.
- ❏ Abnormal epididymis.
- ❏ Abnormal accessory sex glands, e.g. *seminal vesiculitis* results in ejaculates containing large numbers of white cells with no palpable orchitis or epididymitis.
- ❏ Heavy fibre cover – an unshorn Angora with heavy fleece may have reduced fertility due to increase in scrotal temperature and effect on spermatogenesis. Even after shearing, 6 to 8 weeks will be required before return to full fertility.

Further reading

Ahmad, N. and Noakes, D.E. (1996) Seasonal variation in the semen quality of young British goats. *Br. Vet. J.*, **152**, 225–36.

Evans, G. and Maxwell, W.M.C. (1987) *Salamon's Artificial Insemination of Sheep and Goats.* Butterworths, London.

Greig, A. (1987) Infertility in the male goat. *Goat Vet. Soc. J.*, **8** (1), 1–3.

Merman, M.A. (1983) Male infertility. *Vet. Clin. North Am.: Large Animal Practice*, **5** (3), November 1983, 619–35.

4 Periparturient Problems

Preparturient problems

Pregnancy toxaemia

See Chapter 8.

Dead kids without immediate abortion

Retention of a dead or mummified kid is not uncommon in goats. Kids may be retained for several months before the doe produces a macerated kid or bones. Small pieces of bone may be retained in the uterus and cause infertility. Occasionally, mummified kids are found incidentally at postmortem.

Retention of a non-mummified kid will produce an acute toxaemia with pyrexia, anorexia, abdominal pain and usually death within about 3 days. Intermittent straining may occur terminally. If the cervix is closed internal examination is not possible; radiography will confirm the diagnosis.

Abortion

See Chapter 2.

Vaginal prolapse

> Adequate analgesia and control of straining should be primary considerations when dealing with periparturient problems.

Vaginal prolapse is relatively common and likely to recur during subsequent pregnancies with probable increasing severity, but some goats prolapse only once. Most goats generally kid normally without subsequent prolapse of the uterus.

Aetiology

❑ An increase in intrapelvic pressure in late pregnancy initiates straining by the doe, forcing the vagina through the vulva. Factors implicated in increasing the likelihood of prolapse include:
  ■ multiple fetuses
  ■ conformation of dam – musculature, pelvic anatomy, possible hereditary component. In goats, overfatness is generally not significant.

Clinical signs

❑ The degree of prolapse is variable, from a minor protrusion of the vagina through the vulval lips when lying down to a complete prolapse of the vagina and cervix in which the bladder may also be prolapsed.
❑ The contents of the vaginal prolapse can be visualised using real-time B-mode ultrasonography with a 5-MHz transducer and either a linear array or sector scanner.

Treatment

❑ Minor prolapses – if the area is clean, untraumatised and returns to its normal position when the doe stands up, no treatment is necessary.
❑ Larger prolapses will need replacing after thorough cleaning. Analgesia with a suitable NSAID, e.g.
  Flunixin meglumine, 2.2 mg/kg, 2 ml/45 kg (Finadyne, Schering-Plough),
  and use of caudal epidural anaesthesia (Chapter 21) to provide analgesia and control straining are essential before replacement of the prolapse is attempted.
❑ Various retention techniques have been used. Plastic or alloy intravaginal retainers are commonly used in sheep but often cause vaginitis and further straining and are difficult to attach to short-coated dairy breeds. The Buhner suture (Figure 4.1) uses 5-mm umbilical tape which is laid down subcutaneously both sides of the vulva, using a large half-curved needle, starting below the ventral vulval commissure, passing through the lateral fibrous tissue to emerge dorsal to the dorsal commissure, then passing down through the fibrous tissue of the opposite side to emerge below the ventral commissure again, where it is tied with a double bow. The retaining suture must be released to allow kidding to take place, so the doe needs regular checks once the pelvic ligaments relax.

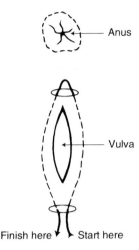

Figure 4.1 Buhner suture

❏ Post surgically, broad-spectrum antibiotic cover should be given for 5 days.
❏ Consider early induced parturition with prostaglandins if the goat is distressed. Induction of parturition also allows the retaining suture to be removed at the optimum time.
❏ *Prolapse of the intestines through a vaginal rupture* may occur if a portion of the intestines is forced into the pelvis.

Rectal prolapse

Rectal prolapse is rare, but may occur on its own or follow vaginal prolapse if straining continues. Effective caudal analgesia often allows the rectal tissue to return to its normal position. Larger prolapses may need manual reduction, with a purse string suture of umbilical tape placed subcutaneously, leaving an anus of about 1.5 cm diameter. Very large rectal prolapses may need amputating under caudal epidural anaesthesia (Chapter 21).

Prolonged gestation

The normal gestation period is 150 days (145 to 154 days). Single kids are often carried longer than multiples. If parturition has not occurred by 155 days, parturition should be induced with prostaglandins (qv) and will result in kidding in about 36 hours. Hypocalcaemia (qv) should always be considered and treated where necessary.

Common causes of prolonged gestation are:

❑ Non-pregnancy!
❑ False pregnancy (qv).
❑ A single large kid.
❑ Dead kids.
❑ Hypocalcaemia.

Dystocia

> The uterus tears easily. If the correction of a malpresentation is prolonged or delivery difficult, a caesarian section is indicated.

Generally, dystocia is due to malpresentation (particularly with multiple fetuses), and occasionally to an oversize fetus or to overfat does, particularly goatlings. The uterus of the goat is more readily damaged than that of the ewe. Adequate lubrication and dilatation of the canal is essential or rupture of the cervix with dorsal tearing of the uterus and possibly uterine haemorrhage will occur.

   Clenbuterol, 0.8 µg/kg, 1.25 ml/50 kg (Planipart, Ventipulmin, Boehringer Ingelheim)

can be used to produce myometrial relaxation during kidding or caesarian section. Goats tolerate caesarian section far better than prolonged manipulation of the fetuses. Opting for early surgery may save the life of the dam and the kids. Techniques for caesarian section are discussed in Chapter 23.

Ringwomb

True ringwomb, where the cervix fails to dilate sufficiently to allow parturition, is rare, but gentle manual dilation of the vulva, vagina and cervix may be necessary where the fetus has not engaged correctly in the pelvis, e.g. with a transverse presentation. Hypocalcaemia (see Chapter 11) may result in apparent failure of cervical dilation and should always be considered, but is not common in goats at the time of parturition. It has been suggested that one cause of ringwomb may be the absence of the final preparturient surge of prostaglandin. Treatment with prostaglandins may produce kidding in about 4 hours:

   Dinaprost, 2 ml i.m. or s.c. (Lutalyse, Pharmacia & Upjohn)

   Clorprostenol, 0.5 ml i.m. or s.c. (Estrumate, Schering-Plough).

Dilation may be promoted by treatment with:

   Vetrabutine hydrochloride, 2 mg/kg, 1 ml/50 kg i.m. (Monzaldon, Boehringer Ingelheim).

Hypocalcaemia

See Chapter 11.

Hypomagnesaemia

See Chapter 11.

Transit tetany

See Chapter 11.

Postparturient problems

Metritis

> A light, odourless, reddish vaginal discharge (Lochia) is normal after kidding for 14 days or more and should not be confused with metritis.

Metritis is indicated by a darker, sticky, usually smelly discharge which may contain pus. The doe may be pyrexic and anorexic with a reduced milk yield and signs of abdominal pain. Does which progress to chronic metritis may be infertile (see Chapter 1).

Retained placenta

Retained placenta is much less common than in the cow; induction of parturition with prostaglandins does not lead to retention.

In many cases, membranes which are hanging from the vulva a few hours after kidding can be easily removed by slow, gentle traction. Fetal membranes should be passed within 12 hours. After this time immediate veterinary intervention is necessary as contraction of the uterus and closure of the cervix will soon prevent manual removal. Injections of oxytocin or prostaglandin may aid removal of the membranes. Antibiotic cover should be given routinely and tetanus antitoxin given to unvaccinated goats.

Retained kid

> Vaginal examination of a sick doe post kidding should be considered routine.

Retained kids after parturition are more common and potentially more serious than a retained placenta. The kid may be delivered normally after a few days, but most affected does will become lethargic and anorexic, with a dramatic drop in milk yield, and eventually die if the condition is not recognised. Some does will strain, but many will not and a manual examination of any sick doe post kidding should be considered routine.

Rupture of the uterus

Rupture of the uterus usually occurs dorsally in the body of the uterus just cranial to the cervix. Repair of a dorsal tear is extremely difficult either by a left flank abdominal incision or vaginally. However, in many cases, contraction of the uterus will seal the defect and the doe may not only survive but breed and kid satisfactorily in subsequent years. The main dangers are shock and peritonitis – the fetal membranes should be removed as completely as possible, high levels of intravenous antibiotics given and pain relief given as:

Isopyrin/phenylbutazone, 3–5 ml i.v. (**Tomanol**, Intervet)
or
Flunixin meglumine, 2 ml/45 kg i.v. (**Finadyne**, Schering-Plough)
or
Aspirin, 50–100 mg/kg orally t.i.d.

Intravenous fluid therapy will increase the goat's chance of survival.

Ruptured uterine artery

Ruptured uterine artery is rare but may accompany a ventral tear of the uterus or occur during a difficult kidding. Fatal intraperitoneal haemorrhage can occur without obvious vaginal haemorrhage.

Uterine prolapse

Uterine prolapse is also rare, but may occur a few hours after kidding, often subsequent to a retained placenta. If the placenta is still attached, it should be gently removed before thorough cleaning and replacement under epidural anaesthesia. The horns of the uterus must be fully extended when replaced. Retention sutures are not generally necessary if the replacement is complete, but a purse string suture is sometimes used (see 'Vaginal prolapse', this chapter).

Hypocalcaemia

See Chapter 11.

Mastitis

See Chapter 12.

Postparturient toxaemia

See Chapter 8.

Laminitis

See Chapter 6.

Further reading

Baxendell, S.A. (1984) Caprine obstetrics. *Proc. Univ. Sydney. Post Grad. Comm. Vet Sci.*, **73**, 363–6.

Brain, L.T.A. (1985) Dystocia in the goat – a practitioner's view. *Goat Vet. Soc. J.*, **6** (2), 57–60.

East, N.E. (1983) Pregnancy toxaemia, abortions and periparturient diseases. *Vet. Clin. North Am.: Large Animal Practice*, **5** (3), November 1983, 601–618.

Noakes, D.E. (1985) Surgical answers to reproductive problems in the female goat. *Goat Vet. Soc. J.*, **6** (2), 61–3.

Scott, P. and Gessert, M. (1998) Management of ovine vaginal prolapse. *In Practice*, **20** (1), 28–34.

5 Weak Kids

> Weak kids arise from multiple causes, which may be interrelated.

Initial assessment

The preliminary history should consider:

- ❏ Individual or flock/herd problem.
- ❏ Kidding routine.
- ❏ Post kidding management.
- ❏ Beginning or end of kidding period.
- ❏ Feeding.

If a flock/herd problem consider:

- ❏ Associated abortions/stillbirths.
- ❏ Possible nutritional deficiencies.

If an individual problem, specific enquiries should cover:

- ❏ Weak since birth or developed since?
- ❏ Seen to suckle or not.
- ❏ Difficult or prolonged birth.
- ❏ Kidded inside or outside – possibility of exposure.

Clinical examination

Observe kid and dam together in their normal surroundings

- ❏ Mismothering – particularly first kidders.
- ❏ Behaviour of siblings.
- ❏ Sucking reflex.

Examine dam

- ❏ Udder conformation/teat abnormalities.
- ❏ Milk let-down.

❏ Mastitis.
❏ Vaginal discharges.

Examine kid

❏ Alert?
❏ Check for congenital lesions.
❏ Nervous signs.

Prematurity/low birth weight

Birth weights of kids are very variable, ranging from over 7 kg for a single male down to 2 or 3 kg in multiple births. Birth weight is important as the larger the kid at birth the faster the growth rate.

Kids up to 14 days premature have a good chance of survival and kids up to 21 days premature can often be reared. Premature kids may have respiratory problems due to inadequate lung surfactant being produced. This is particularly the case if parturition is induced with prostaglandins before about day 144 of gestation.

Birth injury

At birth the kid undergoes some quite profound changes to enable it to adapt to its new environment. With the exception of the development of the rumen the major physiological changes are over in a few days after birth and any associated signs of maladjustment appear by this time. It is quite possible that the kid will have to compensate for the deleterious effects of parturition itself:

❏ *Trauma* from the physical forces of parturition or from traction in an assisted birth.
❏ *Compression* of the kid's thorax as it passes through the pelvis, causing compression of the lungs.
❏ *Asphyxia* from pressure on the umbilical cord during passage through the pelvic cavity or from reduced efficiency of the placenta during uterine contractions.

Birth injury can result directly in the death of a kid if the damage is severe enough, e.g. from abdominal haemorrhage due to liver rupture, or difficulty in breathing, or may lead to death from starvation/hypothermia by impairing feeding and movement.

Intrauterine malnutrition

Inadequate placental development, as a result of maternal malnutrition, intrauterine infection or other cause, will result in poor fetal development and low birth weights because of poor transfer of oxygen, electrolytes and nutrients. The newborn kid is also more prone to hypothermia as chronic fetal hypoxia inhibits the capacity for thermoregulation.

Maternal malnutrition

Correct feeding of the doe throughout pregnancy is essential. Placental development is directly related to the nutrition of the doe, so that low birth weights follow directly from maternal underfeeding. Underfeeding, particularly during the final 6 weeks of pregnancy, will result in small kids with low levels of fetal liver glycogen and fat and the birth of hypoglycaemic kids with poor energy reserves. Gross underfeeding may result in abortion or stillbirths.

Trace element deficiencies

Copper deficiency (enzootic ataxia, swayback)

Aetiology

❏ Copper deficiency is either the result of copper-deficient soils or generally in the UK as a result of a conditioned deficiency with reduced copper utilisation by the grazing animals, e.g. pasture topdressing with molybdenum and sulphur which reduce the availability of copper, or heavy lime applications which increase pasture molybdenum intake and thus reduce the copper intake. It is a disease of grazing animals or animals fed grass-based diets and home-produced cereals. Zero grazed animals receiving a concentrate ration are unlikely to be affected.
❏ Although the clinical signs and pathological lesions are similar to those in lambs, in goat herds clinical cases tend to be sporadic rather than a flock problem as in sheep and there is less correlation between copper levels and clinical disease.
❏ Fibre goats are more susceptible to deficiency than dairy goats (and are also more prone to copper toxicity).

Clinical signs

(1) Congenital form
  ❏ Kid is affected at birth. Some kids may be of low viability and

succumb to hypothermia without showing marked neurological signs.

(2) Delayed form
- ❏ Clinical signs do not appear until the kid is several weeks or
  even months old.
- ❏ Bright, alert, willing to suck and eat.
- ❏ Muscle tremors, head shaking.
- ❏ Progressive hind limb ataxia, progressing to paralysis.
- ❏ Adult goats in the same herd may have anaemia, decreased
  milk production, discoloured hair, diarrhoea, poor fleece
  quality and fail to thrive.
- ❏ Other kids may show growth retardation, increased susceptibility to infections, poor fleece quality and susceptibility to
  fractures (distinguish from parasitism, cobalt deficiency or
  inadequate nutrition).

Diagnosis

- ❏ Clinical signs.
- ❏ Plasma copper levels > 9 μmol/l adequate.
- ❏ Cerebrospinal fluid (CSF) within normal limits.
- ❏ Histological examination of the CNS.
- ❏ Liver copper levels (normal > 40 mg/kg DM).

Low liver copper levels may occur in some kids without enzootic ataxia
and some apparently affected kids appear to have normal levels (due
to subsequent supplementation?).

Postmortem findings

- ❏ Generally no gross pathology of the nervous system.
- ❏ Demyelination of cerebellar and spinal cord tracts.
- ❏ Cerebellar corticol hypoplasia; necrosis and loss of Purkinje cells of
  cerebellum.
- ❏ Chromatolytic necrosis in brain stem nuclei and spinal cord.
- ❏ May be skeletal abnormalities – brittle bones, healing rib fractures.

Treatment

- ❏ Often unsuccessful except early in the disease; may prevent further
  deterioration in delayed form.
  - ■ Injection: **Coppaclear** (Crown); **Cuvine** (C-Vet); **Swaycop**
    (Young's)
    Adult goats: **25 mg**, i.e. **2 ml i.m.**
    If kids are injected, small doses (< 5 mg or 0.4 ml), repeated if
    necessary, are safer than a single large dose.

- Oral: **Copper oxide needles, 1 g/10 kg** in gelatin capsules (**Copacaps**, Merial; **Copporal**, Pfizer), i.e. one 2.5- or 2-g gelatin capsule for kids of 20 to 40 kg body weight and two 2.5- or 2-g capsules or one 4-g capsule for 50-kg adult.
- ❏ Overdosage with copper causes toxicity (qv) so supplementation should be used with care. Copper oxide needles given orally are generally safer than injections.
- ❏ Copper sulphate solutions given by mouth should be mixed with milk to minimise the astringent effects on the gastric mucosa.

Prevention

- ❏ Soil and plant analysis for copper and its antagonists molybdenum, sulphur and iron and correction by fertiliser applications under professional advice.
- ❏ Copper supplementation to does during pregnancy:
  - Injection: **Coppaclear** (Crown); **Cuvine** (C-Vet); **Swaycop** (Young's), **25 mg, 2 ml i.m.** 10 weeks prior to kidding.
  - Oral: **copper oxide needles, 1 g/10 kg** in gelatin capsules (**Copacaps**, Merial; **Copporal**, Pfizer), i.e. one 2.5- or 2-g gelatin capsule for kids of 20 to 40 kg body weight and two 2.5- or 2-g capsules or one 4-g capsule for 50-kg adult.

  The copper oxide particles become trapped in the abomasum for several months, slowly releasing absorbable copper. Liver reserves are increased much more effectively than by copper injections.
  - Water additives: **Aquatrace copper tablets** (Denis Brinicombe).
  - Food supplements: **copper sulphate** (UKASTA) (G), for addition to feed at **254 g/kg**; dose: up to **2 g/head**.

  Supplementation of the doe will prevent swayback, reduce kid mortality and improve early growth rates, but to ensure adequate later growth and prevent delayed swayback, kids should be dosed at about 2 to 3 weeks of age.

Iodine deficiency (goitre)

> Enlarged thymic glands are common in dairy kids and must be distinguished from goitre.

Goitre is commonly misdiagnosed by goatkeepers when kids have any enlargement in the throat region (see Chapter 9). In particular, thymic swellings, which are common, regularly lead to a misdiagnosis. True iodine deficiency is probably rare in the UK. Angoras are more susceptible than dairy goats or sheep.

Aetiology

❏ Natural deficiencies of iodine.
❏ Goitrogenic feeds, e.g. kale and cabbage, produce a secondary iodine deficiency by accumulation of isothiocyanates which prevent the accumulation of iodine in the thyroid gland.

Clinical signs

❏ Abortion.
❏ Stillbirths or very weak kids born at term or slightly early with thin sparse hair coat; susceptible to cold stress, respiratory problems.
❏ Enlarged thyroid glands (goitre) in the affected kids produce palpable swellings posterior and ventral to the larynx (more discrete than thymic glands involving the distal rather than proximal cervical region). The thyroid may weigh between 10 and 50 g compared to the normal weight of 2 g.
❏ A subclinical deficiency may result in small weak kids without obvious goitre.
❏ Older goats in the herd may show decreased production, poor growth rate and reduced appetite.
❏ Iodine deficiency may also result in subfertility.

Diagnosis

❏ Blood thyroxine assay.

Prevention and treatment

❏ Iodised saltlicks or loose iodised salt in the diets of older goats will prevent development of iodine deficiency. Alternatively, dose with potassium iodide 2 months and 2 weeks before kidding – dissolve 20 g of potassium iodide in 1 l of water and dose at a rate of 10 ml per 20 kg body weight.
❏ Affected kids can be treated with 3 to 5 drops of Lugol's iodine in milk daily for 1 week.
❏ Avoid goitrogenic feeds such as kale.

Iodine toxicity: treatment of goats incorrectly diagnosed by the owner as being iodine deficient can lead to iodine toxicity, which produces anorexia, lacrimation, coughing, dandruff in the coat and weight loss.

Selenium deficiency

Kids may occasionally show signs of white muscle disease (qv) at birth.

Congenital infections

Weak kids may be born as part of clinical syndromes involving abortions and stillbirths, such as toxoplasmosis, chlamydiosis and campylobacter (see Chapter 2). Infection of the pregnant doe causes a placentitis which impairs transfer of nutrients to the fetus. Where the infectious agent crosses the placental barrier, as with toxoplasmosis, further signs of disease such as abnormal sucking behaviour may also impair the ability of the kid to survive.

Postnatal malnutrition

Unless the kid is removed at birth and hand reared, it is completely dependent on the doe for food. The kid has very limited energy reserves and a high energy requirement and so is totally dependent on the early intake of colostrum to maintain life. If the kid is unable to suckle easily, or the doe is unable or unwilling to feed the kid, the kid should be removed, dried, stomach tubed and then bottle fed as necessary.

Congenital defects

Congenital defects are relatively uncommon in goats. Some, such as atresia ani and cleft palate, will be incompatible with satisfactory growth and development, unless they can be surgically corrected. Others will limit the ability of the kid to suckle and may lead to starvation, unless the condition is recognised and remedial measures taken.

Contracted tendons as a result of positional constraints in utero are relatively common. Except in severe cases, physiotherapy is usually sufficient to correct the problem. Excessive laxity and overextension of the leg joints is also a common temporary problem, which is usually self correcting in a few days.

Beta mannosidosis (qv) of Nubian and Nubian cross goats and *myelofibrosis* (qv) of Pygmy goats are inherited diseases, attributable to autosomal recessive genes.

Postnatal infections

In the first few hours after birth, the kid is susceptible to infection from a number of infective agents which gain access via the navel or mouth resulting in infection of the navel, septicaemia, pyaemia, enteritis and joint ill. Possible organisms involved include *Escherichia coli*, *Clos-*

tridium perfringens type B, *Staphylococcus aureus*, *Streptococcus* spp., *Corynebacterium* spp., *Salmonella* and rotavirus.

Many other organisms are potential pathogens. Infection is more likely in intensive kidding systems, particularly towards the end of the kidding period.

Floppy kid syndrome (metabolic acidosis without dehydration in kids)

Aetiology

❏ The cause is unknown; many kids may be affected at one time, but it is not known if the condition is infectious or contagious. Most cases occur late in the kidding season. The condition is reversible, suggesting a transient initiating cause.
❏ It is increasingly common in the USA; there have been isolated reports but as yet it is unconfirmed in the UK.
❏ Affected kids have a profound metabolic acidosis with a pH as low as 7 (normal 7.4 to 7.44), low bicarbonate and a base deficit of 20 mmol or more; sodium and chloride levels are normal but potassium is decreased.
❏ Morbidity ranges from 10 to > 50% in affected herds.

Clinical signs

❏ The kid is normal at birth but develops sudden onset of profound muscular weakness (flaccid paresis or paralysis) or ataxia at 3 to 10 days of age.
❏ Affected kids show no signs of diarrhoea, respiratory disease or other signs referable to a specific organ system.
❏ The kids cannot use their tongues but can swallow.
❏ Spontaneous recovery, even of severely affected kids, may occur, but mortality can reach 30 to 50% in untreated cases.
❏ Most kids respond well to treatment, but there may be delayed recovery (4 to 6 weeks) of neuromuscular function. Occasional relapses may occur.

Note: any other profoundly weak or acidotic kid will appear floppy or limp so that the condition needs differentiating from white muscle disease, botulism, colibacillosis, septicaemia and enterotoxaemia.

Treatment
❏ Correction of the acidosis by administration of sodium bicarbonate or liquid antacid such as Peptobismol or Gaviscon.

❏ Mildly affected kids respond to oral bicarbonate or antacids if given at the onset of the disease. Some kids respond to one treatment, but others may require repeated administration of bicarbonate with supportive care and nursing. Milk can be fed by stomach tube.

❏ More severely affected kids require intravenous isotonic (1.26%) sodium bicarbonate to correct the electrolyte imbalance, following electrolyte estimation where possible.

> [body weight in kg] × 0.5 × base deficit = mmol bicarbonate required
>
> where 0.5 is the extracellular fluid volume [ECFV];
>
> base deficit = normal serum bicarbonate – patient's serum bicarbonate;
>
> normal serum level = 25 nmol/l;
>
> and 1 ml of 1.26% sodium bicarbonate = 0.15 mmol bicarbonate.

If the serum bicarbonate level is not known, the correction must be empirical. In mild acidosis, the base deficit is about 5 mmol/l; in severe acidosis, the base deficit is 10 nmol/l or more. The volume of 1.26% bicarbonate required may range from 125 to 200 ml and this should be given over 1 to 3 hours. Overtreatment with intravenous bicarbonate causes clinical depression so it is better to be conservative when estimating the base deficit and finish correcting the acidosis with oral sodium bicarbonate.

Exposure

Primary hypothermia

Primary hypothermia is caused by direct exposure of kids to cold, wet, windy weather so that heat loss exceeds heat production. Small kids have a relatively large surface area relative to body weight and relatively small energy reserves and so are more prone to hypothermia than large kids.

Secondary hypothermia

Most kids who die from hypothermia succumb to secondary hypothermia, where the neonates are unable to suckle and replenish their body reserves in weather which is insufficiently cold to kill through primary hypothermia. Thus, mismothering, agalactia, birth injury, etc. can all lead to death from secondary hypothermia.

Colostrum

Each kid should receive colostrum within the first 6 hours after birth, preferably during the first hour. Colostrum should be fed at a rate of **50 to 75 ml/kg** three times during the first day. Anything which increases the kid's requirement for heat production, such as bad weather or chilling, increases the demand for colostrum. Housed kids require about 210 ml/kg during the first day, while kids outside in inclement weather require around 280 ml/kg.

A housed kid of:

3 kg requires 150 to 200 ml at its first feed and 600 ml daily;
4 kg requires 200 to 300 ml at its first feed and 850 ml daily;
5 kg requires 250 to 475 ml at its first feed and 1100 ml daily.

Hypothermic kids under 5 hours old will require thorough drying and warming to $>37°C$, over 30 to 60 minutes, before being given colostrum. Hypothermic kids over 5 hours old will be hypoglycaemic and must have the hypoglycaemia reversed by intraperitoneal administration of glucose (see below) before warming. If the hypoglycaemia is not reversed, the increased cerebral metabolism, produced by warming, will lead to convulsions and death.

Feeding by stomach tube

Attempting to bottle feed a weak or comatose kid may lead to regurgitation and inhalation pneumonia. Any kids which are not sucking well should be fed by stomach tube using a lamb stomach tube and 60-ml syringe. An 18-French feeding tube or a urethral catheter long enough to reach the last rib can be utilised in an emergency. Kids should be fed at the rate of 50 ml/kg or until the stomach feels full.

Wherever possible the kid should receive its mother's colostrum, but if this is not available, frozen stored colostrum, cow's colostrum or commercial lamb colostrum substitute can be used. Colostrum or milk from other herds should never be used if there is a danger of introducing diseases such as caprine arthritis encephalitis virus. After the first day, the kid can receive goat's milk or milk replacer. Cow, lamb and calf milk replacers can all be successfully used to rear kids.

Intraperitoneal glucose injections

Hypothermic kids over 5 hours old will be hypoglycaemic and must have the hypoglycaemia reversed before warming by an intraperitoneal injection of a **20% glucose solution** at a rate of **10 ml/kg**. Holding the kid by its front legs, inject 1 cm to the side and 2 cm behind the umbilicus (i.e. towards the anus), with the needle directed at a 45° angle towards the rump, using a 50-ml syringe and 19-g 25-mm needle.

Further reading

Anon (1982) Detection and treatment of hypothermia in newborn lambs. *In Practice*, January 1982, 20–22.

Eales, A. (1987) Feeding lambs by stomach tube. *In Practice*, January 1987, 18–20.

Eales, A. and Small, J. (1986) *Practical Lambing*. Longman, London.

Matthews, J.G. (1985) Care of the newborn kid. *Goat Vet. Soc. J.*, **6** (2), 64–7.

Papworth, S.M. (1981) The young kid. *Goat Vet. Soc. J.*, **2** (2), 12–15.

White, D.G. (1993) Colostral supplementation in ruminants. *Comp. Cont. Ed. Pract. Vet.*, **15** (2), 335–42.

6 Lameness in Adult Goats

> The most common cause of lameness and most important welfare issue is poor foot care.

As in most other farm animals, the majority of cases of lameness in goats involve the foot. *Conformation problems* such as weak pasterns or cowhocks will predispose to uneven hoof growth, and environmental factors such as excessively wet conditions which soften the horn may lead to excessive horn growth and increase susceptibility to infection. However, the cornerstone of lameness prevention within a herd remains regular routine foot trimming. Tetanus is a possible sequel to any penetrating infection, particularly of the foot, and adequate anti-tetanus cover should always be given.

Initial assessment

The preliminary history should consider:

❏ Individual or flock/herd problem.
❏ Sudden or gradual onset of lameness.
❏ Duration of lameness.
❏ Static or progressive lameness.
❏ Any predisposing factors, such as excessively wet conditions.

Clinical examination

The animal should be examined at rest and while moving from a distance of a few feet for:

❏ Weight bearing.
❏ Stance.
❏ Obvious wounds, swellings, etc.
❏ Conformation.
❏ Overgrown feet.

A detailed examination should then localise the seat of the lameness by:

❏ Cleaning and trimming the feet where necessary.
❏ Palpation
❏ Manipulation.

Additional information can be obtained from radiography or laboratory examination as indicated.

Treatment

❏ Specific treatment should be instigated as soon as a diagnosis has been made.
❏ Ensure feet are correctly trimmed.
❏ Instigate pain relief/anti-inflammatory treatment as indicated.
❏ Non-steroidal anti-inflammatory drugs:
    Aspirin, 50–100 mg/kg orally every 12 hours (aspirin is poorly absorbed from the rumen so relatively high doses are needed).
    Carprofen, 1.4 mg/kg, 1 ml/35 kg s.c. or **i.v.** (**Zenecarp solution**, Pfizer) every 36 to 48 hours.
    Carprofen, 1.4 mg/kg, 0.5 sachet/75 kg orally (**Zenecarp granules**, Pfizer) once daily.
    Flunixin meglumine, 2 mg/kg, 2 ml/45 kg i.v. or **i.m.** (**Finadyne solution**, Schering-Plough; **Flunixin**, Norbrook; **Binixin**, Bayer, **Meflosyl 5%**, Fort Dodge; **Resprixin**, Intervet) daily for up to 5 days.
    Flunixin meglumine, 2 mg/kg, 100 kg horse calibration/50 kg orally (**Finadyne paste**, Schering-Plough) daily for up to 5 days.
    Flunixin meglumine, 2 mg/kg, 0.5 sachet/50 kg orally (**Finadyne granules**, Schering-Plough) daily for up to 5 days.
    Ketoprofen, 3 mg/kg, 1 ml/33 kg i.v. or **i.m.** (**Ketofen**, Merial) daily for up to 3 days.
    Meloxicam, 0.5 mg/kg, 1 ml/10 kg i.v. or **s.c.** (**Metacam 5 mg solution**, Boehringer Ingelheim) every 36 to 48 hours.
    Phenylbutazone, 4 mg/kg i.v. or **10 mg/kg, orally**. Phenylbutazone can be given orally twice daily for 2 days, then once daily for 3 days, then every other day or as needed.
    Note: Phenylbutazone is banned from use in food-producing animals in the EU.
❏ Corticosteroids:
    Betamethasone, 0.04–0.08 mg/kg, 1 ml/30 kg (**Betsolan** (G); **Betsolan soluble** (G), Schering-Plough).
    Dexamethasone, 0.1 mg/kg, 1 ml/20 kg i.v. (**Azium**, Schering-Plough; **Colvasone**, Norbrook; **Dexadreson**, Intervet.

Non-infectious diseases of the foot

Overgrown feet

> The cornerstone of lameness prevention is regular foot trimming.

White line disease

White line disease involves separation of a portion of the horny outer wall from the underlying sensitive laminae at the white line. Early lesions include thickening, softening and slight separation of the wall from the laminae and this later progresses to complete *horn separation*, with the formation of a pocket which becomes filled with dirt and debris, eventually putting pressure on the laminae. The condition is often noticed at routine foot trimming, particularly during the wetter months of the year. Early foot trimming to pare away loose horn, leaving a characteristic half-moon shape of keratinised laminae, will resolve the problem before lameness occurs. Where foot care is deficient, the condition may progress until the animal is lame. If infection occurs in the area, pus will collect and track to the coronary band, forming a foot abscess (qv).

The aetiological causes of white line disease are not clear – the white line is the cemented junction of the wall and the sole and so is an area of weakness. Minor trauma to the area by stones, rough concrete or gravel may lead to damage and a slight separation, which is then increased by dirt being forced into the space. Wet conditions underfoot will soften the hooves and make damage more likely. If the separation between wall and sole is not marked, normal hoof growth may carry debris back to the surface, where it is shed, and the lesion can resolve. If further impaction of dirt occurs, the lesion will progress until the horn of the hoof wall in the adjacent area separates completely from the sole.

Horn separation

In most cases, horn separation is probably a sequel to white line disease (see above), but the exact relationship between the two conditions requires clarification. Horn separation can also follow trauma to the wall of the hoof.

Bruising/trauma to the hoof

Foreign body penetration of the sole

Puncture of the sole by a foreign body such as a stone or nail results in immediate lameness in the affected leg and occasionally a goat is presented with a foreign body still embedded in the foot or interdigital area. If the foreign body is removed, the penetration site opened up and drainage established, recovery will occur rapidly, but neglect may lead to abscess formation (qv).

Abscess of the sole

Abscess of the sole is an uncommon, painful lesion of uncertain aetiology, probably as a result of trauma to the sole and possibly a precursor to sole ulceration and the formation of a granulomatous lesion. Pain is evident over an area of the sole and pus is released when the foot is trimmed. Treatment consists of careful foot trimming, cleaning of the area and topical or parenteral use of antibiotics.

Granulomatous lesions of the sole

Granulomatous lesions of the sole have been described in a herd of milking goats. Although the aetiology is unclear, it is probable that granulomatous lesions are a sequel to direct trauma to the sole and subsequent ulceration, which is slow to heal. Treatment consists of resection of the granulation tissue at the level of the solar horn, removing all underrun horn and careful foot trimming.

Fracture of the distal phalanx

A fracture of the distal phalanx or pedal bone produces an acute lameness in one foot. Radiography is required to confirm the diagnosis. Resolution may occur if movement is restricted for at least 6 weeks by a waterproof plaster cast.

Laminitis (aseptic pododermatitis)

Aetiology
Laminitis is a metabolic disorder of the corium and germinal layer of the foot, produced by a degeneration of the vascular supply to the corium.

❏ *Acute laminitis* occurs in response to endotoxin release during ruminal acidosis or toxic conditions.

❑ *Subacute* and *subclinical laminitis* are produced by overfeeding over a longer period.
❑ *Chronic laminitis* develops where acute or subacute laminitis is not recognised or satisfactorily treated because horn formation is disturbed.
❑ Trauma to the hoof may also predispose to laminitis.
❑ A genetic predisposition may exist in some families.

Occurrence

Acute laminitis may occur:

❑ After any toxic condition, such as mastitis, metritis, retained fetal membranes or pneumonia.
❑ A few days after kidding with or without one of the above conditions.
❑ As a sequel to acidosis
 ■ in females fed high-energy diets
 ■ in silage-fed goats with continued ingestion of acid silage.

Subacute and *subclinical laminitis* occur:

❑ In goatlings and kids as young as 8 weeks where high protein/ energy concentrate rations (together with inadequate fibre?) are fed.
❑ In does overfed for the level of production.
❑ In male goats fed on milking rations, particularly during the summer months when they are not working. Mammary development and milk production in bucks, particularly British Saanens, or Saanens from high-yielding families, are also accentuated at this time by overfeeding and there is a danger of mastitis developing.

Chronic laminitis occurs as a sequel to acute, subacute or subclinical laminitis.

Clinical signs

Acute laminitis – sudden onset of tender foot or feet (generally both front feet but occasionally all four feet), with a disinclination to walk, prolonged recumbency or walking on knees, and a shifting of weight distribution when standing to spare the affected feet, teeth grinding and other signs of pain, pyrexia, and a fall in milk yield. The coronet of the affected foot feels hot, but the toe cold.

> Subclinical laminitis is a common and often unrecognised disease of dairy goats.

Subacute and *subclinical laminitis* are only differentiated by degree. In subacute laminitis minor gait abnormalities occur whereas in the subclinical condition no gait changes are present and the feet do not feel hot. *Subclinical laminitis is a common and underdiagnosed disease of dairy goats, particularly kids and goatlings, which leads to the development of hoof abnormalities in older animals.*

Haemorrhage of the wall, heel and particularly the sole is evident on routine foot trimming as a fine reddish discoloration which, unlike bruising, is generally not painful.

As in cattle, subclinical laminitis leads to the development of other lamenesses because poor quality horn is produced with changes in horn growth, particularly of the sole, so that the shape of the claw is changed and there may be marked differences in height and width between the lateral and medial claws.

> Chronic laminitis produces very hard feet with thick 'platform soles'.

Chronic laminitis produces a chronically lame goat with feet that, at first glance, appear relatively normal in shape. However, the horn is extremely solid, with failure to differentiate clearly into wall and sole, and may be impossible to trim with ordinary foot shears. The feet are extremely deep, often 5 cm or more (hence the term 'platform soles'). A rock-hard, very deep foot is pathognomonic of the disease. Front feet are more commonly affected than back feet and both front feet are usually affected. Anglo-Nubian and Anglo-Nubian crosses seem more prone to the disease than the Swiss breeds of dairy goats. Severely affected animals have a characteristic goose-stepping walk and spend a lot of time on their knees. Unlike cattle, overgrown 'sledge runner' feet ('slippering') is not a feature of the disease in goats. 'Slippering' in goats is produced by foot overgrowth due to lack of routine foot care. In severe cases of laminitis, the wall and sole may loosen from the corium, with concomitant downward rotation of the pedal bone, but this is much rarer than in the horse.

Treatment and control

❑ Most cases of laminitis can be prevented by better management, particularly by correct feeding practice.
❑ Acute cases should be placed on a reduced protein/energy diet, i.e. hay with a very reduced or no concentrate ration, and a deep bed provided.

❏ Antibiotic cover should be given to combat any infectious or toxic cause of the condition.

❏ Pain relief with an NSAID is essential ('Treatment', this chapter).

❏ The value of antihistamines is uncertain and the use of corticosteroids controversial and possibly contraindicated, as in the horse.

❏ Heat treatment of the feet will help restore the circulation if used during the first few hours when vasoconstriction is occurring. Cold water treatment is of benefit later, and for about 7 days, to reduce the subsequent vasodilation.

❏ Chronic cases need careful foot trimming to relieve pain by reducing pressure on the sensitive areas. Regular repeat foot care is needed when the foot is grossly overgrown or misshapen.

Zinc deficiency

Although more usually recognised as a proliferative dermatitis (parakeratosis; see Chapter 10), zinc-deficient goats may have skeletal and hoof abnormalities, resulting in abnormal posture with the back arched and feet close together. The feet may be painful on palpation with deep transverse ridges around the hoof wall.

Infectious diseases of the foot

> Goats' feet are more severely affected by wet conditions than those of sheep.

Interdigital dermatitis and footrot

Predisposing conditions:

❏ Prolonged grazing of wet, muddy pastures, or housing in wet, dirty yards.

❏ Overcrowding.

❏ Introduction of new stock – infection may be introduced by clinical or subclinical carriers (goats, sheep, cattle or deer).

❏ Poor foot care.

❏ Poor foot conformation.

Aetiology

❏ Continuous wetting of the foot and interdigital skin damages the tissues and allows the invasion of the casual organism of interdigital dermatitis, *Fusobacterium necrophorum*, which is widespread in the environment and cannot penetrate healthy, intact skin. Its penetration is aided by other bacteria such as *Corynebacterium pyogenes.*

❑ Interdigital dermatitis may exist as a distinct condition, but in the presence of *Dichelobacter (Bacteriodes) nodosus*, which is introduced by carrier animals, there is a rapid spread of the infection to the hoof and the sole and *benign footrot* or *virulent footrot* becomes established. *Dichelobacter nodosus*, which acts synergistically with *F. necrophorum*, has a varying keratinolytic activity which destroys the hoof, permitting further invasion of the foot. When strains with low keratinolytic activity are present damage will be limited and only the mild lesions of benign footrot seen. When the strains have high keratinolytic activity, damage is much more severe and virulent footrot occurs.

❑ Spirochaetes of the *Treponema* genus have been implicated in the aetiology of digital dermatitis (papillomatous digital dermatitis) of cattle and a new severe form of virulent footrot of sheep. The possible role of spirochaetes in caprine footrot has not been investigated.

Interdigital dermatitis (scald)

Goats, with longer digits and a deeper interdigital area, show more severe clinical signs of interdigital dermatitis than sheep.

Clinical signs

❑ A mild to severe lameness in one or more goats with a rapid spread throughout the flock or herd if the predisposing conditions are suitable; animals will be lame in one or more feet, or walking on their knees. Affected animals will lose condition, with drop in milk yield or shedding of fleece.

❑ The interdigital area between the claws is inflamed, often with considerable swelling, and there is a characteristic smell. There is no damage to the horn of the hoof. In severe cases there will be ulceration with a purulent discharge.

Footrot

Clinical signs

❑ As for interdigital dermatitis, but there are lesions in the hoof and sole, with separation of the horn, caused by underrunning. In severe cases the hoof will only be attached at the coronet. Pus is present beneath the underrun horn and the horn can be pared away, revealing greyish soft horn with a characteristic foul odour of decomposing tissue.

Secondary complications may arise from fly strike or tetanus.

Treatment and control

❏ Regular examination and foot trimming of the whole herd.

❏ Uncomplicated cases of interdigital dermatitis will resolve quickly if the animals are moved from wet pasture to dry ground or housed and the lesions treated with an antibiotic spray or footbath.

❏ If footrot is present the feet of infected goats should be trimmed separately and the footrot shears disinfected between goats. All infected and underrun tissue should be removed. Foot parings should be disposed of carefully.

❏ If an individual goat is affected, dip the feet in a footbath solution daily for 3 days and then weekly for several weeks. Local antibiotic aerosol sprays, together with parenteral antibiotic therapy, are sometimes useful and a severely affected foot can be bandaged. A zinc sulphate/vaseline mixture can be applied locally inter-digitally.

❏ With a herd problem, the goats should be run through a footbath on a weekly basis. Goats need to be closely supervised as they are much more adept at avoiding the bath than sheep. The bath should be at least 4 cm deep and the goats should stand in the bath for at least 2 minutes routinely and for 30 minutes when the infection is severe.

Three solutions are commonly used:

Copper sulphate 10% (Bluestone):	**10 kg copper sulphate to 100 l water.**
Formalin 5–10%:	**5–10 l commercial formalin (formalin 40%) to 100 l water.**
Zinc sulphate 10%:	**10 kg zinc sulphate to 100 l water.**

Formalin is very effective but stings raw tissue and makes the goats less amenable to adequate bathing and also hardens the skin and hoof, possibly preventing the penetration of further solutions.Copper sulphate may stain fleeces and may also cause toxicity in goats that drink from the footbath. Zinc sulphate solution is thus the preferred treatment, although a longer bathing period is required than with formalin and the solution is more expensive. Footrite (Veterinary Pharmaceuticals) is a zinc preparation containing a penetrating agent to increase the deposition of zinc in the hoof.

The goats should be penned on dry ground until their feet are dry.

❏ Parenteral chemotherapy – advisable in severe cases; use penicillin/streptomycin or tetracyclines.
❏ Vaccination – sheep footrot vaccines have been used with very mixed results:

> **Footvax** (Schering-Plough) or **Vaxall Norot** (Fort Dodge), **1 ml s.c.**, two doses at intervals of 4 to 8 weeks; booster doses every 4 to 6 months as required.

Pregnant does should not be vaccinated 4 weeks before or after kidding; kids can be vaccinated at 4 weeks of age. Vaccination alone will not control the disease.

Note: severe local reactions to these oil adjuvanted vaccines have been reported.

❏ Select for resistance. There is some evidence that there are family and breed differences in the incidence of footrot, possibly related to foot conformation.

Foot abscess

Predisposing conditions:

❏ Injury to the foot from stones, overzealous trimming, puncture wounds, etc.
❏ The presence of interdigital dermatitis/footrot.
❏ White line disease.
❏ Sandcracks in the hoof wall (particularly lateral side of hoof).

Aetiology

❏ As a sequel to interdigital dermatitis/footrot or a penetration wound of the foot, deep infection by *C. pyogenes*, *F. necrophorum* or other bacteria produces an abscess in the heel or more commonly the toe of one claw. The abscess may burst out at the coronet or interdigital space.

Clinical signs

❏ Usually affects individual goats, involving one foot. The animal is very lame, often spending long periods lying down. There is considerable painful swelling of the affected claw, particularly in the interdigital space, with bloody pus discharging between the digits or from the coronet.
❏ Pyrexia, anorexia.

Treatment

❏ Early treatment by paring to release the pus, bathing with antiseptic solution and poultice, together with systemic antibiotic therapy for about 10 days, will be successful provided the deeper tissues and joints are not involved.

❏ Where the condition is more severe, considerable deformity of the foot may occur and amputation of the digit should be considered.

Orf (contagious pustular dermatitis)

Lesions of orf (Chapter 9) occasionally occur around the coronet or on the legs from licking and may result in lameness.

Mycotic dermatitis (strawberry footrot)

Dermatophilus congolense causes '*lumpy wool*' and *strawberry footrot* in sheep and goats. The incidence of both conditions appears to be very low in goats in the UK, although the condition is easily produced experimentally.

Initially there are raised (paint brush) tufts of hair followed by crusting with pus under the crusts. Removal of the crusts leaves circular, raised, red, granulating lesions on the coronet interdigital space and lower leg as well as on the body, scrotum and head. Lesions on the nose and ears must be distinguished from orf (qv) and those on the feet and lower leg from chorioptic mange (qv). Predisposing conditions are wet, unhygienic conditions and ectoparasites which transfer zoospores between animals. Zoospores are generally carried in scabs between animals.

Diagnosis

❏ Smears, skin biopsy or culture on blood agar.

Treatment

❏ Dry conditions, broad-spectrum antibiotics; topical applications of **10% zinc sulphate solution** or **1% potash alum**.

Foot-and-mouth disease

Foot-and-mouth disease produces vesicular lesions at the coronet, heel and interdigitally resulting in acute lameness, generally in all four feet. There are generally only occasional small lesions in the mouth, but the teats may be affected. Other clinical signs include pyrexia, lethargy and anorexia.

Lameness above the foot

Weak pasterns

'Weak pasterns' have been a longstanding problem in some families of dairy goats, particularly among Saanens, British Saanens and their crosses. More recently, Angora goats imported from Tasmania and New Zealand have shown similar weaknesses. The condition appears to be inherited as a recessive gene and accentuated by inbreeding.

Weak pasterns produce excessive wear on the heels and a long foot with an overgrown toe.

Aetiology

❏ Weakness of the flexor tendons attached to the pastern joint, the degree of deformity depending on the degree of involvement of the superficial digital flexor tendon, deep digital flexor tendon and the suspensory ligament (see Figure 6.1). Traumatic damage and rupture of the flexor tendons and suspensory ligament (see below) will produce similar conformational changes.

❏ The condition is accentuated by badly trimmed feet where the heels are cut short and the toes left long. Conversely, well trimmed feet will ameliorate the condition to some extent. Poor trimming of the feet over a long period will produce the condition even in goats which are genetically sound.

❏ Older multiparous milking goats often show weakness of the superficial digital tendon.

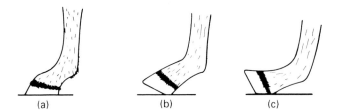

(a)   (b)   (c)

Figure 6.1   Weak pasterns. (a) Superficial digital flexor tendon weakness; (b) superficial and deep digital flexor tendons, weak or ruptured; (c) flexor tendons and suspensory ligament ruptured.

Clinical signs

❏ Affected animals may show weakness by the time they are 6 months old, with the condition worsening as the goat gets heavier through growth and pregnancy. Suspect animals will roll on their heels slightly, lifting the toe from the ground when encouraged to shift their weight backwards by pressing on the brisket. The hind legs are more commonly involved, but some goats show marked weakness in the front legs.

❏ As the condition progresses, the joint adopts a characteristic right-angled bend because of weakness of the superficial flexor tendon, with excessive wear on the heels. With the involvement of the deep flexor tendon the weight is shifted back onto the heels so the toes are raised from the ground, resulting in bruising to the heels. With complete collapse of the joint the weight is carried on the back of the foot without the sole touching the ground.

Accident or trauma

Fractures

Fractures of the limbs are more common in kids than adult goats (see Chapter 7).

Soft tissue damage

A number of specific causes of lameness have been described.

(1) Rupture of the superficial and deep digital flexor tendons

Aetiology

❏ Trauma to the metacarpal or metatarsal region. A common cause of this injury is a tether becoming entangled around the leg and biting into the flesh – gross infection of the wound may be present as these cases are often neglected and severe restriction of the blood supply to the distal limb may lead to gangrene.

❏ Complete rupture of both flexor tendons produces a permanent unsoundness unless surgical repair is carried out. Severe lameness occurs and the animal is unwilling to bear weight as there is overflexion of the fetlock which touches the ground.

❏ A complete rupture of the superficial flexor tendon alone leads to slight lameness, with a dropped fetlock and reasonable weight bearing.

❏ Incomplete rupture of the superficial tendon does not alter the ability to bear weight.

Treatment

❏ The wound should be thoroughly cleaned and the damage to the tendons assessed.

❏ Tendon repair can be carried out in a valuable animal using wire, carbon fibre or other suture material. The prognosis is good if only the superficial tendon is involved and poor if the deep tendon is damaged.

❏ The leg should be immobilised in a suitable external cast for at least a month.

(2) Rupture of the peroneus tertius muscle

Aetiology

❏ Trauma from a fall, etc. results in rupture of the muscle, generally at its proximal origin on the stifle.

Clinical signs

❏ At rest, the limb is weight bearing, but there is a characteristic gait when walking, with the foot dragged and the limb pulled backwards as the hock is extended with the stifle flexed and the Achilles tendon slack and loose.

❏ There is a painful swelling on the lateral side of the stifle.

Treatment and prognosis

❏ The progress is favourable, complete rest for about 6 weeks often resulting in recovery.

(3) Rupture of the cranial cruciate ligament

Aetiology

❏ Trauma to the stifle region.

Clinical signs

❏ During walking, the stifle is fixed, with the heel raised from the ground and weight carried on the tip of the toe. A positive draw forward sign is present.

Treatment

❏ Surgical treatment is essential or secondary damage to the joint may result in permanent lameness. Similar procedures to those used in the dog are satisfactory.

(4) Rupture of the calcaneal tendon

Rupture of the calcaneal tendon results in acute lameness with swelling over the caudal area of the Achilles tendon. Successful primary repair of the tendon has been reported in a kid. In an adult goat repair has been carried out by transposition of the tendon of the peroneus longus muscle.

(5) Luxation of the scapulohumeral joint

Clinical signs

❏ The affected fore limb is carried in a semiflexed position, abducted and rotated outward. Attempts at flexion are painful.

Treatment

❏ Surgery to stabilise the joint.

(6) Luxating patella

Patella luxation may be:

❏ Lateral, congenital and obvious in the young goat (see Chapter 7).
❏ Medial, acquired as a result of trauma; acquired lateral luxation may occur but is less common than medial luxation.

(7) Radial nerve injury

Aetiology

❏ Trauma in the area of the upper limb or axilla.
❏ Lateral recumbency on a hard surface, e.g. during anaesthesia.

Clinical signs

❏ Dropped elbow with flexion of the carpus and fetlock.
❏ The foot is dragged as the carpus and fetlock cannot be extended.

Treatment

❏ Corticosteroids and diuretics to reduce the swelling around the nerve.
❏ Tendon transplantation has been used when the nerve injury was permanent.

Lameness after injection

> Extreme care should be taken with intramuscular injections as permanent lameness can result.

Temporary lameness in goats is common after injections with irritant substances, e.g. tetracyclines, enroflaxacin, because of the relatively small muscular masses in the hind leg, particularly in the gluteal region. A more permanent lameness may result from damage to the sciatic or peroneal nerves. Because of the dangers involved in injecting into the limbs, the mid neck region has been recommended as a more suitable injection site (see Appendix 2).

Lameness may also be produced by painful swellings following the subcutaneous injection of irritant drugs (e.g. some oil adjuvanted vaccines) behind the elbow. Intramuscular injections should be avoided wherever possible and the subcutaneous route used for all drugs where so licensed.

Sciatic nerve injury

Aetiology

❑   Injections in the gluteal muscle mass.

Clinical signs

❑   Loss of function in almost all of the hind limb, with loss of skin sensation on the lateral surface of the tibial region and the hock and below.
❑   The foot is dragged. With each step the leg is pulled upward and forward by contraction of the quadriceps muscles which are innervated by the femoral nerve.

Treatment and prognosis

❑   Even severe cases may resolve, but the prognosis is guarded.

Peroneal nerve injury

Aetiology

❑   Injections in the caudal thigh region.
❑   Trauma to the lateral surface of the thigh.

Clinical signs

❏ Paralysis of the muscles flexing the hock and extending the digits so that when the foot is brought forward there is knuckling at the fetlock and the hoof is dragged along the ground. If the foot is placed in position, normal weight bearing can occur.

Treatment and prognosis

❏ Prognosis is generally favourable, with some improvement being seen in about a week.
❏ Anti-inflammatory drugs and diuretics will reduce swelling in the area of the nerve.
❏ In cases of permanent injury the fetlock joint can be ankylosed.

Carpal hygroma

Aetiology

❏ Persistent trauma to the carpal area results in the development of a bursa.
❏ Common from the routine wear and tear of life but may form part of the caprine arthritis encephalitis syndrome (qv).

Clinical signs

❏ A firm, non-painful swelling, often bilateral, on the dorsal aspect of the carpal joint.
❏ The animal is generally not lame.

Treatment

❏ Acute lesions may resolve without treatment, but chronic conditions are unlikely to resolve.
❏ Aspiration of the bursal fluid may introduce infection if aseptic precautions are not carefully followed and is likely to produce only a temporary reduction in size.
❏ Injection with Lugol's iodine will destroy the membrane of the bursa.
❏ Surgical removal of the bursal sac can be undertaken for cosmetic reasons.

Osteopetrosis

Excessive calcium intake causing deposition in the bones and lameness in bucks and older does has been reported from the USA where large amounts of alfalfa hay are fed. In the UK where grass hay is normally fed, osteopetrosis is unlikely to present a problem.

Degenerative arthritis (osteoarthritis)

Aetiology

❏ A non-infectious arthritis resulting from degenerative changes in articular cartilage, together with hypertrophy of cartilage and bone.

Clinical signs

❏ A chronic lameness of gradual onset in older animals. The joints most commonly affected are the carpus, elbow, hock and stifle and these joints may be palpably enlarged, with crepitus evident on manipulation.
❏ The goat may have difficulty rising or if only one leg is affected may continuously rest the limb.
❏ With lack of use, muscle wasting of the affected limb may be evident.

Treatment

❏ The response to anti-inflammatory drugs and analgesics (see 'Treatment', this chapter, for dosages) is often disappointing and will often only provide temporary relief, if any.

The following have all been used empirically in non-lactating pet goats with dose rates extrapolated from those for other species as there are no published results of clinical trials in goats:

Pentosan polysulphate sodium, 3 mg/kg s.c. (Cartrophen Vet, Arthropharm) weekly for 4 weeks, then a single injection every 4 to 6 months. Do not use concurrently with steroids or non-steroidal anti-inflammatory drugs, including aspirin and phenyl-butazone.

Polysulphated glycosaminoglycan, 125 mg, 1.25 ml i.m. (Adequan, Janssen) for 50- to 80-kg doe (large animals may need increased amount), weekly for 4 weeks, then a single injection every 4 to 6 months.

Sodium hyaluronate, 20 mg, 2 ml i.v. (Hyonate, Bayer).

Once an animal can move with a minimum of pain, it is important to provide exercise on a daily basis.

Caprine arthritis encephalitis

Caprine arthritis encephalitis (CAE) is a disease of major importance in many parts of the world including France, Australia and the USA. In the UK, estimates of the level of infection are now less than 2% and there are only a few reported clinical cases. Since 1983, many goat-keepers have been regularly blood testing for the virus and have adopted suitable control measures, thus drastically limiting the spread of the disease. However, failure to maintain control measures could rapidly lead to an increased incidence of infection.

Aetiology

❑ A lentivirus, caprine arthritis encephalitis virus, exists as a domi-nant DNA provirus in circulating monocytes. The virus is closely related to maedi-visna virus in sheep.

Transmission

❑ Through the colostrum or milk of infected does. The practice of feeding milk pooled from several does will facilitate spread of the disease throughout the kid population.
❑ By direct contact between goats, although prolonged contact is probably necessary, by virus shed in body fluids such as saliva, urogenital secretions, faeces and/or respiratory tract secretions.
❑ By transfer of blood from an infected to a non-infected goat, e.g. by tattooing or multiple use of needles.
❑ *In-utero* transmission probably does not occur, or is at a very low level.
❑ The virus is very labile in the environment and transmission via pasture or buildings, etc., will not occur.
❑ Direct cross species transmission between sheep and goats has not been demonstrated, but lambs fed milk from CAE-positive goats become infected with the virus and sheep inoculated with virus experimentally became infected and developed lesions of the disease.
❑ Goats infected with CAE remain virus carriers for life and many symptomless carriers exist in the population. The virus can thus be unwittingly spread throughout the flock or herd, particularly to the young stock, without the owners being aware of a carrier being present.

Clinical signs

❑ Many goats remain symptomless carriers of the virus.
❑ The disease occurs in five clinical forms.

(1) Arthritis

❑ Generally seen only in yearlings or adult goats, although occa-sionally in kids as young as 6 months.

- ❏ CAE virus affects all synovial membranes including those of joints, tendons and bursae and produces a chronic, progressive synovitis and arthritis with excess synovial fluid.
- ❏ Afebrile.
- ❏ Good appetite.
- ❏ Variable lameness, from slight stiffness to extreme pain on standing.
- ❏ Gradual loss of condition depending on the degree of lameness.
- ❏ The carpal (knee) joints are primarily affected and may be grossly enlarged.
- ❏ Any other joint may be affected, particularly the shoulder, stifle, hock and fetlock, and the atlantal and supraspinous bursae are often enlarged later in the course of the disease.
- ❏ The course of the disease is variable, some animals merely showing slight lameness for a number of years, others showing an acute onset rapidly progressing to restriction of movement.

(2) Hard udder

See Chapter 12.

(3) Pneumonia

See Chapter 16.

(4) Encephalitis

See Chapter 16.

(5) Progressive weight loss

See Chapter 8.

Laboratory confirmation

(1) Serology
- ❏ Virus carriers are identified using an agar gel immunodiffusion test (AGIDT) or an enzyme-linked immunosorbent assay (ELISA) to detect antibody to CAE. Antigens prepared from either CAE or maedi-visna viruses can be used in these tests.
- ❏ The antibodies detected are not protective against disease, but merely an indicator of infection, as only very low levels of neutralising antibodies are produced in response to infection.

❑ Any goat which is seropositive on a CAE test is infected for life. Infection persists even in the presence of neutralising antibodies because of the ability of the virus to exist as latent proviral DNA.

Conversely, however, a goat which is tested seronegative cannot be assumed free from infection, because: (1) current tests are relatively insensitive; and (2) the period between infection with the virus and seroconversion (i.e. production of detectable antibody) may be prolonged. Goats infected by contact or by drinking infected milk when adults may take 3 or more years to become seropositive. Kids infected postnatally generally seroconvert between 6 and 12 months of age. Some seropositive goats will periodically test seronegative.

❑ Many goats seroconvert after a period of stress or at parturition. Testing in late pregnancy will not necessarily detect all does which seroconvert after kidding and these animals will produce infected kids.

❑ Kids which have received infected colostrum have detectable levels of colostral antibody for 2 or 3 months but will subsequently test negative until they seroconvert and produce their own antibodies several months or even years later.

❑ Antibody levels may fall as the disease progresses so even a clinically diseased animal may test seronegative.

❑ More sensitive tests are available in specialised laboratories but not for routine screening:
   ■ Virus isolation
   ■ Detection of viral nucleic acid [polymerase chain reaction (PCR)]
   ■ Western blotting (sensitive test for antibody detection).

The use of these more sensitive tests in the future may lead to the ability to detect latently infected animals, thus greatly facilitating eradication programmes.

(2) Examination of synovial fluid
   ❑ Reddish brown synovial fluid with large numbers of cells 1000 to 2000/mm), mainly mononuclear cells (cf. normal goats <500 cells/mm); may contain fibrin tags.
   ❑ Locally produced antibody may be detectable in the fluid.

(3) Histological examination – joints
   ❑ Subsynovial mononuclear cell infiltration and hyperplasia.
   ❑ Synovial villus hypertrophy.
   ❑ Focal areas of necrosis within the synovial membrane or surrounding connective tissue.

Gross postmortem findings – joints

❑ Hyperplasia of synovial membranes with thickening, fibrosis and, in chronic cases, calcification of joint capsule, tendons and ligaments.
❑ Periosteal reaction with periarticular osteophyte production.
❑ Degenerative joint disease with ulceration and erosion of the articular cartilages and destruction of subchondral bone.

Diagnosis
Diagnosis should be based on:

❑ Serum antibody levels to CAE virus.
❑ Clinical signs.
❑ Postmortem lesions.
❑ Histopathological change.
❑ Virus isolation from synovial or brain cells.
❑ Radiology may aid in determining the severity or progression of arthritic lesions in individual animals and demonstrate pneumonia.

Treatment

❑ There is no treatment at present for CAE.
❑ Non-steroidal anti-inflammatory drugs such as flunixin meglamine (Finadyne, Schering-Plough) and Carprofen (Zenecarp, Pfizer) can be used to relieve the pain of arthritis.

Prevention and control

> Although the level of CAE in the UK is now very low, the potential remains for a rapid increase, unless routine control measures are maintained.

❑ Routine tests at 6- to 12-monthly intervals for a minimum of 5 years and preferably more, with no evidence of infection in the herd during that time, are required before a herd can be said to be 'CAE virus free'.
❑ No kid should receive unpasteurised goats' milk or colostrum from any animal except its dam. Pooled milk should *never* be fed to kids. If a doe subsequently proves to be a virus carrier only her own kids will have been infected.
❑ All adult goats (or in the case of a kid, its dam) should be blood tested before entry into the herd.

❏ No milk from another herd should be fed under any circumstances.

The infected herd/flock

❏ Cull or isolate all reactors.
❏ Cull or isolate the offspring of all reactors.
❏ Infected goats should be separated from non-infected goats by at least 1.8 m. Separate feeding/water utensils should be used.
❏ Milk infected goats last; keep milk separate from any non-infected milk used for feeding kids.
❏ As the virus is labile in the environment, infected goats can graze the same pastures as non-infected goats provided the groups are kept separate, i.e. graze non-infected goats in the morning and infected goats in the afternoon.
❏ Because the incidence of uterine infection by the virus is very low, removing the kids at birth from reactors by 'snatching', i.e. preventing suckling or licking by the dam, enables a non-infected kid to be produced in the vast majority of cases.
❏ Batch-mate and induce parturition using prostaglandins (qv) or delay parturition by use of Clenbuterol hydrochloride (Planipart, Boehringer Ingelheim).
❏ Isolate kids, house separately from infected goats, and rear on cows' colostrum and milk or calf or kid milk replacer. If goats' milk or colostrum is fed, it must be pasteurised even if it comes from a supposedly seronegative doe. Milk can be pasteurised by heating for 1 hour at 56°C, but this will *not* ensure 100% death of the virus and pasteurised milk from known carriers should never be fed. Haemolysis very occasionally occurs in kids fed cows' milk (see Chapter 18). The dangers of producing kids with low colostral antibodies must be weighed against the possible dangers of CAE infection in each herd.
❏ Blood sample kids shortly after birth to detect any possible passive transfer of antibody if the snatching was not done efficiently, then at 6 months and at 3-monthly intervals thereafter to detect possible virus carriers.

Control schemes

❏ Individual herd scheme – tailored to control the disease within one herd along the lines previously described.
❏ British Goat Society Monitored Herd Scheme – a scheme for monitoring the disease status of goat herds by testing but with no restrictions on the movement of goats.

❏ The Scottish Agricultural College Sheep and Goat Health Scheme – monitors the disease status of the herd by regular blood tests and, by restricting movement between herds, aims to maintain herds as CAE free. (Sheep and Goat Health Schemes, P.O. Box 604, Milton Keynes, MK6 1ZZ. Tel 01908 844312.)

Further reading

General

Adams, D.S. (1983) Infectious causes of lameness above the foot. *Vet. Clin. North Am.: Large Animal Practice*, **5** (3), November, 1983, 499–510.
Cottom, D.S. and Pinsent, P.J.N. (1988) Lameness in the goat. *Goat Vet. Soc. J.*, **9** (1/2), 14–23.
Hill, N.P. (1997) Lameness and foot lesions in adult British dairy goats. *Vet. Rec.*, **141**, 412–16.
Merrall, M. (1985) Lameness in goats. In: *Proc. of a Course in Goat Husbandry and Medicine.* Massey University, November 1985, Publ. No. 106, 66–77.
Nelson, D.R. (1983) Non-infectious causes of lameness above the foot. *Vet. Clin. North Am.: Large Animal Practice*, **5** (3), November, 1983, 491–8.
Smith, M.C. (1983) Foot problems in goats. *Vet. Clin. North Am.: Large Animal Practice*, **5** (3), November, 1983, 489–90.

Arthritis

Smith, J., *et al.* (1989) Drug therapy for arthritis in food producing animals. *Comp. Cont. Ed. Pract. Vet.*, **II** (1), 89–93.

Caprine arthritis encephalitis

Adams, D.S., *et al.* (1983) Transmission and control of CAE virus. *Am. J. Vet. Res.*, **44** (9), 1670–75.
Dawson, M. (1987) Caprine arthritis encephalitis. *In Practice*, January, 1987, 8–11.
Knight, A.P. and Jokinen, M.P. (1982) Caprine arthritis encephalitis. *Comp. Cont. Ed. Pract. Vet*, **4** (6), S263–9.
Rowe, J.D. and East, N.E. (1997) Risk factors for transmission and methods for control of caprine arthritis encephalitis virus infection. *Vet. Clin. North Am.: Large Animal Practice*, **13** (1), 35–53.

Footrot

Hay, L.A. (1990) Footrot and related conditions. *Goat Vet. Soc. J.*, **II** (1), 1–6.

Surgery

Baron, R.J. (1987) Laterally luxating patella in a goat. *J. Am. Vet. Med. Assoc.*, **191**, 1471–2.

Hunt, R.J., Allen, D. and Thomas, K. (1991) Repair of a ruptured calcaneal tendon by transposition of the tendon of the peroneus longus muscle in a goat. *J. Am. Vet. Med. Assoc.*, **198** (9), 1640–42.

Purohit, N.R., Choudhary, R.J., Chouhan, D.S. and Sharma, C.K. (1985) Surgical repair of scapulohumeral luxation in goats. *Mod. Vet. Pract.*, **66**, 758–9.

Sack, W.O. and Cottrell, W. (1984) Puncture of shoulder, elbow and carpal joints in goats and sheep. *J. Am. Vet. Med. Assoc.*, **185**, 63–5.

7 Lameness in Kids

Trauma

> The kid is an 'accident waiting to happen'.

The most common lamenesses in kids are the result of accident or trauma, resulting in bruising, sprains, strains or fractures, particularly of the front legs.

Fractures

Fractures occur most frequently in the metacarpal region, followed by the radius/ulna, tibia and metatarsus. In many cases, palpation permits identification of the site of the fracture, but radiography may be required for confirmation if there is little bone displacement.

External fixation with plaster or lightweight resin material is extremely well tolerated. If necessary, internal fixation, using pin or plate, can be undertaken using techniques similar to those used in the dog. Where possible, additional external support is indicated because of the robust use of the leg which will occur as the fracture heals.

Foreign bodies

Foreign bodies, e.g. thorns, may penetrate the hoof more easily in kids than in adult goats.

Congenital abnormalities

Overextension of the stifle and hock

Aetiology

❑ Overextension of the hock and stifle is common in newly born kids and is usually bilateral, although one leg is often more severely affected than the other.

Clinical signs

❏ The kid has difficulty walking as the leg tends to bow and the stifle and hock joints are unstable.

Treatment

❏ No treatment is generally necessary as the condition normally corrects itself within a few days, but it is necessary to ensure that the kid is mobile enough to suckle adequately from its dam.

Contracted flexor tendons of the forelimbs

Congenital, bilateral contraction of the flexor tendons of the forelimbs is common and results in flexion of the fetlocks so that the animal walks on its fetlocks or with partially flexed fetlocks.

Treatment

❏ Mild cases with only partial flexion of the fetlocks will resolve on their own as the tendons stretch with movement.
❏ More severe cases may need splinting to stretch the tendons and allow weight bearing on the foot.

Angular limb deformities and arthrogryposis

Congenital limb deformities involving the bones and joints are occasionally seen in newborn goats and generally result in a bilateral articular rigidity, particularly flexion of phalangeal, metacarpophalangeal and carpal joints.

Aetiology

❏ In the UK, usually as the result of contracted tendons caused by positional constraints *in utero*; outwith the UK, congenital Akabane disease and congenital lupinosis may produce limb deformities. An inherited tendon shortening has been reported in Australian Angora goats.
❏ *Beta mannosidosis* is an inherited lysosomal disease of Nubian goats attributable to an autosomal recessive gene, which has been reported in Australia, New Zealand, the USA, Fiji and Canada but not the UK. Because of the absence of the enzyme betamannosidase, kids are unable to stand from birth due to carpal contractures and hyperextended fetlocks. Withdrawal reflexes are normal, but movement is accompanied by an intention tremor. Kids may show domed skulls, narrow muzzles and palpebral fissures.

Treatment

❏ Cases of mild articular rigidity may correct themselves with weight bearing. Surgical treatment of severe retractions can be attempted in valuable animals.

Luxation of the patella

Aetiology

❏ Lateral luxation of the patella is an uncommon problem in goats and is usually congenital. Anglo-Nubian goats are more prone to the condition because of the upright conformation of their hind legs. In Swiss breeds, luxation occasionally occurs as the result of acute trauma in the adult goat and is generally *medial.*

Clinical signs

❏ The luxation may be bilateral or unilateral, permanent or inter-mittent. In its severest form, the stifles will remain permanently flexed, so that the animal adopts a crouching stance and has dif-ficulty in standing. Where the condition is intermittent there will be periods of acute lameness which is relieved when the patella is returned to the normal position by manipulation.

Treatment

❏ Mild intermittent luxation requires no treatment, more severe luxations can be corrected surgically using similar techniques to those used in the dog, and severe congenital luxations may necessitate euthanasia.

Infections

Joint ill

Joint ill is a bacterial arthritis of young kids under 3 months of age.

Aetiology

❏ A number of bacteria may be involved. These are usually environmental contaminants, particularly haemolytic *Strepto-coccus* spp. and *Staphylococcus* spp. but also *Corynebacterium* spp. and *E. coli.* Infection occurs through the umbilical cord shortly after birth.

Clinical signs

❑ Pain and swelling in one or more joints of a neonatal kid, especially carpus, shoulder, hock and stifle. Occasionally pronounced lameness with minimum joint swelling. In more chronic cases, the affected joint will be stiff or even ankylosed.
❑ The kid may or may not be pyrexic depending on the stage and type of infection.
❑ The umbilicus is often inflamed.

Laboratory investigation

❑ Joint fluid or umbilical swabs can be cultured for bacteria if indicated.

Prevention, control and treatment

❑ A clean environment at kidding.
❑ Treat umbilical cord with Lugol's iodine or antibiotic spray as soon after birth as possible and then check regularly for signs of inflammation or infection.
❑ Adequate colostrum, i.e. about 300 ml within 6 hours of birth.
❑ Broad-spectrum antibiotics parenterally and intra-articularly, but the response to treatment is often poor.
❑ Intra-articular lavage may remove pus and reduce damage to the joint surfaces.

Tick pyaemia (enzootic staphylococcal infection)

Aetiology

❑ *Staphylococcus aureus*; the tick *Ixodes ricinus* damages the kid's skin, permitting penetration of the bacteria which are already present on the skin surface.
❑ Infection with tickborne fever (qv) may exacerbate the pathogenicity of tick pyaemia.

Clinical signs

❑ Variable depending on the site of abscesses, which form in various parts of the body, e.g. liver, spinal cord, following the introduction of the bacteria and the resulting pyaemia.
❑ Hot, swollen, painful joints (particularly carpal joints and hocks); lameness; eventually chronic arthritis, with permanent lameness and poor growth rates.
❑ Various neurological signs – blindness, incoordination, posterior paraplegia.

Treatment

❏ Early cases can be treated with penicillin.
❏ Superficial abscesses can be lanced and drained.
❏ Once severe joint lesions are present, treatment is not successful.

Mycoplasma

Mycoplasma spp. have been reported to cause arthritis in goats (usually kids under 6 months) in Europe, Australia and the USA, and with increasing numbers of goats being imported into the UK, mycoplasma should be regarded as a possible importation hazard.

Aetiology

❏ *Mycoplasma* spp. such as *M. capricolum*, and *M. mycoides* subsp. *mycoides*.

Clinical signs

❏ Outbreaks of arthritis generally in kids and young goats, with acutely swollen joints and pyrexia with or without pneumonia.

Postmortem findings

❏ Purulent or fibropurulent arthritis with haemorrhagic erosions of articular surfaces.
❏ Lungs collapsed and rubbery.

Diagnosis

❏ Serology (complement fixation test).
❏ Isolation of the organism from joint fluid in mycoplasma medium.

Chlamydia

Chlamydia psittaci has been reported to cause polyarthritis in young goats in parts of Europe and the USA but not in the UK, although the organism has been isolated from sheep joints in this country.

Clinical signs

❏ Polyarthritis and stiffness as part of an acute febrile illness in a number of kids.

Postmortem findings

❏ Fibrinous arthritis with no changes to the cartilage.

Diagnosis

❑ Smears of joint exudate stained with Giemsa.
❑ Immunofluorescence.
❑ Isolation of chlamydia in embryonating yolk sacs.

Erysipelas

Erysipelas polyarthritis has been occasionally reported in kids under 2 months of age.

Aetiology

❑ The bacterium *Erysipelothrix insidiosa* enters through breaks in the skin, e.g. castration wounds, or via the umbilicus.

Clinical signs

❑ Pyrexia, anorexia and lethargy, with hot, swollen, painful joints in the acute stage. The disease often becomes chronic.

Diagnosis

❑ Isolation of the organism from joints in acute cases.

Treatment

❑ High doses of penicillin.

Other bacterial arthritides

Other bacteria may occasionally cause arthritis as a result of either septicaemia or direct penetration into the joint from a puncture wound.

Footrot/interdigital dermatitis

See Chapter 6. Infection with *Fusobacterium necrophorum* and *Dichelobacter nodosus* may become significant in older kids.

Nutritional causes

Calcium, phosphorus and vitamin D deficiency or imbalance

Kids are susceptible to imbalances in the calcium:phosphorus ratio. The calcium:phosphorus ratio in goat diets should not drop below

1.2:1 and should ideally be around 2:1. Vitamin D is essential for the absorption and metabolism of calcium and phosphorus. On typical diets in the UK a relative calcium deficiency is more likely than a calcium excess.

Table 7.1 gives the daily requirements for calcium and phosphorous.

Table 7.1 Daily calcium/phosphorus requirements. (After Tomas and Turner, 1979; quoted in Baxendell, 1984.)

	Gain (g/day)	Calcium (g)	Phosphorus (g)
Maintenance			
50 kg		2.5	1.5
80 kg		4.0	2.4
Production requirements/kg milk		4.0	3.0
Gestation requirements last 2 months		1.5	1.8
Kid daily requirements			
At 1 month old	175	2.0	1.3
At 2 months old	200	2.7	1.7
At 3 to 5 months old	175	2.9	1.9
At 6 months old	150	3.2	2.0

Angular limb deformities

Angular limb deformities may be present at birth (qv), but mild limb deformities are also the most common manifestation of calcium:phosphorus imbalance in goats in the UK.

Aetiology

❏ Acquired limb deformities occur in a rapidly growing early maturing kid with a calcium:phosphorus imbalance.
❏ Angulation of the limb results in epiphyseal compression, producing increased pressure on the growth plate on that side and retarding growth.

Clinical signs

❏ Outward (lateral) deviation of the fetlock joint (fetlock valgus) is the most common deformity seen in young goats, but more severe imbalances may result in carpal valgus (knock knees) or carpal and stifle varus (bow legs).
❏ Uneven wear of the feet may occur.
❏ Lameness.

Treatment

- ❏ Correct dietary imbalances.
- ❏ Use corrective foot trimming on a fortnightly basis.
- ❏ The application of splints in the early stages of carpal varus and fetlock valgus may correct the problem.
- ❏ Surgical compression of the growth plate with staples or screws and wire will slow the growth on that side and allow the limb to straighten. Early remedial action is necessary before the natural closure of the growth plates.

Rickets

Rickets is a disease of young growing kids characterised by defective calcification of growing bone.

Aetiology

- ❏ Relative or absolute dietary deficiencies of calcium, phosphorus and vitamin D. Rapidly growing kids kept indoors on an otherwise good diet are most likely to be affected.

Clinical signs

- ❏ Enlarged painful epiphyses and costochondral junctions.
- ❏ Poor appetite and unthriftiness.
- ❏ Stiff gait, lameness, unwillingness to stand.
- ❏ Arched back.
- ❏ Possible bending of the long bones.

Prevention

- ❏ Exercise in sunlight with increased vitamin D levels.
- ❏ Feed sun-dried hay.
- ❏ Calcium and phosphorus supplements where necessary.
- ❏ Vitamin D 500 U or vitamins A, D and E 125 000 U.

Treatment

- ❏ Correct any calcium/phosphorus imbalance with supplements as necessary.
- ❏ Vitamin D 500 U injection.

Osteodystrophia fibrosa

Aetiology

- ❏ Like rickets, osteodystrophia fibrosa is caused by an imbalance of calcium and phosphorus and results from a secondary calcium deficiency due to excess phosphorus feeding, giving a calcium : phosphorus ratio of 1 : 2.5 or greater.
- ❏ Cereals and bran are high in phosphorus. Diets low in fresh green food and good hay but high in cereals and bran predispose to the disease.

Clinical signs

- ❏ Unthriftiness.
- ❏ Poor appetite.
- ❏ Lameness.
- ❏ Bilateral swelling of bones of the face and jaw.
- ❏ Molar and premolar teeth rotated and loose.
- ❏ Fractures of long bones.
- ❏ Bones soft.

Prevention and treatment

- ❏ Correct the calcium : phosphorus ratio in the ration.
- ❏ Feed a diet high in green foods; add bonemeal or powdered limestone.
- ❏ Severely affected animals with distortion of the mandible should be culled.

White muscle disease

Vitamin E and selenium both have antioxidant functions and can partially substitute for one another in the diet. Vitamin E requirements of the goat may be higher than those of sheep and cattle.

Aetiology

- ❏ A selenium/vitamin E deficiency produces a degenerative myopathy, particularly in very young kids born to deficient dams. The clinical signs depend on whether the skeletal muscles (skeletal muscle form) or the heart muscle and diaphragm (cardiac form) are affected or both forms may appear together in the same animal.

Predisposing conditions

❑ Selenium-deficient pastures, where animals are fed on locally produced feed without supplementation.

❑ Vitamin E-deficient diets – poor quality hay or straw with little concentrate.

❑ High levels of unsaturated fatty acids, e.g. fish/soya oils, calf milk with added vegetable fat, cause relative vitamin E deficiency.

Clinical signs

❑ Kids are affected at birth or up to 6 months of age but generally between 2 and 16 weeks. The most active kids are often affected first and the disease is often seen 2 to 3 days after turnout.

(1) Skeletal muscle form

❑ Stiffness and reluctance to move; lying down frequently; standing up with difficulty; crying if forced to move.

❑ Skeletal muscles firm and painful on palpation (cf. nervous disease) particularly in the hind limbs.

❑ Non-pyrexic.

❑ Appetite remains good even if the kid is unable to stand.

❑ Older kids and adults may show signs of the skeletal muscle form after stress or exercise.

(2) Cardiac form

❑ Sudden death, typically in kids 2 to 6 months old after or during exercise.

❑ Tachycardia.

❑ Tachypnoea; hyperpnoea.

❑ Weakness.

❑ Severely deficient does may produce stillborn or weak lambs which die of acute heart failure after a few days.

Postmortem findings

❑ Pale or white streaks in the skeletal muscles, particularly of the hind limbs and lumbar area and the subendocardial muscle of the ventricles of the heart.

Laboratory findings

❑ Creatine phosphokinase (CPK) and aspartate transaminase (AST) levels markedly elevated.

❏ Blood selenium levels are below 50 ppb (normal 158 to 160 ppb; marginal 50 to 80 ppb).
❏ Glutathione peroxidase levels low (< 60 U/ml RBCs).
❏ Liver selenium levels below 500 nmol/kg or vitamin E below 2.5 µmol/kg are considered deficient.

Prevention

❏ Dietary concentrations of 0.1 mg/kg dry matter for selenium and 30 to 50 mg/kg dry matter for vitamin E are adequate.
❏ One month before kidding, inject the does with **3 mg/kg Vitamin E** and **0.07 mg/kg selenium, 2 ml/45 kg s.c.** (**Vitesel**, Norbrook; **Dystosel**, Intervet), and/or
❏ Inject the kids at birth and at 3 to 4 weeks of age with **34 mg vitamin E** and **0.75 mg selenium, 0.5 ml s.c.**, and possibly at 12 to 16 weeks of age with **68 mg vitamin E** and **1.5 mg selenium, 1 ml s.c.** (**Vitesel**, Norbrook; **Dystosel**, Intervet). Always use subcutaneous injections, as intramuscular injections cause local reactions.
❏ Slow-release bolus containing selenium (**Zincosel**, Telsol), 4 to 8 weeks before lambing.
❏ Add selenium at 100 ppm to feed.
❏ Oral drench with 5 mg sodium selenite during the last week of pregnancy.
❏ Oral drench with selenium combined with anthelmintics.

Treatment

❏ Affected kids should be treated with **34–68 mg vitamin E** and **0.75–1.5 mg selenium, 0.5–1 ml s.c.** (**Vitesel**, Norbrook; **Dystosel**, Intervet).

Selenium toxicity

Overdosage with selenium supplements may result in selenium poisoning. The minimum toxic dose by injection is about 0.5 mg/kg (i.e. 50 times the therapeutic dose). Acute poisoning produces dyspnoea, diarrhoea, pyrexia, tachycardia, apparent blindness, head pressing, collapse and death from heart failure within 24–48 hours. Chronic poisoning may occur with long-term supplementation or in parts of the world with naturally high selenium levels in the soil, but is unlikely to occur in the UK. Chronic poisoning produces lethargy, weight loss, pica, lameness and neurological signs.

Copper deficiency

The ataxia produced by copper deficiency [swayback or enzootic ataxia (qv)] may be confused with lameness in kids from birth to 4 weeks of age.

Further reading

General

See Chapter 6.
Baxendell, S.A. (1984) Caprine limb and joint conditions. *Proc. Univ. Sydney Post Grad. Comm. Vet. Sci.*, **73**, 370.

Osteodystrophia fibrosa

Andrews, A.H., *et al.* (1983) *Osteodystrophia fibrosa in young goats. Vet. Rec.*, **112**, 494–96.

8 Chronic Weight Loss

Initial assessment

The preliminary history should consider:

- ❏ Individual or herd/flock problem.
- ❏ Similar cases in the herd in the past.
- ❏ Management practices:
    - ■ Housing; availability of shelter; general hygiene
    - ■ Feeding systems
    - ■ Size of groups; age mix of groups; recent mixing of goats?
    - ■ Horned/disbudded goats
    - ■ Grazing history
    - ■ Routine medication – worming, external parasite control.
- ❏ Stage of lactation/pregnancy.
- ❏ Milk yield.

Clinical examination

> Dairy goats have little subcutaneous fat. Most fat is carried internally in the omentum and perirenal tissues.

Body condition should be carefully assessed. *Condition scoring,* using standard techniques to assess lumbar fat and muscle as used routinely in sheep, is difficult to apply to dairy goats as most of the body fat is carried internally. Apparently thin goats may be found to have a large amount of abdominal fat at postmortem examination and obese goats have little subcutaneous fat. In Angora goats, scoring is easier but never so accurate as with cattle or sheep. Angoras always feel thin when compared to dairy goats, because they are more slightly built. Careful palpation in thick-fleeced animals is essential to get an accurate impression of body condition.

A condition scoring system which combines lumbar and sternal measurements is more accurate in dairy goats. Sternal scoring gives a better indication of the amount of fat carried by the goat, while the lumbar score indicates body protein. The body condition score is taken as an average of the lumbar and sternal scores.

(1) Lumbar scoring:

☐ Score 0. Extreme emaciation: bones of the skeleton are apparent; junctions between vertebrae are readily perceptible to the touch; skin seems in direct contact with bones.
☐ Score 1. Very lean: body angular; lumbar vertebrae prominent, with transverse processes readily palpable.
☐ Score 2. Lean: lumbar vertebrae less prominent; transverse processes easily palpated but with some tissue cover.
☐ Score 3. Good condition: lumbar vertebrae and transverse processes palpable but with reasonable cover; moderately rounded appearance to body.
☐ Score 4. Fat: lumbar vertebrae only palpable with gentle pressure and the transverse processes with firm pressure; body smooth and rounded.
☐ Score 5. Obese: vertical processes cannot be detected even with pressure; there is a dimple in the fat layers where the processes should be; transverse processes cannot be detected; loin muscles are very full and covered with very thick fat.

Condition score 2 is adequate during lactation, with condition rising to score 3 at the time of service.

(2) Sternal scoring:

☐ Score 0. Extreme emaciation: chondro-sternal joints are very prominent; bony surfaces of the sternum are very obvious to the touch; the hardened area of skin lacks mobility.
☐ Score 1: Very lean: chondro-sternal joints are rounded but still very easily felt; hollow in the midline of the sternum is not filled in; the hardened area of skin is loose.
☐ Score 2. Lean: chondro-sternal joints are difficult to feel; considerable amount of internal fat which forms a furrow along middle of sternum; subcutaneous fat fills this furrow and extends to lateral borders of sternum and ends posteriorly at hollow of last sternal joint.
☐ Score 3. Good condition: bones of sternum are no longer detectable but the ribs can be felt; thickness of internal fat makes a fatty layer along lateral edge of sternum; subcutaneous fat forms a mobile mass which extends in a thin band to the rear in hollow of last sternal joint; when whole sternum is grasped with the hand, two large depressions between these masses and the bone can be detected on each side.

❏ Score 4. Fat: neither sternum nor ribs are detectable; a shallow depression can be detected on either side by palpation; at the rear, depression on last sternal joint remains.
❏ Score 5. Obese: subcutaneous fatty mass is no longer mobile; contours are rounded without depressions on each side; hollow on last sternal joint is filled in.

Regular weighing is the most accurate way of monitoring condition in a particular flock or herd.

General examination at rest should include skin (lice, mange), mouth (teeth, lesions), feet (footrot, laminitis), mucous membranes (anaemia), abdomen (ascites, rumen function), auscultation of thorax (cardiac/respiratory function) and lymph nodes.

Primary nutritional deficiency

Starvation

Starvation is caused by failure to ensure that the ration provides adequate energy and protein to meet the needs of maintenance, growth and production, together with sufficient minerals and vitamins and clean water. It may occur owing to:

❏ Neglect.
❏ Inexperience:
  ■ inappropriate feedstuffs
  ■ unbalanced ration
  ■ feed shortage at critical times.

Table 8.1 shows the daily requirements for energy and protein. Obvious dietary deficiencies can generally be easily remedied. Less obvious problems can be investigated by analysing feedstuffs or by *metabolic profiles* of a number of goats in the herd. Suggested profiles are:

❏ Energy: glucose, β-hydroxybutyrate, non-esterified fatty acids, ketones.

Table 8.1   Daily requirements for energy and protein.

	Energy (MJ)	Protein (g DCP)
Maintenance (80-kg goat)	10	6.5
Plus milk production per litre (3.5% BF)	5.19	48
Pregnancy (average last 2 months)	6.0	54
Mohair production (6 kg/year)	0.75	18

❏ Protein: total protein, albumin, urea.
❏ Trace elements: copper, zinc, iron, selenium, cobalt.

Trace element deficiency

Cobalt deficiency (pine)

Aetiology

❏ Primary deficiency of cobalt in the diet produces signs of vitamin B_{12} deficiency with inability to metabolise propionic acid.
❏ A secondary vitamin B_{12} deficiency may occur with helminth infection.

Incidence

❏ Certain areas of the UK are known to be cobalt deficient.

Laboratory tests

❏ Blood cobalt or vitamin B_{12} levels are a poor guide to cobalt status (suggested that 150 to 300 pmol vitamin B_{12}/l is considered marginal and over 300 pmol vitamin B_{12}/l adequate).
❏ Liver cobalt and vitamin B_{12} levels provide a useful guide (normal cobalt levels 0.2 to 0.3 ppm DM).
❏ Less than 0.1 ppm DM cobalt on pasture sample suggests cobalt deficiency.
❏ The presence in urine of methylmalonic acid (MMA) and forminoglutamic acid (FIGLU) indicates cobalt deficiency.

Clinical signs

❏ Growing animal more severely affected than the adult.
❏ Unthriftiness.
❏ Inappetence.
❏ Wasting.
❏ Emaciation.
❏ Ocular discharge.
❏ Anaemia (normocytic, normochromic).
❏ Reduced milk production.
❏ Death.

Diagnosis

❏ Response to cobalt or vitamin B_{12}.

Treatment and control

- ❏ **Vitamin B$_{12}$ injections, 250–750 µg, s.c. or i.m.**
- ❏ **Oral cobalt sulphate, 1 mg/kg** at monthly intervals; **50 g cobalt sulphate added to 10 l water**; 5-ml drench to growing lambs, 10 ml to ewes.
- ❏ **Water medication (Aquatrace cobalt tablets**, Dennis Brinicombe).
- ❏ **Trace element boluses (Agrimin** smAll-Trace; **Zincosel**, Telsol), provide several trace elements and vitamins but are an expensive treatment for cobalt alone.
- ❏ Cobalt oxide bullets have previously been used successfully.
- ❏ **Anthelmintic preparations** containing cobalt sulphate (**'SC drenches'**) are an effective prophylaxis if used correctly.
- ❏ Concentrates fed to does should contain appropriate mineral and trace element supplementation.
- ❏ Cobalt sulphate, 2 kg/ha, applied as top dressing to pasture every 3 or 4 years (but expensive).

Copper deficiency

As well as neurological signs (see Chapter 15), copper deficiency may result in growth retardation, emaciation, microcytic anaemia, diarrhoea and increased susceptibility to infection.

Selenium deficiency (see white muscle disease)

Selenium deficiency may occasionally cause illthrift.

Inability to utilise available foodstuffs

Dentition

Figure 8.1 shows the dentition of kids and adult goats with approximate time of eruption of teeth. Goats over 5 years of age kept extensively show increasing wear of the incisor and molar teeth, so prehension and mastication may become difficult. Uneven wear of molar teeth can result in sharp points, leading to ulceration of the buccal cavity and tongue, often complicated by secondary bacterial infections – goats may show reluctance to eat, chewing on one side and pouching or dropping of food. Congenital defects such as overshot/undershot jaws may predispose to dental problems.

Mouth lesions

Painful mouth lesions from infection [e.g. Orf (qv)], toxic material resulting in mouth ulceration (e.g. giant hogweed poisoning), necrotic

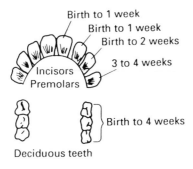

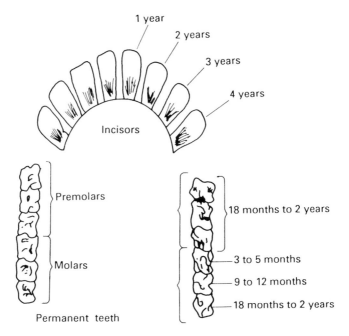

Figure 8.1 Dentition and time of eruption. (From Owen, 1977.)

stomatitis from eating abrasive plant material, drenching-gun injuries or perodontal disease will inhibit eating.

Facial paralysis

For example, listeriosis (qv).

Lameness

See Chapters 6 and 7. Lameness will reduce grazing or feeding at troughs if the pain is severe. This may be caused by in particular:

- ❑ Chronic degenerative joint disease – CAE, osteoarthritis, etc.
- ❑ Footrot or interdigital dermatitis.
- ❑ Laminitis.
- ❑ Overgrown feet.

Blindness (see Chapter 19)

- ❑ Severe keratoconjunctivitis.
- ❑ Vitamin A deficiency.
- ❑ Post cerebrocortical necrosis.
- ❑ Lead.

Bullying

Goats have a well-established rigid social order – the bottom goat(s) may be denied access to food. The problem may be precipitated by:

- ❑ Introducing a new goat into an established group.
- ❑ Providing insufficient space/goat (3.3 to 9.3 m²/goat).
- ❑ Providing insufficient trough space (0.4–0.6 m/goat).
- ❑ Having groups of mixed ages.
- ❑ Running horned goats with polled or disbudded goats.

Unwillingness to utilise available foodstuffs

Unpalatable feed caused by spoilage, mould, etc., will be refused by goats. Even a change in food, e.g. a new batch of concentrates, may result in feed refusal for a week or more.

Male goats at the start of the breeding season will often refuse feed, with consequent weight loss.

Inability to increase feed intake to match production demands

Peak lactation

All heavily lactating goats, particularly young first kidders, will lose weight despite the availability of an adequate diet. On a body weight for weight basis, goats are much heavier producers than cows. 'Running through' these milkers the following year (i.e. allowing a 2-year gap between kidding) allows time for these animals to regain their body reserves and prevents restriction of growth. In the second year of lactation, a good milker will give 80 + % of its first year milk yield.

Periparturient toxaemia

> Overfat does and multiple fetuses rather than
> underfeeding cause most periparturient toxaemias.

Periparturient toxaemia [pregnancy toxaemia, postparturient toxaemia, acetonaemia (ketosis)] occurs in response to insufficient intake
of energy to meet the increasing demands of pregnancy or lactation:

❑ *Before kidding* – in the last 4 to 6 weeks of pregnancy as *pregnancy
toxaemia*, or
❑ *After kidding* – usually about 2 to 4 weeks postpartum. Most does
suffer a mild ketonaemia in early lactation as the demands of the
lactation for energy are not met adequately by the diet. In most
animals an equilibrium is established and the ketosis remains
subclinical. Goats which are not overfat may develop an acute
clinical ketosis or *acetonaemia*. Goats which have large fat deposits
at kidding may develop a *postparturient toxaemia* similar to pregnancy toxaemia or fatty liver disease of cows, presumably in
response to impaired liver function.

Predisposing factors

❑ Multiple fetuses:
  ■ nutritional drain on dam during last 6 weeks of pregnancy;
  ■ compression of the rumen by fetuses decreases voluntary food
    intake. Suboptimum food intake is the main predisposing fac-
    tor in periparturient toxaemia.
❑ Goat overfed as a goatling.
❑ Goat overfed during the dry period at the end of parturition:
  ■ intra-abdominal fat deposits reduce the rumen capacity and
    thus food intake;
  ■ excessive quantities of fat are mobilised from body depots and
    deposited in the liver; fatty infiltration of the liver results in
    hepatic dysfunction.
❑ Lack of exercise.
❑ Undernutrition – undoubtedly a major cause of pregnancy toxaemia and acetonaemia in goats kept extensively, through inadequate food supply, poorly balanced rations or heavy worm
burdens but *not* a major cause of periparturient toxaemia in
intensively kept dairy goats in the UK where most goats which
show the disease are being offered an adequate balanced ration.
❑ Stress factors (fear, weather, housing, etc.) play a part in initiating
the disease in goats on a poor plane of nutrition, but in the majority
of cases in dairy goats there is no obvious stress involved.

Laboratory tests

❏ Ketostix, Multistix, Acetest tablets or Rotheras reagent can be used to detect ketones in urine or milk.
❏ A blood sample can be submitted for an energy profile – glucose, β-hydroxybutyrate, non-esterified fatty acids, ketones.
❏ Changes in liver enzyme levels are not generally useful for diagnosis.

Pregnancy toxaemia

Clinical signs

❏ Initially inappetence (eats browsings/hay, refuses concentrates); later complete anorexia.
❏ Lethargic, unwilling to move; walks with difficulty; legs may swell.
❏ Weight loss.
❏ Occasionally nervous signs – tremor around the head and ears, reduced vision or blindness, head pressing, stargazing, eventually recumbency, coma with or without abortion, death.

Treatment

> Termination of pregnancy is generally the only successful treatment for pregnancy toxaemia.

❏ In the absence of abortion or parturition, treatment is generally unsatisfactory. Terminate pregnancy by inducing parturition (qv) or caesarian section or rapid removal of kids by non-sterile caesarian section under local anaesthesia, followed by euthanasia of the doe. Use dexamethasone rather than prostaglandins to induce parturition – improved survival of kids, plus gluconeogenic effect in the dam. Give calcium borogluconate because hypocalcaemia may coexist with the condition.
❏ If there is doubt concerning the viability of fetuses, fetal movement can be demonstrated during the last month of gestation by real-time β-mode ultrasonography using a 5-MHz sector transducer, although near to term fetal heartbeats can be more difficult to detect.

Postmortem findings

❏ Emaciated carcase or large amounts of abdominal fat.
❏ Yellow–orange enlarged liver which is greasy and friable.
❏ Adrenal glands may be enlarged.

Postparturient toxaemia (fatty liver syndrome)

Clinical signs

❑ Inappetence (eats browsings/hay, refuses concentrates); later complete anorexia.
❑ Milk yield initially depressed and then drops markedly.
❑ Lethargic.
❑ Chronic weight loss over several weeks.
❑ Eventually recumbency, coma and death – most goatkeepers will request euthanasia before this stage is reached.

Postmortem findings

❑ As for pregnancy toxaemia.

Treatment

❑ Encourage the goat to continue eating (anything!) – usually best response to browsings, green food (e.g. ivy in winter). Goats that continue to eat may survive; totally anorexic animals will die.
❑ Stimulate appetite with products such as **B vitamins**, **Rumen stimulant** (Vetoquinol), **Collate Twin Lamb** or **Collate Multilamb Rapid** (Net-Tex Agricultural).
❑ Provide glucogenic agents:
    20% Glucose solution, 200 ml, part **i.v.** or **i.p.**, the rest **s.c.**
    Glycerine (glycerol), 60 ml in warm water orally, twice daily for 4 to 5 days.
    Propylene glycol (Ketol, Intervet; **Ketosaid**, Norbrook), **200 ml** orally twice daily for 4 to 5 days.
❑ Stimulate gluconeogenesis:
    Dexamethasone, 25 mg, 12.5 ml i.m. (**Azium**, Schering-Plough; **Colvasone**, Norbrook; **Dexadreson**, Intervet; **Duphacort Q**, Fort Dodge), will produce abortion in late pregnancy.
    Dexamethasone, 25 mg + protamine zinc insulin, up to **40 U**, **s.c.**, twice daily. Insulin has an antilipolytic effect as well as affecting peripheral glucose utilisation.
    Anabolic steroids (where allowed by regulatory bodies).
❑ Supportive therapy:
    Multivitamins – particularly A/D. Vitamin E/selenium preparations may help hepatic metabolism in postparturient toxaemia.
    Electrolytes –1 to 3 l of a balanced electrolyte solution (plus bicarbonate if respiratory acidosis is present).
    Calcium borogluconate 20%, with **magnesium hypophosphite 5%** and **dextrose 20%, 80–100 ml**, **i.v.** or **s.c.** (**Calciject PMD**, Norbrook), in case of concomitant hypocalcaemia.

Restoration of normal rumen microflora – use natural yoghurt or
probiotics or drench rumen contents from healthy animal.

❏ **Diazepam, 0.05 mg/kg, 0.01 ml/kg i.v. (Valium,** Roche) will
stimulate feeding for about 30 minutes.

Acetonaemia (ketosis)

Clinical signs

❏ Inappetance (eats browsings/hay, refuses concentrates).
❏ Mild ataxia.
❏ Constipation.
❏ Acetone smell to breath.
❏ Milk yield drops.

Note: left-sided displacement of the abomasum (see Chapter 14) produces a
secondary ketosis and clinical signs similar to primary acetonaemia.

Treatment

❏ Corticosteroids.
❏ Other treatments as for postparturient toxaemia.

Prognosis

❏ Good; animals with this form of ketosis respond well to treatment.

Interference with absorption of nutrients/loss of nutrients

Gastrointestinal parasitism (qv)

> Gastrointestinal parasites are a major cause of weight
> loss. Assume infection until proved otherwise.

Trichostrongylus spp. – diarrhoea
Ostertagi ostertagi – ill thrift ± diarrhoea
Haemonchus contortus – anaemia

Gastrointestinal parasitism should be assumed in all goats with
chronic weight loss (consider *underdosing* with anthelmintics, *dosing at
incorrect time* and *resistance*, particularly with Benzamidazole
products).

A single low faecal egg count is not sufficient to eliminate internal
parasitism as a cause of weight loss, as egg counts may not reliably
indicate the number of adult worms present (see Chapter 13).

Johne's disease (paratuberculosis)

> Johne's disease in goats presents as a wasting disease; diarrhoea is not a major sign. In the UK, it is primarily a disease of commercial herds and probably the biggest cause of death or culling.

Johne's disease is of increasing importance in commercial dairy herds in the UK and is a major reason for culling adult goats (up to 20% per annum), with economic loss from poor milk yields and lost genetic potential. However, it is uncommon in goats kept singly or in small herds.

Aetiology

❏ Infection with acidfast bacterium, *Mycobacterium avium* subsp. *paratuberculosis (Mycobacterium johnei)*, producing chronic inflammatory bowel disease.

Epidemiology

❏ Excreted in faeces by clinically ill or symptomless carriers.
❏ Persists in environment for months.
❏ Some animals may be intermittent excretors.
❏ Kids generally infected in first few weeks of life by faecal contamination of the udder or environment or possibly through infected colostrum (intrauterine transmission and infection via semen have also been demonstrated in cattle).
❏ Ingested organisms remain dormant in the gastrointestinal tract and adjacent lymph nodes, often for many years.
❏ Clinical disease may be precipitated by stress such as parturition or introduction to a new herd.
❏ An age-related resistance to infection occurs in cattle and probably also occurs in goats. Animals older than 6 months of age are unlikely to be infected, thus limiting the opportunity for horizontal transmission within a herd. Most infections probably occur within the first 30 days of life.

Clinical signs

❏ Affects adult goats, generally 2 to 3 years old; rarely occurs in younger goats.
❏ Progressive weight loss; may extend from weeks to months, leading to dramatic emaciation.
❏ Appetite maintained initially but later decreases.

❑ Increasing lethargy and depression.
❑ Rough hair coat, loss of fibre, flaky skin.
❑ Diarrhoea only occurs in the terminal stages.
❑ Anaemia develops as the disease progresses.
❑ Signs of hypoproteinaemia, such as intermandibular oedema.

Diagnosis

> The non-specific signs mean it is impossible to diagnose Johne's disease by clinical examination.

❑ Diagnosis is very difficult in the living animal and it is generally considered to be grossly underdiagnosed.
❑ No single bacteriological or serological test is sufficiently accurate to identify all clinical and subclinical cases or has sufficient specificity to avoid false positives.
❑ Identification of acidfast organisms in ileocaecal or mesenteric lymph nodes is the best diagnostic test whether at postmortem or by biopsy.
❑ Faecal culture is the next most reliable antemortem test, but requires 8–12 weeks and will not detect less than 100 organisms/g, thereby missing some carriers.
❑ Agar gel immunodiffusion (AGID) test correlates reasonably well with faecal culture; useful for detecting profuse excretors.
❑ ELISA tests are replacing AGID tests in some laboratories: antibody ELISA measures the level of antibody (humeral response) in plasma or serum; gamma interferon ELISA measures the level of gamma interferon (cell-mediated immune response), which is the host's earliest response.
❑ Various DNA techniques are currently being developed. DNA probes can detect repetitive DNA sequences unique to *M. paratuberculosis* in faeces samples.
❑ Complement fixation tests are inaccurate; false positives and false negatives occur.
❑ Intradermal tests are not recommended; false negatives occur.
❑ Significantly decreased levels of total protein, albumin and calcium occur in sheep and, although not specific to Johne's disease, may provide a useful preliminary diagnostic screen for emaciated goats in the absence of diarrhoea.

Postmortem findings

❑ Postmortem findings in goats are generally not as obvious as in cattle as intestinal lesions are less pronounced.

❏ Emaciation; absence of abdominal fat.
❏ Mesenteric lymph nodes generally enlarged and oedematous in later stages with foci of caseation.
❏ Slight thickening and corrugation of the ileal mucosa and possibly of the mucosa of the caecum and proximal colon.
❏ Even in the absence of gross lesions sections from the mesenteric lymph nodes, distal ileum and ileocaceal valve should be submitted for histological examination.
❏ Characteristic granulomatous lesions in the intestinal tract, lymph nodes and possibly liver.
❏ Massive infiltration of acidfast bacteria and inflammatory cells into the intestinal mucosa.
❏ Architecture of intestine destroyed, with significant villus atrophy and villus fusion, leading to a malabsorption syndrome and protein-losing enteropathy.

Treatment

❏ None.

Control

(1) Identify and remove infected animals from the herd.
   ❏ Frequent testing – faecal culture + AGID or ELISA every 6 months.
   ❏ Cull all positive goats and their offspring.
   ❏ Expensive and will not detect infected non-shedders.
(2) Improve management and hygiene:
   ❏ Clean and rebed pens between kiddings.
   ❏ Snatch kids at birth (see CAE control, Chapter 6); will also help control CAE and *Mycoplasma* spp.).
   ❏ Prevent faecal contamination of water and feed troughs.
   ❏ Clean pens regularly.
   ❏ Prevent overcrowding.
   ❏ Do not spread manure on pasture.
(3) Vaccinate kids
   ❏ Live attenuated adjuvanted vaccine is available from the Central Veterinary Laboratory, New Haw, Weybridge, Surrey. The shelf life of the vaccine is only 14 days, so it must be ordered as required.
   ❏ Vaccinate between 2 and 4 weeks of age, using half the cattle dose, and then rear kids separately.
   ❏ When all goats on the unit have been vaccinated as kids, continue for a further 2 years.
   ❏ Shown to reduce the incidence of clinical disease, but animals

may still become infected and shed bacteria without ever developing the disease.

❏ May cause granulomatous nodule at the injection site – the brisket is generally the recommended site for subcutaneous injection.

❏ Vaccinated kids may develop cross reactivity to *M. tuberculosis* and the use of the vaccine may influence Johne's complement fixation tests and intradermal tests for Johne's disease and tuberculosis.

Public health considerations

There is current debate on the connection between Johne's disease and Crohn's disease in humans. *Mycobacterium* species have been detected in humans with Crohn's disease. There is a possibility of the disease being transmitted in raw or inadequately pasteurised milk.

Liver disease

See Chapter 14.

Chronic fascioliasis

Aetiology

❏ The liver fluke, *Fasciola hepatica,* which has an indirect lifecycle with the water snail, *Lymnea truncatula,* acting as the intermediate host.

Fluke can cause acute, subacute or chronic disease, according to the numbers and stage of development of the parasite in the liver. Acute fascioliasis occurs when large numbers of immature fluke cause massive destruction of liver tissue, resulting in liver failure and haemorrhage. Subacute fascioliasis occurs when large numbers of fluke are ingested over a longer period, so that as well as immature fluke in the liver parenchyma, there are adult fluke in the major bile ducts. Chronic fascioliasis is the result of liver damage caused by migrating fluke and blood loss caused by adult flukes in the bile ducts. The browsing habits of goats mean that large numbers of infective metacercariae are unlikely to be ingested over a short period so that although acute and subacute disease does occur, the chronic form is more common. There is no immunity to reinfection with *F. hepatica.*

Clinical signs

❏ See Table 8.2.

❏ The main period for chronic infection is late winter, January to

Table 8.2 Fascioliasis.

Type		Clinical signs	Fluke number	Eggs/g faeces	Clinical pathology	Postmortem
Chronic	January to April June to July	Progressive weight loss Anaemia Oedema, ascites	250+ (adults)	100+	Hypochromic macrocytic anaemia Eosinophilia, hypoalbuminaemia AST (other liver enzymes normal)	Hepatic fibrosis Hyperplastic cholangitis
Acute	October to January	Sudden death Abdominal pain Dyspnoea, ascites	1000+ (mainly immature)	0	Nomochromic normocytic anaemia Eosinophilia, hypoalbuminaemia AST, GGT, SDH, LDH	Liver enlarged and haemorrhagic Tracts of migrating fluke Fibrinous peritonitis
Subacute	October to January	Rapid weight loss Anaemia Submandibular oedema, ascites	500–1500 (adults + immature)	<100	Hypochromic macrocytic anaemia Eosinophilia, hypoalbuminaemia	As acute + bile ducts distended by adult fluke

AST, apartate aminotransferase; GGT, gamma-glutamyltransferase; SDH, sorbitol dehydrogenase; LDH, lactate dehydrogenase.

March, from summer infection of snails, or June to July, from winter infection of snails producing metacercariae in the spring.

Diagnosis

❏ Clinical signs of severe loss of body condition, anaemia and subcutaneous oedema.
❏ Faecal egg counts.
❏ Postmortem signs of ascites and liver fibrosis, with low to moderate numbers of adult fluke.

Treatment

❏ Treat the whole herd/flock.
    Chronic fascioliasis:
        Oxyclozanide, **15 mg/kg orally** (**Zanil**, Schering-Plough)
        Albendazole, **7.5 mg/kg orally** (**Valbazan**, Pfizer), also effective against intestinal worms and tapeworms
        Triclabendazole, **10 mg/kg orally** (**Fasinex**, Novartis)
        Netobimin, **20 mg/kg orally** (**Hapadex**, Schering-Plough)
        Closantel, **10 mg/kg orally** (**Flukiver**, Janssen)
        Nitroxynil, **10 mg/kg s.c.** (**Trodax**, Merial).
    Acute and subacute fascioliasis:
        Triclabendazole, **10 mg/kg orally** (**Fasinex**, Novartis) is active against all stages of fluke from 2 days old to adults.
        Closantel, **10 mg/kg orally** (**Flukiver**, Janssen) is moderately effective against fluke from 3 to 4 weeks old and highly effective against adult fluke.
        Nitroxynil, **10 mg/kg s.c.** (**Trodax**, Merial) is moderately effective against fluke from 8 to 9 weeks old and highly effective against mature fluke.

Control

❏ Reduce availability of snail populations – by drainage, fencing, molluscicides.
❏ Prophylactic use of fluke anthelmintics – in non-lactating animals use of triclabendazole in March and May will prevent pasture contamination with fluke eggs.

MAFF produce annual fluke forecasts based on the temperature and rainfall in the spring and early summer, so that specific control measures can be varied according to the predicted incidence of disease.

Dicrocoelium dentricum

Dicrocoelium dentricum, the lancet fluke, is found in the UK only on islands off the west coast of Scotland. This fluke is less pathogenic than *F. hepatica* because it remains in the bile ducts, rather than migrating through the liver parenchyma, and very large numbers of fluke can be carried by individual animals. Goats may have subclinical or chronic infections, with a history of weight loss, lethargy and possibly signs of anaemia and hypoprotienaemia. There are two intermediate hosts: eggs are ingested by various species of land snail and ants eat the slime balls, containing cercariae, expelled by the snails. Because the intermediate hosts are widespread and do not depend on water, control measures adopted for *F. hepatica* are not applicable and the only practicable control measure is the strategic use of anthelmintics, such as netobomin.

Abscess

In adult goats, liver abscesses are an occasional finding at slaughter, generally associated with a variety of other concurrent diseases, e.g. septicaemia or caseous lymphadenitis (see Chapter 9). Liver abscesses may arise in kids following a navel infection.

Tumour

Primary tumours of the liver are rare; secondary tumours occasionally occur.

Ragwort poisoning

See Chapter 20.

Visceral cysticercosis

Cystercus tenuicollis is the metacestode of the carnivore tapeworm *Taenia hydatigena*. After ingestion, migrating cysts pass through the liver. Infection with small numbers is unapparent, but large numbers of cysts will cause widespread damage to the liver parenchyma (hepatitis cysticercosa) and result in depression, anorexia, pyrexia, weight loss, abdominal discomfort and occasionally death in kids. Acute disease is rarely seen in animals over 6 months of age.

The migrating cysts may lead to infection with *Clostridium novyi* (*Clostridium oedematiens* type B, 'black disease', see Chapter 18).

Hydatid disease

Hydatid cysts are the metacestode stage of the carnivore tapeworm *Echinococcus granulosus*. The cysts initially develop in the liver and in high numbers may cause vascular of biliary obstruction in the liver. A local host response may lead to necrosis and infection of the liver. However, clinical disease is uncommon, large numbers of cysts being carried by apparently healthy animals. A proportion of cysts reach the lungs and may produce respiratory signs, particularly if a secondary infection, e.g. pasteurellosis, occurs.

Public health considerations
Hydatid cysts can also infect man. Although the goat is not a direct source of human infection, an infected animal would indicate environmental contamination, and control of tapeworm infection in dogs should be instigated.

Aflatoxicosis

Goats are relatively resistant to aflatoxins – the clinical signs are similar to those caused by other hepatotoxins such as pyrrolizidone alkaloids, e.g. ragwort.

Diabetes mellitus

There is a single report of naturally occurring diabetes mellitus in a Pygmy goat, which showed chronic weight loss, polydipsia and polyuria.

Interference with rumen/intestinal mobility

- ❑ Chronic rumen impaction (see Chapter 14).
- ❑ Ascites – chronic fascioliasis (qv); passive congestion of the liver.
- ❑ Ruminoreticular ulceration.
- ❑ Adhesions following surgery (e.g. caesarian section).
- ❑ Tumour – carcinomas (rare, older goats).
- ❑ Cestode infection? (see Chapter 13); if present in sufficient numbers could occlude intestinal lumen, otherwise unlikely to cause weight loss.
- ❑ Left-sided displacement of the abomasum – see Chapter 14 and periparturient toxaemia.

Presence of chronic disorders

Recurrent bouts of pyrexia, toxaemia and lethargy or painful conditions will lead to progressive weight loss.

- ❏ Chronic pneumonia
    - ■ pasteurella
    - ■ CAE
    - ■ lungworm infection
    - ■ viruses
    - ■ caseous lymphadenitis
    - ■ mycoplasma.
- ❏ Chronic peritonitis.
- ❏ Chronic enteritis
    - ■ salmonella
    - ■ chronic enterotoxaemia?
- ❏ Chronic mastitis (see Chapter 12).
- ❏ Metritis.
- ❏ Tuberculosis.

Tuberculosis

Tuberculosis is rare and notifiable.

Aetiology

- ❏ Goats generally infected with *Mycobacterium bovis* but are also susceptible to infection with *M. tuberculosis* and *M. avium* subsp. *avium*.

Transmission

- ❏ Infection can occur by inhalation or ingestion.

Clinical signs

- ❏ Goats may have extensive lesions without obvious clinical signs.
- ❏ Occurs as a disseminated disease involving the thorax (mediastinal lymph nodes, lungs, pleura) and abdomen (peritoneum, liver, spleen, mesenteric lymph nodes); occasionally superficial lymph nodes are enlarged and palpable.
- ❏ Chronic weight loss ± diarrhoea.
- ❏ Chronic cough due to bronchopneumonia.
- ❏ Skin lesions occasionally present – fistulae, ulcers and nodules.

Postmortem findings

❏ Tuberculosis granulomas in one or more lymph nodes.
❏ Caseous tubercles in lung, liver or spleen.

Diagnosis

❏ Single intradermal or comparative intradermal test as for cattle.
❏ False positives and false negatives occur.

Public health considerations

Mycobacterium bovis can be excreted in milk, faeces, urine, vaginal discharges, expired air and discharges from skin lesions or lymph nodes.

Pruritic conditions

❏ Lice (see Chapter 10) – often present in large numbers in chronically wasted goats, either (1) as secondary opportunists when a goat is in poor condition from any other cause, or (2) very occasionally as a primary cause of weight loss through pruritis and anaemia when there is a heavy infestation.
❏ Sarcoptic mange (see Chapter 10).
❏ Scrapie (see Chapter 11).

Further reading

General

Buchan, G.A.G. (1988) The wasting goat. *Goat Vet. Soc. J.*, **10** (2), 58–63.
East, N.E. (1982) Chronic weight loss in adult dairy goats. *Comp. Cont. Ed. Pract. Vet*, **4** (10), S419–24.
Owen, N.L. (1977) *The Illustrated Standard of the Dairy Goat*. Dairy Goat Journal Publishing Corporation, Scottsdale, Arizona.
Sherman, D.M. (1983) Unexplained weight loss in sheep and goats. *Vet. Clin. North Am.: Large Animal Practice*, **5** (3), November 1983, 571–90.

Condition scoring

Morand-Fehr, P., Hervieu, J. and Santucci, P. (1989) Notation de létat corporel: à vos stylos. *La Chèvre*, **175**, 39–42.

Johne's disease

Baxendell, S.A. (1984) Johne's disease in goats. *Proc. Univ. Sydney Post Grad. Comm. Vet. Sci.*, **73**, 508–10.

Saxegaard, F. and Fodstad, F.H. (1985) Control of paratuberculosis in goats by vaccination. *Vet. Rec.*, **116**, 439–41.
Sweeney, R.W. (1996) Paratuberculosis (Johne's disease). *Vet. Clin. North Am.: Food Animal Practice*, **12** (2).
Thomas, G.W. (1983) Paratuberculosis in a large goat herd. *Vet. Rec.*, **113**, 464–6.

Liver fluke

Taylor, M. (1987) Liverfluke treatment. *In Practice*, September 1987, 163–6.

Nutrition

Oldham, J.D. and Mowlem, A. (1981) Feeding goats for milk production. *Goat Vet. Soc. J.*, **2** (1), 13–19.
Randall, E.M. (1985) Nutrition in late pregnancy and early lactation. *Goat Vet. Soc. J.*, **6** (2), 51–5.
Randall, E.M. (1988) Caprine nutrition. *Goat Vet. Soc. J.*, **10** (1), 28–33.
Suttle, N.F. (1989) Predicting risks of mineral disorders in goats. *Goat Vet. Soc. J.*, **10** (1), 19–27.
Webster, A.J.F. (1988) Goat nutrition. *Goat Vet. Soc. J.*, **10**, 46–9.

Periparturient toxaemia

Andrews, A.M. (1985) Some metabolic conditions in the doe. *Goat Vet. Soc. J.*, **6**, 70–72.
Baxendell, S.A. (1984) Pregnancy toxaemia. *Proc. Univ. Sydney Post. Grad. Comm. Vet. Sci.*, **73**, 548–56.
Merrall, M. (1985) Nutritional and metabolic diseases. In: *Proc. Course in Goat Husbandry and Medicine*, Massey University, November 1985, 126–51.
Pinsent, J. and Cottom, D.S. (1987) Metabolic diseases of goats. *Goat Vet. Soc. J.*, **8** (1), 40–42.

9 External Swellings

Throat swellings

The differential diagnosis for throat swellings should include the following.

Thymus enlargement

Thymic hyperplasia/non-regression of the thymus

Thymic hyperplasia is a common condition in kids, resulting in soft swellings in the ventral neck region. It is probably a normal developmental occurrence – often confused by owners with 'goitre' (qv). It occurs as early as 2 weeks of age and regresses spontaneously by about 6 months.

Thymoma

Thymoma is a relatively common tumour in adult goats. It is operable if relatively small but may extend into the chest cavity, preventing swallowing and regurgitation by pressure on the oesophagus at the thoracic inlet or producing respiratory or cardiac dysfunction.

Multicentric lymphosarcoma

Thymic tumours may form part of a multicentric lymphosarcoma complex.

Wattle cysts

Wattle cysts are an inherited fault occurring particularly in British Alpine and Anglo-Nubian goats, resulting in a swelling at the base of one or both wattles, varying from peasize to several centimetres diameter. Surgical removal may be requested if the cyst is unsightly, particularly in show goats.

Diagnosis

❑ The position of the cyst is diagnostic.
❑ Histopathology is confirmatory, revealing walls of stratified squamous epithelium with mature hair follicles.

Salivary cysts

Salivary cysts are relatively common, as developmental abnormalities, in Anglo-Nubian goats, resulting in painless fluid-filled swellings in the submandibular region or side of the face. Damage to the submandibular or parotid salivary glands or their ducts can also lead to the formation of a mucocoele containing saliva.

Treatment

❑ Drainage or lancing of the cysts is unsatisfactory.
❑ Surgical excision is straightforward, provided the salivary duct is occluded by ligation; excision of the gland itself is not necessary.

Thyroid enlargement

Thyroid enlargement presents as swellings either side of the trachea.

Goitre (see Chapter 5)

Owners commonly associate *any* throat swelling with 'goitre', treat with iodine and risk iodine overdose. Genuine goitre is rare.

Iodine excess (see Chapter 5)

Iodine overdosage will in itself produce enlarged thyroid glands.

Tumours

Lymphosarcoma

Multicentric lymphosarcomas usually involve generalised enlargement of the lymph nodes, particularly in the face and shoulder region, with lesions in the spleen, liver, kidney or intestines. Occasionally the disease is more localised, with the jaw region a predilection site.

Malignant melanoma

Malignant melanomas (qv) often spread rapidly via the lymphatic system to involve the lymph nodes of the neck.

Other swellings around the head and neck

Abscess

Abscessation or cellulitis may arise occasionally as the result of pene-trating wounds. A variety of bacteria, including *Streptococcus* spp., *Staphylococcus* spp., *Actinomyces* (*Corynebacterium*) *pyogenes* and *Mor-axella* spp., have been isolated. These present as an individual problem in individual animals.

An injection abscess may arise at the site of vaccination or other injection because of faulty injection techniques (but most swellings produced by vaccination are sterile – see below).

Caseous lymphadenitis

> Caseous lymphadenitis is an emerging disease in the UK. All goats with abscesses should be handled carefully.

Aetiology

❏ *Corynebacterium pseudotuberculosis* (*C. ovis*), a gram-positive rod-shaped bacterium.

Incidence

❏ Occurs in many countries on all continents. Introduced into the UK with an importation of Boer goats in 1987. The condition is still rare but probably more common than reported at present and continuing vigilance is required to stop the spread of the disease.

Transmission

❏ Contamination of open wounds is the main cause of infection; inhalation is also possible, the tonsils can be infected after ingestion of the organism and kids can be infected by bacteria in milk. Flies can spread the disease.
❏ Following discharge from an abscess, the organism survives in the environment for many months.
❏ Spread between farms occurs by purchase of infected animals, by use of equipment (shearing, tattooing, ear-tagging) or by sharing facilities (handling, dipping).
❏ Spread between animals occurs when the skin is broken by any

method, including castration, vaccination, fighting, head butting and browsing, allowing bacteria to enter.

❏ The incubation period until abscesses are visible in superficial lymph nodes is 2 to 6 months or longer. After introduction into a clean herd, a high incidence of disease in the herd develops within 2 to 3 years.

Clinical signs

❏ Enlarged and abscessed peripheral lymph nodes, particularly of the head and neck (parotid, mandibular and prescapular nodes) but occasionally other sites such as popliteal nodes, depending where the organism gained entry to the body.

❏ The generalised (visceral) form of the disease causes abscessation of almost any organ and internal lymph nodes following haematogenous spread, but is less common in goats than sheep Goats with internal abscesses do not always have enlarged peripheral nodes.

❏ Although goats with external abscesses often show no other clinical signs of disease, goats with internal abscesses may become progressively emaciated and involvement of the thoracic lymph nodes can lead to respiratory signs.

Diagnosis

❏ Clinical examination – encapsulated abscesses, primarily at lymph nodes.

❏ Culture of aspirated abscess contents – use a sterile needle through shaved, disinfected skin, avoiding contamination of the environment.

❏ In goats, the pus is more commonly creamy white or yellow, rather than green as in sheep, and, although there may be caseation and a greenish tinge in older lesions, calcification is rare and the concentric 'onion ring' appearance, seen in sheep, is generally absent. The pus is thick and clinging. If the pus is freely flowing, it is unlikely to be caused by *C. pseudotuberculosis.*

❏ Serology – a variety of serological tests have been used in eradication and control programmes. Although of value in detecting infected herds, they have limited value in detecting individual infected animals. Most tests are accurate during the period of active abscess formation, but false negatives occur during the early stages of the disease and after abscess rupture, although the animals remain carriers. An ELISA test has been used in The Netherlands as part of their CL eradication programme.

❏ Postmortem examination may reveal internal abscesses.

Treatment

❏ Consider culling an infected animal to limit spread of the infection within the herd.
❏ Once abscess formation has occurred, treatment with antibiotics is unsuccessful.
❏ Surgical drainage, or removal of superficial nodes, will remove visible abscessation but will not necessarily prevent abscesses appearing elsewhere.
❏ Care should be taken to avoid contamination of the environment with pus; the abscess cavity should be flushed with a strong povidone iodine solution, all pus collected and burnt and the animal isolated until the lesion is completely healed. Gloves should be worn as the disease is potentially zoonotic.
❏ Alternatively, the pus can be aspirated using a large-gauge needle and 60-ml syringe, containing 25 ml of 10% formalin. Repeat aspirations and flushing will allow all the pus to be removed.

Eradication

❏ Cull or isolate all infected goats; an infected goat is infected for life.
❏ Never allow abscesses to spontaneously rupture.
❏ Remove kids from the adult herd at birth, and feed heat-treated colostrum, cow colostrum or colostrum substitute, then milk replacer.
❏ Rear kids separately from other animals.
❏ Vaccines are available in the USA, Canada and Australia but not the UK. Use of vaccines will decrease the level of abscesses in a herd but will not eradicate the disease.
❏ If abscess contents contaminate the environment, the whole area, including walls, floors, troughs, water bowls and gates, should be thoroughly cleaned to remove organic material and then disinfected. Most commercial disinfectants are effective.

Public health considerations

The disease is rarely transmissable to man. Most cases have involved shearers or abattoir workers. Milk from infected animals should be considered a possible risk.

Vaccination reaction

Sterile swellings commonly occur as a reaction to the clostridial vaccine adjuvant (particularly if oil-based) and may range in size from small nodules to several centimetres in diameter. Some animals seem particularly sensitive to any clostridial vaccine; others will react to only one particular product. In show animals vaccination on the sternum may be preferable to the neck or scapular regions.

Tooth root abscess

Tooth root abscesses present as a lump on the upper or lower jaw, often closely associated with the bone, sometimes with an associated cellulitis. An abscess of the lower jaw may track to the outside on the mandible; an abscess of the upper jaw may discharge into the mouth or sinuses of the skull.

Dentigerous cysts

Dentigerous cysts are sterile fluid-filled spaces surrounding the crown of an unerupted incisor tooth, or sometimes the whole tooth, causing localised enlargement of the mandible with varying degrees of bone destruction or remodelling.

Bottle jaw

'Bottle jaw' is a soft fluid-filled swelling under the jaw as a result of anaemia, particularly haemonchosis. Other signs of anaemia will also be present.

Impacted cud

Dental abnormalities, such as worn or poorly aligned molars in older goats, may result in retention and impaction of cud in the mouth, producing swollen cheeks. Cud retention can also occur with facial nerve paralysis in listeriosis (see Chapter 11), otitis media or trauma to the facial nerve.

Osteodystrophia fibrosa

Osteodystrophia fibrosa (see Chapter 7) in growing kids causes marked bilateral enlargement of the mandibles.

'Big head'

Clostridial infections (*C. novyi* or *C. oedematiens*) in bucks which have been fighting produce a swollen head ('big head') as part of an acute illness associated with lethargy, anorexia and pyrexia.

Tumours

Skin tumours

The incidence of skin tumours is very low in the UK. The major tumours – papillomas, squamous cell carcinomas and malignant melanomas – occur most commonly in white dairy or Angora goats with non-pigmented skin exposed to strong sunlight, so the incidence is likely to remain low unless the greenhouse effect produces a dramatic climate change!

Cutaneous papillomas
Papillomatosis is caused by a virus of the papovirus group. Three types of papillomas have been described in the goat:

❏ Mammary.
❏ Cutaneous.
❏ Genital.

Cutaneous papillomas occur particularly on the head, neck and thoracic limb and are flat, circumscribed with a crusty surface and ringwormlike in appearance.

Generally, a spontaneous resolution occurs in a few months. Occasionally, surgical removal or the use of autogenous vaccines is indicated.

Squamous cell carcinomas
Squamous cell carcinomas occur particularly perianally, around the vulva and udder and on the eyelid and nictitating membrane in areas of non-pigmented skin in response to stimulation by ultraviolet irradiation. In the early stages the tumours appear as thickened areas of skin, enlarging rapidly and becoming ulcerated and often coalescing to form large masses.

Malignant melanoma
Malignant melanomas commonly occur on the head and ears, and occasionally on the vulva or perianally, arising as small firm nodules from black pigmented areas and enlarging rapidly to form a black mass. Rapid spread via the lymphatic system may occur to involve the regional lymph nodes. Some melanomas may be unpigmented and resemble squamous cell carcinomas.

Mouth tumours

Lymphosarcoma
The goat appears unique in that lymphosarcoma commonly involves bony tissues of the face, with the mandible and maxilla being pre-

dilection sites. Affected animals present with varying degrees of mouth pain, dysphagia, inability to graze and weight loss. Most affected animals are between 2 and 4 years of age.

Other tumours

A variety of other tumours – sarcoma, adenocarcinoma, osteoma, fibrosarcoma, fibroma – are occasionally found in the mouths of goats and cause localised swelling.

Orf (contagious ecthyma; contagious pustular dermatitis)

Orf is a poxvirus infection causing pustules and then crusty, scabby lesions on the commissures of the lips, gums, nostrils, buccal mucosa and occasionally the udder, feet or tail. Unlike papillomas which are firmly attached to the skin, orf scabs can be picked off, revealing inflamed, granulating areas.

Debilitation and even death may occur if painful lesions prevent feeding. Local secondary bacterial infections may occur.

Diagnosis

❏ The virus can be demonstrated in fresh scabs by electron microscopy. Submit scabs from fresh lesions to the laboratory in a screwtopped container.

Treatment

❏ Secondary bacterial infection can be controlled with antibiotic sprays.

Prevention

❏ In infected herds, vaccination can be considered. Vaccinated animals develop mild lesions of orf at the site of vaccination which is usually the inside of the ear or the underside of the tail and live virus will be shed for 3 or 4 weeks, so the vaccine should only be used on farms where there is an existing problem.

Scabivax (Schering-Plough) or **Vaxall Orf** (Fort Dodge) by scarification of the skin.

Adults and kids should be vaccinated 3 to 4 weeks before the period of disease risk, with revaccination every 5 to 12 months. Kids can be vaccinated from 1 to 2 days of age. The vaccine should not be used during the last 2 months of pregnancy.

Public health considerations
Orf causes localised lesions on hands or forearms.

Herpes virus

Herpes viruses have been identified as causing wart-like lesions on the eyelid and proliferative lesions around the mouth and hard palate as well as vulvovaginitis, abortion, ulcerative enteritis and pneumonia (not confirmed but possibly present in the UK).

Diagnosis

❏   Culture of virus; serology.

Mycotic dermatitis (dermatophilosis)

See Chapter 6.

Ringworm

See Chapter 10.

Actinomycosis ('lumpy jaw')

Actinomycosis occurs rarely in goats, mimicking the bovine disease and producing hard painful swellings on the mandible and maxilla.

Diagnosis

❏   Direct smears, culture in anaerobic conditions or biopsy show the gram-positive filamentous organism *Actinomyces bovis.*

Treatment

❏   Intramuscular/local antibiotics; surgical excision and drainage.

Body swellings

❏   Abscess.
❏   Haematoma/seroma.
❏   Tumour – reported tumours include squamous cell carcinoma, melanoma, lymphosarcoma, papilloma, haemangioma and histio-cytoma.
❏   Hernia
  ■   umbilical

- ■ scrotal
- ■ perineal
- ■ ventral.
❑ Prolapse
  - ■ rectal (see Chapter 4)
  - ■ vaginal (see Chapter 4).
❑ Umbilical abscess – associated with joint ill.
❑ Ectopic mammary tissue – may result in a bilateral enlargement of the vulva lips in late pregnancy.
❑ Ticks – the sheep tick *Ixodes ricinus* is sometimes found on goats grazing sheep pastures. The hedgehog tick, *I. hexagonus*, is also occasionally identified.
❑ Keds – the sheep ked, *Melophagus ovinus*, occasionally infects goats.
❑ *Coenurus* cyst of *Taenia multiceps* can occur as a subcutaneous cyst.
❑ Warble flies – typical swellings under the skin on the back have been reported, although not from the UK.

Leg swellings

❑ Orf – see 'Other swellings around the head and neck'.
❑ Chorioptic mange – see Chapter 10.
❑ Mycotic dermatitis (strawberry footrot) – see Chapter 10.

Further reading

General

Fubini, S.L. and Campbell, S.G. (1983) External lumps on sheep and goats. *Vet. Clin. North Am.: Large Animal Practice*, **5** (3), November 1983, 457–76.

Caseous lymphadenitis

Brown, C.C. and Olander, H.J. (1987) Caseous lymphadenitis of goats and sheep, a review. *Vet. Bull.*, **57** (1), 1–12.
Lloyd, S., Lindsay, H.J., Slater, J.D. and Jackson, P.G.G. (1990) *Corynebacterium pseudotuberculosis* infection (caseous lymphadenitis) in goats. *Goat Vet. Soc. J.*, **11** (2), 55–65.
Williams, C.S.F. (1980) Differential diagnosis of caseous lymphadenitis in the goat. *Vet. Med. Small Animal Clin.*, **75**, 1165.

Dentigerous cyst

Miller, C.C., Selcer, B.A., Williamson, L.H. and Mahaffey, E.A. (1997) Surgical treatment of a septic dentigerous cyst in a goat. *Vet. Rec.*, **140**, 528–30.

Developmental cysts

Brown, P.J., *et al.* (1989) Developmental cysts in the upper neck of Anglo-Nubian goats. *Vet. Rec.,* **125**, 256–8.

Hypothyroidism

Rijnberk, A., *et al.* (1977) Congenital defect in iodothyronine synthesis; clinical aspects of iodine metabolism in goats with congenital goitre and hypothyroidism. *Br. Vet. J.,* **133**, 495–503.

Lymphosarcoma

Guedes, R.M.C., Facury Filho, E.J. and Lago, L.A. (1998) Mandibular lymphosarcoma in a goat. *Vet. Rec.,* **143**, 51–2.

Thymic hyperplasia

Pritchard, G.C. (1988) Throat swellings in goats. *Goat Vet. Soc. J.,* **10** (1), 34–7.

Thymoma

Parish, S.M., Middleton, J.R. and Baldwin, T.J. (1996) Clinical megaoesophagus in a goat with thymoma. *Vet. Rec.,* **139**, 94.

10 Skin Disease

Initial assessment

The preliminary history should consider:

- Clinical signs observed by owner and how long present.
- Individual or herd problem.
- Contact with goats and other animals.
- General health of affected goat and of herd.
- Response to any treatment given.
- Management (feeding, worming, etc.).

Clinical examination

The goat should be carefully examined:

- For signs of intercurrent disease, e.g. helminthiasis.
- To assess its behaviour (rubbing, nibbling, pruritis, etc.); study the goat, preferably in its own surroundings.
- To assess the general condition of the animal – weight etc.; evidence of malnutrition. Malnourished goats will have dry scaly skin often with a heavy lice burden.

Examination of skin

- Head/neck – particularly periorbital area and pinnae; mouth and mucocutaneous junction of lips.
- Thorax/abdomen – particularly axillae, udder and inguinal regions.
- Perineal region.
- Legs and feet.

Table 10.1 shows the common distribution of lesions in skin diseases. Table 10.2 lists the external parasites that cause skin disease, together with their effects and treatment.

Record

- Distribution of lesions (use sketches if indicated).
- Type and size of lesions.

Table 10.1   Distribution of lesions.

Lips, face and neck
- ❏ Staphyloccocal dermatitis
- ❏ Ringworm
- ❏ Sarcoptic mange
- ❏ Dermatophilosis
- ❏ Orf
- ❏ Zinc deficiency
- ❏ Pemphigus foliaceus

Ears
- ❏ Sarcoptic mange
- ❏ Dermatophilosis
- ❏ Ringworm
- ❏ Ear mites
- ❏ Photodermatitis
- ❏ Frostbite
- ❏ Pemphigus foliaceus

Feet
- ❏ Chorioptic mange
- ❏ Staphylococcal dermatitis
- ❏ Fly worry
- ❏ Dermatophilosis
- ❏ Sarcoptic mange
- ❏ Orf
- ❏ Zinc deficiency
- ❏ Contact dermatitis
- ❏ Pemphigus foliaceus
- ❏ Foot-and-mouth disease

Udder
- ❏ Staphylococcal dermatitis
- ❏ Fly worry
- ❏ Orf
- ❏ Zinc deficiency
- ❏ Sunburn
- ❏ Tumours

Perineum
- ❏ Orf
- ❏ Staphylococcal dermatitis
- ❏ Tumours
- ❏ Ectopic mammary gland
- ❏ (Caprine herpes virus)

❏ Quality of skin – colour, elasticity, odour, temperature.
❏ Response of animal to palpation of lesions.
❏ Hair loss or damage to follicles.
❏ Skin secretions.
❏ Self-inflicted damage.

Laboratory investigation

❏ *Hair sample* – pluck with tweezers from edge of active lesion.
   ■ Direct microscopy – identification of ringworm.
Note: Wood's lamp normally *negative* in goats with ringworm.
   ■ Culture
     – fungal media (ringworm)
     – blood agar (*Dermatophilus congolensis*).
❏ *Skin swab* – from active lesion near scaly or scabby area.
   ■ Culture on blood agar – *Staph. aureus* in pure culture is generally significant, but may be a secondary infection.
❏ *Impression smear* – of pus under a crust.
   ■ Stain with Dip Quick, Giemsa or new methylene blue.
   ■ Useful for *Dermatophilus congolensis* and candidiasis.
❏ *Skin scrapings* – essential for diagnosis of some manges. Scraping taken from each of a number of active lesions, collected and covered with potassium hydroxide before being warmed in a waterbath overnight.
   ■ Sarcoptic mange – mites difficult to find; diagnosis difficult from scrape; repeated deep scrapings required.
   ■ Demodectic mange – many mites found when nodule expressed.
   ■ Chorioptic and psoroptic mange – mites easily found in scrapes from legs and ears respectively.
❏ *Skin biopsy* – whole thickness skin strips taken under local anaesthesia; preferably from normal, marginal and abnormal areas; fix in formol saline.
❏ *Electron microscopy* – useful in diagnosis of orf; scabs fixed in buffered gluteraldehyde.
❏ *Blood sample*
   ■ Anaemia (lice infestation, etc.).
   ■ Neutrophilia (bacterial infection).
   ■ Eosinophilia (allergic, parasitic infestation).

Table 10.2 External parasites causing skin disease.

	Causal agent	Incidence	Distribution of lesions	Clinical signs	Pruritus	Diagnosis	Treatment
Lice	*Damalinia caprae* (biting) *Linognathus stenopsis* (**sucking**)	+++	Head, neck, back	Hair loss Broken hairs Moth-eaten coat	++	Naked eye	Amitraz Pyrethrins and synthetic pyrethroids Avermectins Moxidectin Fipronil Phosmet Dips
Sarcoptic mange	*Sarcoptes scabiei*	+	Head, ears, body Lymph nodes	Alopecia Crusting lesions Self-inflicted damage Weight loss	+++	Skin biopsy (skin scraping)	Avermectins Moxidectin Amitraz Phosmet
Harvest mites, forage mites, Cheyletiella		Rare	Legs, face, lower body	Exudative patches	++	Naked eye	As for lice
Psoroptic mange	*Psoroptes cuniculi*	Rare	Ear (head, body)	Head shaking	++	Skin scraping	Canine ear preparations Avermectins Moxidectin Amitraz Phosmet

Chorioptic mange	*Chorioptes caprae*	+++	Lower posterior limb Occasionally ventral abdomen, sternum	Crusting lesions Erythema	–	Skin scraping	Avermectins Moxidectin Amitraz Phosmet Fipronil
Demodectic mange	*Demodex caprae*	++	Head, neck, body	Hard nodules with yellow caseous material	–	Microscopy on expressed material Skin biopsy	Amitraz
Pustular dermatitis	*Staphylococcus aureus*	+++	Udder, teats[a], ventral abdomen, groin, body	Pustular scabs Dry scaly coat	–	Culture[b]	Local/ parenteral antibiotics or udder washes
Ringworm	*Trichophyton verrucosum Microsporum canis Trichophyton mentagrophytes*	Rare	Head, body	Raised, circular crusty lesions	–	Microscopy culture	Topical preparations *Griseofulvin in feed* (but not legal in the EU)

[a] See 'Staphylococcal dermatitis', this chapter.
[b] *Staphylococcus aureus* is often a secondary invader in other skin conditions, e.g. mange.

Treatment of external parasites

> There are no drugs licensed for the treatment of ectoparasites in goats in the UK.

Rational treatment involves extrapolation from products licensed for use in cattle and sheep, preferably, or, outwith the EU, from dogs and cats where no other suitable products exist, if permitted by regulatory authorities. All of these preparations have a mandatory withholding time for milk of at least 7 days and for meat of 28 days, which can cause major difficulties in formulating control strategies for milking herds and may lead to welfare problems. Wherever possible, the opportunity should be taken to treat young stock and dry goats. Table 10.3 lists the treatments available.

Pruritic skin disease

Lice

The biting louse *Damalinia caprae* and the blood-sucking louse *Linognathus stenopsis* affect goats, producing pruritus and hair loss particularly on the head, neck and back. Lice are very common and in particular will multiply where animals are debilitated for any reason and may complicate the problem by producing anaemia (qv). The damage to fleece can cause financial loss in Angora goats.

Diagnosis

❏ Lice are visible to the naked eye. Under magnification, biting lice are seen to have broad heads with wide mouth parts, whereas sucking lice have pointed heads to enable them to pierce the skin and suck blood.

Treatment

❏ As lice dislike warm weather and ultraviolet light, lice numbers decrease in summer and rise in winter. The best time for treatment is thus late summer or autumn when lice numbers are lowest. The whole herd should preferably be treated at the same time.

❏ Most treatments are not effective against nits, so treatment should be repeated after 10 to 14 days to kill young lice before they mature.

Table 10.3 Treatment of external parasites.

		Lice		Chorioptic mange	Sarcoptic mange	Demodectic mange	Psoroptic mange	Ticks/keds
		Sucking	Biting					
Amitraz	Taktic Aludex	+	+	+	+	+	+	+
Cypermethrin	Crovect	–	+				+	+
	Provinec	–	+					
	Vector	–	+					
Deltamethrin	Spot On	+	+					+
Permethrin	Dog/cat shampoos and powders	+	+					
Pyrethrin/ pironyl peroxide	Dog/cat sprays and powders	+	+					
Abamectin	Enzec	+	–	+	+		+	
Doramectin	Dectomax	+	+ –	+	+		+	
Eprinomectin	Eprinex	+	+ –	+	+		+	
Ivermectin	Ivomec Panomec	+	+ –	+	+		+	
Moxidectin	Cydectin	+	+ –	+	+		+	
Fipronil	Frontline	+	+	+	+			
Phosmet	Vet-Kem	+	+	+	+			
	Sponge-On Dermol Plus Poron						+	
Flumethrin	Bayticol	+	+				+	+

Note: none of these products is licensed for use in goats in the UK. Particular care should be taken when treating goats producing milk for human consumption.

(1)   Amidines
    Biting and sucking lice:
        Amitraz, 0.025% solution, by **spray** or **wash** (**Taktic**, Hoechst Roussel), dilute 1 volume in 250 volumes of water; or (**Aludex**, Hoechst Roussel), dilute 1 volume in 200 volumes of water.

(2)   Pyrethrins and synthetic pyrethroids
    Biting lice only:
        Cypermethrin 1.25% solution, **0.25 ml/kg** (maximum 20 ml) by **pour-on** (**Crovect**, Crown; **Provinec**, C-Vet; **Vector**, Young).
    Sucking and biting lice:
        Deltamethrin 1%, 'spot-on' (**Spot On**, Schering-Plough).
        Permethrin
        Permethrin 4%, 'pour-on' (**Ridect**, Pfizer; **Ryposect**, C-Vet; **Swift**, Young's).
        There are also many preparations, containing permethrin, marketed for use in dogs and cats as shampoos and powders which can be used on pet and Pygmy goats.
        Pyrethrins
        As with permethrin, dog and cat sprays and powders containing pyrethrins and piperonyl butoxide can be used on pet and Pygmy goats.

(3)   Avermectins and milbemycin
    Sucking lice:
        Abamectin, 10 mg/50 kg, 1 ml/50 kg s.c. (**Enzec**, Janssen).
    Sucking lice and partial control of biting lice:
        Doramectin, 10 mg/50 kg, 1 ml/50 kg s.c. (**Dectomax**, Pfizer).
        Eprinomectin, 0.5 mg/kg, 5 ml/50 kg 'pour-on' (**Eprinex**, Merial).
        Ivermectin, 10 mg/50 kg, 1 ml/50 kg s.c. (**Ivomec, Panomec**, Merial).
        Moxidectin, 10 mg/50 kg, 1 ml/50 kg s.c. (**Cydectin 1%**, Fort Dodge).

(4)   Fipronil
    Biting and sucking lice:
        Fipronil (**Frontline Spray**, Merial).
        Suitable for Pygmy goats or individual pet goats as expensive! Not licensed in the UK for food producing animals.

(5) Phosmet
     Biting and sucking lice:
     Phosmet, 0.09% solution (**Vet-Kem Sponge-On**, Sanoffi), dilute
         30 ml with 3.8 l water.
     Phosmet, 200 mg/ml, **20 mg/kg**, 'pour-on' (**Dermol Plus**,
         Crown; **Poron 20**, Young's).

(6) Dips
     Fibre goats can be dipped, using products approved for sheep.
     The body should be immersed for at least 30 seconds, until the
     coat is completely saturated. The head should be immersed once
     or twice, allowing the animal to breathe between immersions.
         Amitraz (**Taktic**, Hoechst Roussel), **pyrethroids – cyperme-
         thrin** (**Crovect**, Crown; **Provinec**, C-Vet), flumethrin (**Bayti-
         col Scab and Tick Dip**, Bayer).

Sarcoptic mange

Sarcoptic mange is a relatively common disease affecting goats of all
ages. It is transmitted primarily by direct contact but also by indirect
contact such as milking, handling, etc.

Clinical signs

❏ Lesions start around the eyes and ears with erythema and small
   nodules, progressing to hair loss, thickening and wrinkling of the
   skin, in response to intense pruritus and scratching over the head,
   neck and body. Secondary infection with *Staph. aureus* is common.
❏ Affected goats often lose condition and the milk yield falls because
   of the intensity of the irritation.

Diagnosis

❏ Demonstration of the mite, *Sarcoptes scabiei*, in deep skin scrapings
   may be extremely difficult as very few mites can be found even
   with severe lesions; skin biopsy may demonstrate mites.

Treatment

(1) Avermectins and milbemycin
     Abamectin, 10 mg/50 kg, 1 ml/50 kg s.c. (**Enzec**, Janssen).
     Doramectin, 10 mg/33 kg, 1 ml/33 kg s.c. (**Dectomax**, Pfizer).
     Ivermectin, 10 mg/50 kg, 1 ml/50 kg s.c. (**Ivomec, Panomec**,
         Merial).

> **Moxidectin,** 10 mg/50 kg, 1 ml/50 kg s.c. (**Cydectin** 1%, Fort Dodge).
> Moxidectin and doramectin are more persistent than ivermectin. Treatment with ivermectin should be repeated after 7 days.

(2) Amidines

> **Amitraz** 0.025% solution, by **spray** or **wash** (**Taktic** Hoechst Roussel), dilute 1 volume in 250 volumes of water or (**Aludex**, Hoechst Roussel), dilute 1 volume in 200 volumes of water.

(3) Phosmet

> **Phosmet,** 0.09% solution (**Vet-Kem Sponge-On**, Sanoffi), dilute 30 ml with 3.8 l water.
> **Phosmet,** 200 mg/ml, **20 mg/kg,** 'pour-on' (**Dermol Plus,** Crown; **Poron 20,** Young's).

Use of a soap and water or antiseborrhoeic shampoo to remove crusts before using amitraz or phosmet will ensure better penetration of the drug. Washes can be repeated after 7 to 14 days as necessary.

Fly worry

Biting flies are particularly worrying to housed goats in the summer, producing quite severe lesions resembling superficially staphylococcal dermatitis on the udder but generally more pruritic. Topical creams and washes will ease the lesions. Control of flies in the goat house will help prevent the problem, e.g. Golden Malrin (Sanoffi).

Myiasis (*blowfly strike*) is much less common than in sheep but may occur around the head following fights, in wounds in soiled areas around the tail, breech and penis, or on the feet of animals with footrot/ scald. **Cyromazine** (**Vetrazin**, Novartis) can be used in animals at risk.

Other external parasites

Harvest mites are the reddish or orange larvae of the free-living trombiculid mite which attaches to the pasterns, muzzle, ears or ventral abdomen when goats are exposed to infested fields or woods or contaminated fodder in the late summer. The mites produce severe localised pruritis and exudative patches and even anorexia in severe cases. Other mites such as **Cheyletiella** and **poultry mites** (*Dermanyssus gallinae*) are also occasionally reported. The small red poultry mites are nocturnal feeders and so are rarely actually seen on the goat, but the combination of a pruritic goat housed with poultry or roosting birds, particularly in the late summer months, would suggest a provisional diagnosis of infestation *Forage mites* (*Tyroglyphidae* spp.) are chance contaminants from bedding, food, etc. which are occasionally associated with a dermatitis. Most lice treatments will also kill mites.

Flea infestations are uncommon in temperate climates, although both cat and dog fleas (*Ctenophalides* spp.) are found occasionally on goats. Lice treatments are suitable for control of fleas, but environmental control is as important as treatment of individual animals.

Scrapie

See Chapter 11. Scrapie causes pruritus and self-mutilation but is not as pruritic in goats as in sheep.

Psoroptic mange

Psoroptes cuniculi parasitises the ear, generally without clinical signs, occasionally producing head shaking and scratching. Scaly lesions may be found on the inside of the pinnae and occasionally on the head, neck or body. Kids are infected by their dams and may show clinical signs by 3 weeks of age. Severe vestibular disease and facial nerve paralysis may occur if the tympanic membrane ruptures.

Note: Railettia caprae is a mite affecting the ears of goats in Australia, Mexico and the USA, but not in the UK.

Diagnosis

❑ Identification of mite; larger than *Chorioptes* with long jointed pedicel and trumpet-shaped suckers.

Treatment

❑ Canine ear mite preparations can be used where the mites are confined to the ears, but removal of wax plugs and crusting is necessary to allow penetration of the drug. Several weekly treatments are necessary.
❑ Subcutaneous injections of avermectins or moxidectin will kill the mites but cannot be used in lactating goats.
❑ Body mange can be treated with avermectin, or moxidectin, injection or by amitraz or phosmet washes.

Strongyloidiasis

A localised dermatitis can occur as part of the immune response to the larvae of *Strongyloides papillosus*. Strongyloidiasis affects the lower limbs, causing pruritus, with stamping and nibbling.

Onchocerca

Onchocerca produces fine skin nodules particularly in the neck and shoulder region with mild pruritus.

Autoimmune skin disease

Pemphigus foliaceus has been diagnosed in goats showing crusty pruritic lesions on the skin in the perineal and scrotal regions and on the ventral abdomen. Diagnosis is confirmed by skin biopsy.

Treatment

❑ Remission has been achieved with an immunosuppressive induction dose of **prednisolone, 1 mg/kg i.m. every 12 hours** followed by a maintenance dose of **1 mg/kg i.m. every 48 hours**.

Photosensitisation

Photosensitisation causes pruritus, erythema, oedema and swelling of the skin, with blistering and scab formation.

❑ Primary – due to ingestion of St. John's wort (*Hypericum perforatum*) or buckwheat (*Fagopyrum esculentum*).
❑ Secondary – in animals with hepatic dysfunction due to accumulation of phylloerythrin, a breakdown derivative of chlorophyll. Any liver damage affecting bile excretion may be implicated – liver disease, hepatotoxic drugs, chemicals, mycotoxins or plant toxins, e.g. bog asphodel (*Northecium ossifragum*).

Treatment

❑ Prevent access to any photosensitising plant.
❑ Protect from sunlight.
❑ Symptomatic and supportive therapy.

Non-pruritic skin disease

Chorioptic mange

Chorioptic mange is a very common infection of goats in the UK, particularly in housed goats in the winter but occurring throughout the year. Legs should always be checked for chorioptic mange during routine foot trimming.

Clinical signs

❏ White/brown scabby lesions generally at the back of the pasterns but occasionally extending as far as the knee or hock in severe infection. Very occasionally lesions may be found on the ventral abdomen, sternum or even upper body. Lesions may be complicated with a *Staph. aureus* infection.

Diagnosis

❏ Microscopical identification of non-burrowing mite *Chorioptes caprae*. Mites generally easily found; short pedicel with flask-shaped suckers on legs.

Treatment

Treatment of chorioptic mange is extremely frustrating because of lack of effective drugs and the necessity to treat milking animals with drugs with long withholding times.

❏ Success of treatment with injectable *avermectins* and *moxidectin* (see treatment of lice) is variable because of the superficial location and the feeding habits of the mites, so repeat injections at 7- to 10-day intervals are necessary, particularly with less persistent drugs like ivermectin.
❏ Before topical treatments are used, the skin should be thoroughly washed to remove crusts and scabs. Topical treatments include **amitraz**, **phosmet**, **ivermectin**, **moxidectin** and **fipronil** (see treatment of lice). At least two treatments at 10- to 14-day intervals will be required.
❏ Secondary bacterial infections should be treated with systemic antibiotics.

Demodectic mange (*Demodex caprae*)

Demodectic mange is relatively common. Goatlings most commonly show clinical disease following infection as a kid. It is usually an individual rather than a herd problem.

Clinical signs

❏ Small nodules (generally about 1 to 2 cm) in the skin of the head, neck and body due to multiplication of the mite in individual sebaceous glands. Yellow caseous material, containing numerous mites, can be expressed from the nodules.

Diagnosis

❏ Microscopical identification of mites in caseous material from nodules. Very easy to find in smears. Cigar-shaped body with bluntly pointed abdomen.

Treatment

❏ Where the lesions are widespread or generalised, topical treatment with **amitraz** (see treatment of lice) is necessary. Nodules will persist for a considerable time after the mites have died, so it is difficult to know when a clinical cure is achieved.
❏ If there are only a small number of lesions, they can be treated by lancing each nodule and squeezing out the contents. The area can be washed with amitraz after the nodules have been expressed.

Staphylococcal dermatitis (pustular dermatitis)

Staphylococcus aureus infection is very common, causing pustules of variable size up to 4 cm especially on the udder, teats and groin but also on the ventral abdomen and occasionally any part of the body. First kidders are particularly affected soon after parturition. Pustules are easily broken and spread, healing as a scabby or impetigo-like lesion, and infection may be spread between goats at milking by hands, cloths or milking dusters. The lesions are generally non-painful and milk yield is not affected.

The disease is colloquially known as 'goat pox' but true 'goat pox' caused by capripoxvirus does not occur in the UK.

Note: Staphylococcus aureus is a common secondary invader of other skin lesions.

Orf

See Chapter 9.

Zinc deficiency

Zinc deficiency is probably more common than generally recognised. Diets should usually be adequate in zinc, but (1) an excess of copper will interfere with zinc uptake as will a high calcium intake (e.g. lucerne); (2) individual goats may not absorb adequate amounts; and (3) some male goats may have higher requirements.

Clinical signs

❑ Hair loss; hyperkeratosis and parakeratosis with thickened, wrinkled skin particularly on the hind limbs, scrotum, neck and head.

❑ Hair loss on the ears of Anglo-Nubian kids has also responded empirically to zinc supplements.

Note: zinc deficiency may also result in infertility with low conception rates.

Laboratory tests

❑ Zinc blood levels can be estimated using a sample taken into a sodium citrate vacutainer, but correlation between serum and dietary zinc levels may be poor.

Treatment

❑ **Zinc sulphate drench 1% or zinc sulphate tables, 250 mg to 1 g daily, orally for 2 to 4 weeks.**

❑ **Zincosel bolus** (Telsol Ltd.) is a slow-release bolus containing zinc, cobalt and selenium.

Urine scald

Male goats urinate on themselves during the breeding season, particularly down the back of the forelegs, face and beard, and this will result in staining, hair loss and possibly scalding of the skin.

Similarly, staining will occur on goats that are recumbent or housed in dirty conditions.

Alopecia/skin thickening in older male goats

Older male goats (particularly British Toggenburg and British Alpine) commonly have thickened scaly skin especially over the head and back, possibly due in part to urine scald, nutritional deficiency during the breeding season (zinc related?) and as a response to rubbing, although the exact aetiology is unknown.

Treatment with baby oils or olive oil thinned with surgical spirit has been suggested as suitable for removing excess scaling to allow new hair to grow, following thorough shampooing. Zinc sulphate supplements should also be considered.

Labial dermatitis in artificially reared kids

Kids reared artificially may develop erythema and hair loss around the face and mouth due to wetting. Occasionally, a secondary infection with *Staph. aureus* occurs (see 'Staphylococcal dermatitis'). Labial dermatitis needs distinguishing from the early stages of orf (see Chapter 9) and from dermatophilosis (see Chapter 6).

Ringworm

Ringworm is an uncommon infection acquired from other hosts. *Trichophyton verrucosum* from cattle is seen most frequently, occasionally *T. mentagrophytes* from rodents and *Microsporum canis* from dogs or cats.

Lesions are initially circular, crusty and raised, later irregular in shape, often occurring on the head, ears and neck.

Diagnosis

❏ Microscopy and culture.
❏ *Trichophyton* species do *not* fluoresce under a Wood's lamp.

Treatment

❏ Topical fungicides
    Copper naphthenate (**Kopertox**, Crown)
    Eniliconazole (**Imaverol**, Janssen), 0.2% solution by wash or spray, every 3 days for three or four applications.
    Natamycin (**Mycophyt**, Intervet), 0.01% solution locally, repeat after 4 or 5 days and again after 14 days if required.
❏ **Griseofulvin, 7.5 mg/kg orally** for 7 days.
    Under present EU legislation, griseofulvin cannot be used in food-producing animals as no official residue limits have been set.

Pygmy goat syndrome (Seborrhoeic dermatitis)

Certain families of Pygmy goats develop non-pruritic crusty lesions around the eyes, ears, nose and head and in the axilla, groin and perineal region. Aetiology unknown.

Treatment

❏ Topical treatment with combination corticosteroid and antibiotic ointments or parenteral treatment with corticosteroids and antibiotics produces complete resolution for up to 4 weeks, but the lesions recur.

Golden Guernsey goat syndrome ('sticky kid')

Golden Guernsey goat syndrome is an hereditary disease caused by an autosomal recessive gene. Affected kids are born with sticky, greasy, matted coats which remain abnormal throughout life.

Mycotic dermatitis (dermatophilosis)

See Chapter 6.

Iodine deficiency

See Chapter 5. Iodine deficiency may result in weak kids born with thin sparse hair coats, as part of a syndrome of abortion, weak kids and stillbirths. Older goats may show poor growth rate and dry scabby skin as a result of general malnutrition.

Selenium/vitamin E deficiency

A deficiency of selenium/vitamin E may produce a dry coat and dandruff.

Skin disease presenting as swellings (qv)

❏ Neoplasia
  ■ papillomatosis
  ■ melanoma
  ■ squamous cell carcinoma
  ■ haemangioma.
❏ Orf (see Chapter 9).
❏ Ticks – several species of ticks have been reported from goats in the UK. *Ixodes ricinus*, the caster bean tick, occurs widely throughout the country and the hedgehog tick, *Ixodes hexaganus*, is also occasionally found. *Ixodes* is a three host tick, with all three stages – larva, nymph and adult – feeding on a different mammalian host.

Heavy tick burdens will cause loss of condition, but the most important consequence of tick infestation is the transmission of bacterial, viral or protozoal diseases in endemic areas. These include *tickborne fever* (see Chapter 2) and *tick pyaemia* (see Chapter 7).
❏ Keds – *Melophagus ovinus* is a wingless bloodsucking fly that infests both sheep and goats, with the whole life cycle completed on the host. Heavy infestation may cause anaemia and irritation, but keds are generally of limited pathological significance. Keds are often present with lice.
❏ Abscess (see Chapter 9).

Further reading

Jackson, P. (1982) Skin disease in goats. *Goat Vet. Soc. J.*, **3** (1), 7–11.

Jackson, P. (1986) Skin diseases in goats. *In Practice*, January 1986, 5–10.

Jackson, P., Richards, H.W. and Lloyds, S. (1983) Sarcoptic mange in goats. *Vet. Rec.*, **112**, 330.

Jefferies, A.R., Casas, F.C., Hall, S.J.G. and Jackson, P.G.G. (1991) Seborrhoeic dermatitis in Pygmy goats. *Vet. Dermatol.*, **2** (3/4), 109–117.

Scott, D.W., Smith, M.C. and Manning, T.O. (1984) Caprine dermatology. Part I. Normal skin and bacterial and fungal disorders. *Cont. Ed. Pract. Vet.*, **6** (4), S190–211.

Scott, D.W., Smith, M.C. and Manning, T.O. (1984) Caprine dermatology. Part II. Viral, nutritional, environmental and congenitohereditary disorders. *Cont. Ed. Pract. Vet.*, **6** (8), S473–85.

Scott, D.W., Smith, M.C. and Manning, T.O. (1984) Caprine dermatology. Part III. Parasitic, allergic, hormonal and neoplastic disorders. *Cont. Ed. Pract. Vet.*, **7** (8), S437–52.

Smith, M.C. (1981) Caprine dermatologic problems: a review. *J. Am. Vet. Med. Assoc.*, **178**, 724.

Smith, M.C. (1983) Dermatologic diseases of goats. *Vet. Clin. North Am.: Large Animal Practice*, **5** (3), November 1983, 449–56.

Valdez, A., Gelberg, H.B., Morin, E.L. and Zuckermann, F.A. (1995) Use of corticosteroids and aurothioglucose in a Pygmy goat with pemphigus foliaceus. *J. Am. Vet. Med. Assoc.*, **207** (6), 761–5.

Walton, G.S. (1980) Skin lesions and goats. *Goat Vet. Soc. J.*, **1** (2), 15–16.

Wright, A.I. (1989) Dermatology. *Goat Vet. Soc. J.*, **10** (2), 64–6.

11 Nervous Diseases

> Animals with severe anaemia, liver, kidney, lung or myocardial disease may present with apparent nervous dysfunction.

Initial assessment

The preliminary history should consider:

❏ Herd/flock or individual problem.
❏ Age.
❏ Sex.
❏ Stage of pregnancy/lactation.
❏ Diet/dietary changes.

Specific management practices should be discussed:

❏ Disbudding, castration, dipping.
❏ Prophylactic therapies – coccidiostats, anthelmintics.
❏ Feeding/grazing routine.

A careful study of the environment should be made:

❏ Feed sources – silage, grazing.
❏ Water sources.
❏ Fertilisers/weed killers.
❏ Trace element availability.
❏ Possible sources of poison.

Clinical examination

❏ Examine the animal(s) undisturbed in their usual surroundings – are they bright, alert, responsive or dull and depressed?
❏ Response to approach – apprehension, trembling, etc.
❏ Head carriage
  ■ hyperaesthesia
  ■ defective vision

- ■ head tilt
- ■ tremors
- ■ head pressing
- ■ lateral deviation
- ■ circling movements.
- ❏ Ability to rise – opisthotonus, coma, semicoma.
- ❏ Locomotion – move animal slowly at first, then faster. Watch for knuckling, circling, incoordination, ataxia, aimless wandering.
- ❏ Physical examination – general examination plus specific features referable to neurological disorders, e.g. drooping of ear or eyelid, facial paralysis, retention of cud, nystagmus, size of pupils.
- ❏ Examine eye with ophthalmoscope.
- ❏ Specific neurological examination – refer to appropriate textbook; techniques applicable to dog or cat can be used in goats.

Table 11.1 gives some indication of how clinical signs relate to sites of lesions and possible aetiologies.

Laboratory investigation

- ❏ Complete blood count.
- ❏ Specific tests as indicated.
- ❏ Cerebrospinal fluid analysis and culture.

Cerebrospinal fluid collection

Lumbosacral space

Restrain animal in lateral recumbency with hind legs pulled forward to flex the spine; prepare site surgically and block with local anaesthetic.

Insert a 0.9 × 38 mm spinal or disposable needle into the depression between the last lumbar and first sacrodorsal spinous process, advancing the needle slowly until a slight pop is felt when the dura mater is penetrated. Approximately 1 ml of CSF per 5 kg body weight can be collected.

Atlanto-occipital site

Samples obtained from the atlanto-occipital site are more likely to represent accurately intracranial lesions, but sedation or general anaesthesia is necessary – use lumbosacral space if the animal is too ill to risk sedation.

Prepare site surgically and place animal in lateral recumbency with head at right angles to neck and horizontal to ground. Insert a 0.9 × 38

Table 11.1 Nervous diseases.

Clinical sign	Site of lesion	Possible aetiology

Convulsions	Cerebrum	Infectious
		  meningioencephalitis
		  enterotoxaemia
		  tetanus
		  pseudorabies
		Parasitic
		  coenurosis (gid)
		  Oestrus ovis
		Metabolic
		  cerebrocortical necrosis
		  periparturient toxaemia
		  hypomagnesaemia
		  hypoglycaemia
		  hepatoencephalopathy
		Toxic
		  organophosphates
		  lead
		  levamisole overdose
		Epilepsy

Muscle tremors	Cerebrum	Infectious
		  meningoencephalitis
		  scrapie
		  louping ill
		  border disease
		  CAE
		  rabies
		Metabolic
		  hypoglycaemia
		  cerebrocortical necrosis
		  hypocalcaemia
		  hypomagnesaemia
		  hepatoencephalopathy
		  enzootic ataxia
		Poisoning
		  Prunus (cyanide)
		  laburnum
		  hemlock
		  nitrate, nitrite
		  oxalate
		  urea
		  organophosphates
		  levamisole overdose

Contd.

Table 11.1 *Contd.*

Clinical sign	Site of lesion	Possible aetiology

Coma	Cerebrum
	Midbrain
		Infection
		    meningoencephalitis
		    enterotoxaemia
		    pseudorabies
		Metabolic
		    cerebrocortical necrosis
		    periparturient toxaemia
		    hypocalcaemia
		    hepatoencephalopathy
		    uraemia
		Poisoning
		    organophosphates
		    salt poisoning
		    oxalate

Excitability
Aimless wandering
Head pressing
Hyperaesthesia
Constant chewing
Fear or aggression
	Cerebrum	Infection
		    meningioencephalitis
		    pseudorabies
		    rabies
		Parasitic
		    coenurosis (gid)
		    Oestrus ovis
		Metabolic
		    cerebrocortical necrosis
		    periparturient toxaemia
		    hypomagnesaemia
		    hepatoencephalopathy
		Poisoning
		    organophosphates
		    Prunus (cyanide)
		    nitrates (rape, beet tops)

Opisthotonus	Cerebrum
	Cerebellum
	Midbrain
	Pons
		Infectious
		    enterotoxaemia
		    tetanus
		    meningoencephalitis
		    brain abscess
		    CAE
		    rabies
		Metabolic
		    cerebrocortical necrosis
		    hypomagnesaemia
		Any cause of convulsions

Contd.

Table 11.1 *Contd.*

Clinical sign	Site of lesion	Possible aetiology

Circling	Cerebrum	Infectious
		  listeriosis
		  brain abscess
		  CAE
		  rabies
		Parasitic
		  coenurosis (gid)
		  Oestrus ovis
		Metabolic
		  cerebrocortical necrosis

	Vestibular system	Infectious otitis media/interna

Hypermetria	Cerebellum	Parasitic
		  coenurosis (gid)
		  Oestrus ovis
		Metabolic
		  enzootic ataxia

Ataxia	Spinal cord lesions
	Cerebellum
	Vestibular
	Cerebrum
		Infectious
		  listeriosis
		  meningoencephalitis
		  brain abscess
		  scrapie
		  CAE
		  rabies
		Parasitic
		  tick pyaemia
		  cerebrospinal nematodiasis
		  Oestrus ovis
		Metabolic
		  hypocalcaemia
		  hypomagnesaemia
		  cerebrocortical necrosis
		  enzootic ataxia
		Neoplasia
		Congenital vertebral or spinal deformities
		Poisoning
		  oxalate
		  Prunus (cyanide)
		  Fool's parsley

Contd.

Table 11.1 *Contd.*

Clinical sign	Site of lesion	Possible aetiology
Head tilt	Vestibular system	Infectious
		listeriosis
		otitis media/interna
		brain abscess
		CAE
		Parasitic
		ear mites
		cerebral nematodiasis

or 63 mm spinal needle or 0.9 × 38 mm disposable needle with the needle pointing towards the lower jaw and advance *slowly* until the dura mater is penetrated.

Note: trauma to the brain stem may cause death.

Cerebrospinal fluid analysis and culture

Collect CSF in EDTA tube for cytological examination and plain tube for biochemical analysis and bacteriological culture.

❏ *Colour* – should be clear and colourless. Turbidity indicates viral, bacterial, fungal or parasitic infection. Yellowish discoloration (xanthochromia) indicates presence of blood pigments from trauma or vascular damage.
❏ *Protein level* – normal goats have a level of 0 to 0.39 g/l; can be measured with urinary reagent strips; >1+ is abnormal. Protein levels are increased in infective conditions, may be slightly elevated in traumatic conditions and remain normal in degenerative congenital or toxic conditions.
❏ *Cell counts* – use undiluted fluid in a haemocytometer; allow cells to settle for 5 to 10 minutes before counting. Normal goats have counts of 0 to 4 white cells/μl. Elevated white cell counts may be found in viral conditions (mononuclear cells), parasitic conditions (neutrophils, occasionally many eosinophils), and bacterial or fungal infections (usually neutrophils; with listeriosis half neutrophils, half mononuclear cells). Red cells may be found following trauma.
❏ *Glucose levels* – use urinary reagent strip. Normal levels are about 80% the blood glucose level, i.e. about 3.0 to 4.0 mmol/l.
❏ *Blood content* – use urinary reagent strip.
❏ *Gram stain* of CSF smear following sedimentation.
❏ *Bacterial culture.*

Postmortem examination

Many neurological disorders are likely to be fatal or even present as sudden death.

Treatment

> Early aggressive treatment may mean the difference between recovery and death.

Specific treatment should be instigated as soon as a diagnosis is made. Until such time, general supportive therapy is indicated.

❏ Sterilise the CSF with broad-spectrum antibiotics, **intravenously** for the first 4 days.

  Trimethoprim/sulphonamide, 15–24 mg combined/kg (Borgal, Hoechst Roussel; **Trivetrin**, Schering-Plough) every 6 to 12 hours.

  Oxytetracycline, 3–10 mg/kg (Alamycin, Norbrook; **Duphacycline**, Fort Dodge; **Engemycin**, Merial; **Oxytetrin**, Schering-Plough; **Terramycin**, Pfizer) every 12 to 24 hours.

  Benzylpenicillin, 10 mg/kg (Crystapen, Schering-Plough) every 6 hours.

  Ceftiofur, 1 mg/kg, 1 ml of reconstituted vial/50 kg i.m. only (Excenel 1 g Powder, Pharmacia & Upjohn) every 24 hours.

  Ampicillin, 3 mg/kg (Penbritin Veterinary Injectable, Pfizer) every 8 hours.

  Gentamicin, 3 mg/kg every 8 hours, alone or in combination with trimethoprim/sulphonamide combinations.

  Chloramphenicol, 5–10 mg/kg, every 12 to 24 hours (prohibited in food-producing animals in the EU).

  Doses required to penetrate into the CSF are often higher than recommended by the manufacturers – trimethoprim/sulphonamide combinations and chloramphenicol penetrate well, ampicillin penetrates well if the CNS is inflamed, gentamicin and tetracyclines penetrate relatively poorly. Treatment should be continued for at least 48 hours after the goat seems normal and may be required for as long as 10 to 14 days.

❏ Stop convulsions.

  Diazepam, 0.25–0.5 mg/kg, 2–4 ml/40 kg i.v. to effect (**Valium**, Roche)

Phenobarbitone, 0.04 ml/kg i.v. to effect (**Sagatal**, Merial) then **0.22 ml/kg i.v.** every 8 to 12 hours as required.

❏ Correct fluid and electrolyte imbalances, with intravenous fluids, in animals which are not drinking or have collapsed (or subcutaneous fluids if handling stresses the goat). Most animals will be acidotic. If in doubt, use lactated Ringer's solution.

Electrolytes can be given orally by stomach tube – up to 8 l daily will be required.

> A goat may survive the neurological challenge only to die of dehydration.

❏ Resolve CNS inflammation.

Flunixin meglumine, 2 mg/kg, 2 ml/45 kg i.v. or **i.m.** (**Finadyne Solution**, Schering-Plough) every 12 or 24 hours for up to 5 days.

Carprofen, 1.4 mg/kg, 1 ml/35 kg s.c. or **i.v.** (**Zenecarp Solution**, Pfizer) every 36 to 48 hours.

Ketoprofen, 3 mg/kg, 1 ml/33 kg i.v. or **i.m.** (**Ketofen**, Merial) daily for up to 3 days.

Meloxicam, 0.5 mg/kg, 1 ml/10 kg i.v. or **s.c.** (**Metacam 5 mg Solution**, Boehringer Ingelheim) every 36 to 48 hours.

Methylprednisolone, 10–30 mg/kg i.v. (**Solu-medrone**, Pharmacia & Upjohn) every 4 to 6 hours for 24 to 48 hours.

Dimethyl sulphoxide (DMSO), 1 g/kg as 10% solution in i.v. drip over 30 minutes every 24 hours for 3 or 4 days (50 ml DMSO in 500 ml saline/50 kg).

Phenylbutazone, 4 mg/kg, 1 ml/50 kg i.v. (banned from use in food-producing animals in the EU).

❏ Reduce cerebral oedema.

Dexamethasone, 0.1 mg/kg, 1 ml/20 kg i.v. (**Azium**, Schering-Plough; **Colvasone**, Norbrook; **Dexadreson**, Intervet)

Mannitol, 1.5 g/kg slowly **i.v.**

Neonatal kids

See Chapter 5.

❏ Congenital infections.
❏ Hypoglycaemia.
❏ Birth trauma.
❏ Enzootic ataxia (swayback).

Kids up to 1 month old

Kid mentally alert

Spinal abscess

Spinal abscesses and vertebral osteomyelitis occur sporadically in kids, generally following a bacteraemia subsequent to a navel infection.

Aetiology

❏ A number of bacteria including *Staphylococcal* spp., *C. pyogenes*, *Pasteurella* spp. and *Fusobacterium necrophorum* have been implicated.

Clinical signs

❏ A gradual onset of clinical signs may occur where abscessation results in increasing compression of the spinal cord, with signs progressing from slight hind limb ataxia to complete hind limb paralysis, and in these cases long-term broad-spectrum antibiotic therapy or more specific therapy based on CSF culture and sensitivity may be satisfactory. In other cases, acute clinical signs, with paraparesis or tetraparesis and pain around the spinal lesion, may occur some time after the original infection when there is sudden collapse of a vertebra and spinal cord compression.

Diagnosis

❏ Radiography will demonstrate a collapsed vertebra. CSF may appear normal or show increased numbers of neutrophils.

Trauma

In all age groups, trauma to the head or spinal cord may cause neurological signs. Kids are particularly prone to spinal cord and vertebral injuries because of their inquisitive active nature.

Haynets should be avoided and the spacing on hayracks or gates should be chosen carefully. Trauma can also arise from kicks or bites from other species of animals and from fighting, and neck injuries can also occur in tethered goats.

Pathological vertebral fractures can occur in malnourished animals. Exostosis may develop over incomplete fractures of a vertebral body and subsequently produce neurological signs.

Congenital vertebral lesions

Congenital vertebral lesions can result in compression of the spinal cord with resulting neurological clinical signs, which may not become apparent for several weeks after birth.

Tick pyaemia (enzootic staphylococcal infection)

See Chapter 7.

Kid mentally impaired

Bacterial meningitis

Aetiology

❑ Generally secondary to septicaemia, with infection from the navel or intestine; enterotoxigenic *E. coli* is generally the causal organism, but also *Staphylococci*, *Streptococci*, *Pasteurellae*, *Klebsiella* and *Haemophilus* species.

Clinical signs

❑ Variable neurological signs.
❑ Lethargy, drowsiness or hyperaesthesia, pyrexia.
❑ Failure to suck.
❑ Compulsive wandering; head pressing.
❑ Nystagmus, apparent blindness.
❑ Convulsions, coma.
❑ Death.
❑ Often history of diarrhoea or diarrhoea present concurrently.

Treatment

❑ Antibiotic therapy – *E. coli* meningitis is difficult to treat because most bactericidal antibiotics do not penetrate well into the CSF. Trimethoprim-sulphonamide preparations given intravenously at a level of 16 to 24 mg of the combined drugs/kg three times daily alone or in combination with gentamicin 3 mg/kg intramuscularly or intravenously (dilute in equal volumes of saline) have been recommended.
❑ General supportive therapy with fluids, anticonvulsants and anti-inflammatory drugs.

Focal symmetrical encephalomalacia (enterotoxaemia)

Aetiology

❏ The epsilon toxin produce by *Clostridium perfringens* type D (see Chapter 15) affects the cerebral vasculature, producing haemorrhage and oedema.

Clinical signs

❏ Generally affects kids, occasionally adult animals.
❏ Lethargy.
❏ Head pressing, apparent blindness, trembling.
❏ Ataxia.
❏ Opisthotonos, convulsions, coma.
❏ Death.

Note: (1) A similar condition in calves is produced by a labile *coccidial toxin*. It has been suggested that coccidial infections (qv) may be implicated in the condition in kids; (2) Enterotoxigenic *E. coli* (qv) can also produce similar neurological signs – see 'Bacterial meningitis'.

Tetanus

Aetiology

❏ Gram-positive bacillus *Clostridium tetani* produces a neurotoxin responsible for the clinical syndrome.

Epidemiology

❏ *Clostridium tetani* spores enter through wounds following disbudding, castration, shearing, kidding, ear tagging, etc., resulting in clinical signs 4 to 21 days later.

Clinical signs

❏ Variable neurological signs – erect ears, elevated tail, extended neck, rocking-horse stance, rigidity and hyperaesthesia on stimulation.
❏ Prolapsed third eyelid.
❏ Dysphagia, difficulty in opening mouth.
❏ Lateral recumbency, death.

Diagnosis

❏ Clinical signs.
❏ Isolation and identification of *Cl. tetani.*

Treatment

- ❏ Clean any obvious wound, expose to the air, debride, flush with hydrogen peroxide and apply penicillin locally.
- ❏ **Tetanus antitoxin, 10 000–15 000 units i.v.** every 12 hours for at least 24 hours.
- ❏ **Diazepam, 0.5 mg/kg i.v., 5 ml/50 kg (Valium,** Roche) to effect, or **Acepromazine (ACP), 0.05–0.1 mg/kg, 1.25–2.5 ml/50 kg i.v. (ACP 2 mg/ml injection,** C-Vet).
- ❏ **Benzylpenicillin, 10 mg/kg i.v. (Crystapen,** Schering-Plough) every 6 to 12 hours.
- ❏ Supportive therapy – intravenous fluids, nasogastric tube to relieve bloat and for food and fluids, enema, deep bed with regular changes in position.

Prevention

- ❏ Routine vaccination with a multivalent clostridial vaccine (see enterotoxaemia, Chapter 15).

Disbudding meningoencephalitis

Prolonged or excessive pressure with a disbudding iron can cause heat necrosis to bone, meninges and brain.

Clinical signs

- ❏ Sudden death – sometimes within hours but often several days or even weeks after disbudding.
- ❏ Depression, anorexia, pyrexia, fits.

Postmortem findings

- ❏ Focal meningoencephalitis.
- ❏ Meningeal and superficial cerebrocortical necrosis with infiltration by neutrophils and mononuclear cells.

Treatment
As for bacterial meningitis.

Louping ill

Aetiology

- ❏ Acute encephalomyelitis caused by a flavivirus transmitted by the tick vector *Ixodes ricinus*.

Epidemiology

❏ Louping ill is transmitted exclusively by the nymph and adult tick. Virus titres which are high enough for tick infection are only obtained in sheep – infection in the goat is thus irrelevant to the maintenance of the viral cycle.

❏ Strong colostral immunity is imparted to kids so that young animals in endemic areas will be susceptible in their second year of exposure, in contrast to tickborne fever (see Chapter 2) where no colostral protection is conferred, so kids are susceptible during their first season. In endemic areas tickborne fever and louping ill do not simultaneously affect the same animals. However, when goats are moved into endemic areas, all ages of goats could be at risk.

Clinical signs

❏ In adult goats the disease is generally subclinical. Within 24 to 48 hours of infection a febrile reaction occurs and the temperature may remain elevated for several days before returning to normal. Clinical signs are not usually recognised during this period and neurological signs only develop if the virus gains entry to nervous tissue. In other animals, recovery is rapid and the animals remain immune to subsequent infection. Susceptibility to clinical disease is increased by stress factors such as age, cold, nutrition and transportation and in particular by concurrent infection such as toxoplasmosis and tickborne fever.

❏ Severe clinical infection can be produced in kids that drink infected milk.

❏ Lethargy, excessive salivation.

❏ Intermittent head shaking, twitching of lips, nostrils and ears.

❏ Muscle tremors, particularly neck and limbs, followed by muscular rigidity.

❏ Jerky, stiff movement, with progressive incoordination, loss of balance with frequent falling.

❏ Apparent blindness, head pressing.

❏ Convulsions, paralysis, recumbency and death.

Postmortem findings

❏ Non-suppurative encephalomyelitis.

Diagnosis

❏ Serology – detection of IgM antibody is diagnostic, but some animals have little antibody while clinically ill.

❏ Virus isolation from brain tissue.

Treatment

❏ None.

Control

❏ Prevent exposure to ticks:
   ■ improve hill grazing to remove tick habitat;
   ■ pyrethroid dips: **Flumethrin** (**Bayticol Scab and Tick Dip**, Bayer).
❏ Vaccination, 1 ml s.c. (**Louping ill vaccine**, Schering-Plough) at least 4 weeks before exposure to infection, repeat every 2 years. Lambs from vaccinated dams have passive immunity for 2 to 3 months after birth.

Public health considerations
The high titres of virus excreted in goats' milk provide a potential zoonotic risk. Goats in tick areas should be vaccinated to reduce the possible risk to the public.

Kids 2 to 7 months old

Trauma

See earlier this chapter.

Delayed swayback.

See Chapter 5.

Spinal abscess

See earlier this chapter.

Coccidiosis

See Chapter 13. Kids with severe coccidiosis sometimes show nervous signs – dullness, depression, head pressing, opisthotonos and death.

Caprine arthritis encephalitis

See Chapter 6. CAE virus can produce neurological signs in the kid (*caprine leucoencephalitis*) and the adult goat – neurological signs are rarely reported in the UK.

Juvenile form: kids 2 to 4 months old

Consistent with upper motor neurone disease involving an ascending infection of the spinal cord. Spinal reflexes frequently intact (cf. swayback).

Clinical signs

❏ Pyrexia or fluctuating high temperature (*not* always).
❏ Bright and alert, good appetite until recumbent.
❏ Tremor.
❏ Initial lameness and ataxia, progressing over a number of days to hemiplegia or tetraplegia, circling, hyperaesthesia, blindness and recumbency with torticollis (indicate disease involving higher centres, particularly midbrain).

Treatment

❏ None.

Adult form

Neurological signs are often preceded by other clinical signs of CAE (arthritis, pneumonia, mastitis) and may be complicated by painful arthritic lesions. In the absence of arthritis, it may resemble listeriosis.

Clinical signs

❏ Knuckling of fetlocks, circling, progressing to paresis and paralysis.

Laboratory tests

❏ Serology; kids often seronegative at this age, although passive maternal antibodies may be detected. Test kid's dam and any goat used to supply kid with milk.
❏ CSF analysis – generally elevated white cell count (many mononuclear cells) and protein level.

Postmortem findings

❏ Perivascular mononuclear cell infiltration, and perivascular demyelination in the white matter.
❏ Gross lesions may be visible in the spinal cord as swollen brownish areas of malacia that are usually unilateral.

Kids 7 months to adult

Infectious disease

Listeriosis

Aetiology

❑ *Listeria monocytogenes,* a gram-positive, β-haemolytic bacillus.

Transmission

❑ By ingestion of the organism, which is resistant in the environment, surviving in the soil and water for several months and in silage for over 5 years.
❑ Direct contact with the products of abortion by ingestion or via the conjunctivae.
❑ Venereal transmission may occur.
❑ Latent carriers exist and when stressed may excrete the organism.
❑ The incubation period at 10 to 15 days is generally shorter than in sheep.

Clinical signs

(1) Encephalitis
    ❑ Depression, anorexia, pyrexia.
    ❑ Facial paralysis, drooping of ears and eyelids (often asymmetrical), protruding of tongue, drooling of saliva.
    ❑ Dysphagia – cud remains in mouth.
    ❑ Head tilt, nystagmus, circling, head pressing.
    ❑ Progressively uncoordinated movement – knuckling, rigidity, paresis.
    ❑ Recumbency, opisthotonos, convulsions.
    ❑ Death (mortality rate 3 to 30%).

Note: (1) Very acute encephalitis does not always present as the 'circling disease' more typical of sheep. Goats may be presented as dull and uncoordinated, with death occurring in as little as 6 hours. The disease may be mistaken for hypocalcaemia or even pneumonia. (2) Abortion and encephalitis occur in the same goat more commonly than is the case for sheep.

(2) Sudden death
    ❑ Because the disease in goats may be very acute – goats are much more susceptible to listerial encephalitis than sheep –

listeriosis should be considered in the differential diagnosis of sudden death (see Chapter 18).

(3) Septicaemia
- ❏ Lethargy, pyrexia (41°C) and bloody diarrhoea in young animals, with signs lasting from a few days to several weeks.

(4) Abortion
See Chapter 2.

(5) Keratoconjunctivitis
See Chapter 19.

(6) Metritis/vaginal discharge.

Diagnosis

❏ Physical and neurological examination
- ■ clinical signs vary depending on areas of brain involved but include mostly upper motor neurone signs involving ipsilateral limbs.

❏ Laboratory tests
- ■ examination of CSF: elevated white cells (mononuclear cells and neutrophils), elevated protein content;
- ■ examination of urine: glucosuria, ketonuria;
- ■ examination of paired serum samples;
- ■ culture and identification of *L. monocytogenes* from brain, liver, spleen, kidney and heart, fetal stomach, uterine discharges, milk and placenta.

❏ Postmortem examination
- ■ gross brain lesions may be minimal, possibly congested meninges and oedema;
- ■ suppurative meningoencephalitis; microabscesses in the brain stem usually unilateral; vasomeningeal cellular infiltration.

Treatment

❏ See 'Treatment' earlier this chapter.
❏ Early treatment with high doses of antibiotics (ampicillin or tri-methoprim/sulphonamides), intravenous where possible, and with maintenance doses for at least 7 days.
❏ Supportive therapy – vitamins, fluids, flunixin meglumine, phenylbutazone or corticosteroids – where indicated.
❏ It may be advantageous to treat all animals in an affected group with long-acting ampicillin.

Control

❏ Difficult.
❏ Avoid soil-contaminated feed, particularly silage.
❏ Ensure good quality silage is made – do not feed mouldy silage, silage with a pH content >5 or an ash content >70 mg/kg DM; reject silage from damaged bales. Remove any silage not eaten within 24 hours.
❏ Keep food and water containers clean: avoid faecal contamination.
❏ Vaccination – experimental studies have yielded variable results. Sheep vaccine available in parts of Europe.

Public health considerations

Carrier goats may excrete the organism under stress – milk may be infected. Pasteurised cheese has also been implicated in recent outbreaks.

Scrapie

Scrapie is a notifiable disease in the UK. It is a progressive fatal degenerative disease of the central nervous system of sheep and goats, related to bovine spongiform encephalopathy (BSE), transmissable mink encephalopathy and Creutzfeldt-Jakob disease and Kuru of man.

Aetiology

❏ Scrapie is caused by a small infectious agent, the prion, with some of the properties of a virus. Separate strains of the agent exist and the development of clinical disease depends on the scrapie strain and on host genetic factors.
❏ In sheep, the susceptibility to scrapie has been shown to be genetically controlled. To produce disease, the infective agent or prion must be present in the animal and must be able to influence the PrP gene, which encodes a normal neuronal glycoprotein. In animals with scrapie, this neuronal protein is somehow modified and forms a major component of the scrapie associated fibrils (SAFs) found in scrapie brains. Variations in the PrP gene result in differing susceptibilities or resistance to the prion and thus to natural and experimental scrapie. Different strains of scrapie target different alleles of the PrP gene. PrP genotyping in sheep has the potential to be a valuable aid in scrapie control.

   The situation in goats appears different in that no genetic influence is apparent in experimental infection, with goats being almost completely susceptible. However, goats show a similar variation in the length of disease incubation to that described in sheep, suggesting a variation in susceptibility to the disease. Goat PrP is expressed from a single gene, which appears homologous to that of the sheep. Analysis of the caprine PrP gene has revealed several different alleles. Four PrP protein variants have been described, three of them goat-specific with single amino acid changes at codons 142, 143 and 240. The amino acid changes associated with scrapie susceptibility in sheep, i.e. Val at codon 136, have not been described in goats. However, an amino acid change from Ile to Met at codon 142 appears to modulate scrapie susceptibility and result in different incubation periods in goats experimentally infected with scrapie. Further PrP gene sequencing in goats will help to clarify the role of the host in natural scrapie in this species.

❏ An age-related susceptibility means that maximum opportunity for disease spread is from dam to kid between birth and 9 months of age.

Transmission

Possible routes of transmission are:

❏ Doe to kid
- ■ Prenatal?
  - – Transplacental: unlikely; some evidence that snatching kids at birth stops transmission.
  - – Infection of egg: embryo transplant studies suggest egg transmission is unlikely.
- ■ Postnatal – licking or sucking, fetal membranes.

❏ Lateral
- ■ Oral
  - – by ingestion of fetal membranes (known to be heavily infected);
  - – contamination of pasture, troughs, etc. (but very low levels of infection in body fluids);
  - – by goat feed containing scrapie-infected meat and bone meal as with BSE in cattle.
- ■ Conjunctival?
- ■ Direct infection via needles, etc?

Clinical signs

❏ Because of the long incubation period, the disease is rarely seen in goats less than 2 years old. Animals infected close to parturition often first show clinical signs at around 3 or 4 years of age.

❏ Two forms of scrapie, *pruritic* and *nervous*, have been described in the goat, but there is considerable overlap between the two forms and many naturally infected animals show a combination of pruritic and neurological signs.

❏ Initially, clinical signs may be very non-specific – behavioural changes, increased excitability, lethargy or apprehension, weight loss despite a good appetite, reduced milk yield, and in some animals more specific signs may not become apparent, at least for a considerable period. Most goats, however, progressively show more obvious signs.

■ *Pruritic signs*
  - Scratching with hind feet.
  - Rubbing poll, withers and back.
  - Nibbling abdomen, sides or udder when touched.
  - Biting at limbs.
■ *Neurological signs*
  - Behavioural changes.
  - Hyperaesthesia.
  - Tremor of the head and neck or whole body.
  - Incoordination, particularly of hind limbs.
  - Postural and gait changes, e.g. highstepping fore limbs.
  - Ataxia.
  - Ears pricked, tail cocked and carried over back.
  - Excessive salivation with strings of saliva at mouth.
  - Cud dropping.
  - Ocular changes: nystagmus; apparent blindness.
  - Death in weeks or months.

Diagnosis

❏ Clinical signs.
❏ Histological lesions of the central nervous system.

Postmortem findings

❏ No obvious gross pathology.
❏ Histologically there is vacuolation of nerve cells in the medulla, pons and midbrain, with interstitial spongy degeneration.

Goats and bovine spongiform encephalopathy

Bovine spongiform encephalopathy (BSE) has been transmitted experimentally to goats by intracerebral injection and oral dosing with brain homogenate derived from cattle with BSE. No naturally occurring cases have been confirmed.

Louping ill

See this chapter.

Tetanus

See this chapter.

Caprine arthritis encephalitis (CAE)

See this chapter.

Pseudorabies (Aujesky's disease)

Aetiology

❏ Herpes virus occurring mainly in pigs but occasionally in goats, other ruminants, dogs and cats in contact with pigs.

Clinical signs

❏ Intense pruritus.
❏ Mania, ataxia.
❏ Paralysis, death.

Diagnosis

❏ Clinical signs.
❏ History of exposure to pigs.
❏ Viral isolation; fluorescent antibody test.

Treatment

❏ None.

Rabies

Aetiology

❏ Rhabdovirus spread by bite of an infected animal.

Clinical signs
There are two forms:

❏ Furious form – less common. Hyperexcitability, ataxia, sexual excitement, mania, hoarse voice, paralysis, death.
❏ Dumb form – clinically similar to listeriosis. Ataxia, swaying of hindquarters, tenesmus, paralysis of anus, salivation, loss of voice, paralysis, death.

Postmortem findings

❏ Histopathology shows Negri bodies in brain tissue.

Metabolic disease

Cerebrocortical necrosis (CCN, polioencephalomalacia)

Aetiology

❏ Thiamine (vitamin B_1) deficiency. Thiamine (vitamin B_1) is usually produced in adequate amounts by ruminal microflora. Deficiency can arise owing to:
  ■ Thiaminase type 1 production by ruminal bacteria: possibly following ingestion of mouldy or fungal contaminated feed or acidosis resulting in changes in rumen microflora.
  ■ Prolonged diarrhoea, e.g. coccidiosis.
  ■ Drug therapy, e.g. thiabendazole, levamisole and amprolium. *Note:* Take care when treating diarrhoea as may exacerbate CCN.
  ■ Plant thiaminase ingestion, e.g. bracken poisoning (*Pteridium aquilinum*).

Clinical signs

❏ Generally young animals affected, but also older animals.
❏ Stargazing, ataxia, nystagmus, blindness (normal pupillary light reflexes, dorsomedial strabismus), head pressing, collapse $\pm$ convulsions and opisthotonus.
❏ Severe but transient diarrhoea.
❏ Afebrile (except during convulsions).
❏ Death 1 to 2 days after onset of clinical signs.

Laboratory tests

❏ Estimates of thiamine levels can be made: (1) indirectly by erythrocyte transketolase assay on heparinised blood, or (2) directly on samples of frozen brain, liver or heart.
❏ Thiaminase levels can be estimated in frozen faecal or rumen samples.
❏ CSF may show slightly elevated protein levels and white cell count (but relatively acellular compared to pituitary abscess syndrome or listeriosis).
❏ Urine may test positive for glucose due to hyperglycaemia.

Postmortem findings

❏ Cerebral oedema produces a swollen brain with disparity in colour between the normal grey of the cerebellar grey matter and the comparatively pale or yellowish grey cerebral cortex.
❏ Cut surface of cerebral cortex exhibits auto-fluorescence under ultraviolet light.

Treatment

❏ **Thiamine, 10 mg/kg i.v., 1 ml/10 kg (Vitamin B$_1$,** Bimeda) every 6 hours for 24 hours.
❏ Multivitamin preparations can be used if thiamine is not available, but must be given according to the thiamine content (usually 10 or 35 mg/ml).
The response to thiamine is diagnostic but will only be successful if treatment is commenced early; in more advanced cases there may be residual brain damage and blindness.
❏ Unaffected animals in a group should be treated as a preventative.
❏ Support therapy with corticosteroids, diuretics and hypertonic intravenous drips may aid recovery by reducing the cerebral oedema.

Hypocalcaemia (milk fever)

Aetiology

❏ There is a fall in the serum calcium and phosphorus levels in all goats at kidding due to the onset of lactation; a greater fall occurs in goats which develop hypocalcaemia around parturition, due to a failure in the calcium homeostatic mechanisms to meet the increased demand for calcium.
❏ In heavy milking goats, an absolute deficiency of calcium at any stage of lactation will precipitate the disease.

Incidence

❏ Frank clinical signs are *not* common in the UK, although it is probable that subclinical disease is more widespread and many goats will benefit from calcium therapy when presented with other periparturient diseases such as mastitis, metritis, etc.
❏ The disease is most common in young, high-yielding first kidders in the first few weeks after parturition but may occur in late pregnancy, during parturition and *at any stage of lactation*, particularly in heavy milkers, and in any age of adult goat. Older goats are more likely to suffer from hypocalcaemia around and during parturition.

Clinical signs

❏ Often only slight tremors and twitching, with some hyper-excitability and slight ataxia, or even lethargy, inappetence and poor milk yield with no obvious nervous signs.

❏ More severe cases show marked ataxia and incoordination or fits followed by paresis, paraplegia, recumbency and coma which may last several hours.

❏ An eclamptic form occasionally occurs during lactation, e.g. after a change to better pasture, with pyrexia (41.1°C), marked muscular tremors, excitement, rapid panting respirations, collapse and death. *All recumbent or comatose goats should be treated as potentially hypocalcaemic and given calcium.*

Diagnosis

❏ Clinical signs.
❏ Rapid response to calcium therapy.
❏ Serum calcium measurements (normal 2.2 to 2.6 mmol/l).

Treatment

❏ **Calcium borogluconate 20%** (or better calcium borogluconate, magnesium and phosphorus), **80–100 ml** slowly **i.v.**, **s.c.** or half by each route. The response to calcium by the s.c. route is very rapid in the goat and may be preferable if the goat is stressed by handling.

❏ Relapses may occur, in which case extra phosphorus as well as calcium may be beneficial.

Note: Many toxic conditions, e.g. enterotoxaemia and mastitis, may show a temporary response to calcium therapy.

Hypomagnesaemia (grass tetany)

Aetiology

❏ Heavy milking goats grazing lush heavily fertilised grass may receive a diet deficient in magnesium. The disease usually occurs fairly early in lactation soon after starting to graze rich pasture. Pregnant goats on poor pasture in early spring may also develop the disease.

Incidence

❏ The disease is of sporadic occurrence in the UK because most high yielding goats are, at least in part, zero grazed and supplied with hay, browsings and concentrates.

Clinical signs

❏ *Acute* – excitement, tremors, twitching of facial muscles; hyper-aesthesia, aimless wandering, falling over, frothing at the mouth; convulsions, death; some animals may be found dead.
❏ *Subclinical* – inappetence, apprehension, milk yield decreased, mild ataxia, may convulse in response to noise or handling; may be spontaneous recovery or progression to acute phase.
❏ *Chronic* – other animals in an affected herd may show poor growth, reduced milk yield and dullness due to low serum magnesium levels.

Diagnosis

❏ Clinical signs.
❏ Response to treatment.
❏ Serum magnesium levels (normal 0.83 to 1.6 mmol/l).

Treatment

❏ **Calcium borogluconate 20%** with **magnesium** and **phosphorus, 80–100 ml i.v.** or **s.c.,** plus **100 ml magnesium sulphate 25% s.c.**
❏ Oral maintenance dose of at least 7 g calcinated magnesite or equivalent while dietary imbalances are corrected.

Prevention

❏ Correct diet – good quality fibre, adequate energy plus adequate magnesium [supplement where necessary, e.g. **Rumbol magnesium sheep bullets** (Agrimin)].
❏ Avoid grazing heavily fertilised pastures.

Transit tetany

Aetiology

❏ Combined hypocalcaemia/hypomagnesaemia brought on by stress, particularly transport, but also by late pregnancy, fear, etc.
❏ May occur in castrated males.

Clinical signs

❏ As for acute hypomagnesaemia.

Treatment

❏ As for acute hypomagnesaemia.

Periparturient toxaemia

See Chapter 8. Does with *pregnancy toxaemia* and *acetonaemia* occasionally show nervous signs – ataxia, tremors around the head and ears, reduced vision or blindness, head pressing, stargazing and eventually recumbency, coma and death.

Does with *postparturient toxaemia* (fatty liver syndrome) generally only show nervous signs terminally when starvation results in recumbency and coma.

Space-occupying lesions of the brain

Cerebral abscess

Aetiology

❏ Bacterial infection often with *C. pyogenes*, *Staph. aureus* or *Fusobacterium necrophorum*; often follows fight wounds in male goats.

Clinical signs

❏ Variable; may be associated with meningitis or act as a space-occupying lesion with head tilt, visual defects, circling (with head turned towards side of lesion) etc. Brain stem compression may cause ataxia, weakness or asymmetric pupil size.
❏ CSF changes variable – often increased white cell count (neutrophils).

Coenuriasis (gid)

Aetiology

❏ Intracranial pressure from cyst of the tapeworm *Taenia multiceps*, *Coenurus cerebralis*.

Clinical signs

❏ Clinical signs depend on the location of the cyst and the pressure it exerts on the surrounding brain tissue. Pressure on the cerebral hemispheres results in incoordination, blindness, head tilt, head pressing, circling and stargazing. Gait abnormalities occur when the cerebellum is involved. Skull softening as a result of bone rarefaction may occur when the cyst is superficial.

Diagnosis

❏ Intradermal gid test –0.1 ml cyst fluid injected into caudal fold beneath tail or shaved area of skin on neck; 0.1 ml sterile water used

as control. Skin thickening at test site within 24 hours classified as positive. Not very reliable.
❏ Serology and haematology of no diagnostic use; CSF – increased white cell count particularly eosinophils and mononuclear cells.
❏ Surgery or postmortem examination.

Treatment

❏ Surgical removal of the cyst, when it can be located by skull softening, under sedation and local anaesthesia or general anaesthetic. Skin incised and bone removed with trephine or scalpel blade. After the dura mater is penetrated, the cyst will often bulge through and can be removed by applying negative suction pressure by syringe or pipette.
❏ Where there is no skull softening but the cyst site can be approximately located by detailed neurological examination, ultrasound examination via a trephine site may aid localisation.
❏ Radiography can also be used, but interpretation of the results is difficult.

Control

❏ Regular treatment of all dogs on the farm for tapeworm.

Pituitary abscess syndrome

Aetiology

❏ Abscessation of the pituitary gland following lymphatic or blood-borne infection often with *C. pyogenes* but also many other gram-positive (*Streptococcus, Staphylococcus, Actinomyces*) and gram-negative (*Fusobacterium, Bacteroides, Pasteurella, Pseudomonas, Actinobacillus*) bacteria from another infected focus in the body, e.g. mastitis, arthritis, lung abscess, sinusitis or intracranial damage with secondary sepsis after fighting.

Pressure by the enlarging abscess acts as a space-occupying lesion affecting the adjacent areas of the brain and brain stem and producing various neurological signs depending on the extent of the abscess. Cranial nerve functions are progressively affected, usually asymmetrically.

Incidence

❏ Generally adult animals; more commonly males.

Clinical signs
Varying clinical signs but commonly:

❏ Anorexia, depression.
❏ Bradycardia (see below).
❏ Dysphagia.
❏ Head pressing.
❏ Blindness (pupillary light reflexes often absent; ventrolateral strabismus, cf. cerebrocortical necrosis).
❏ Nystagmus.
❏ Ataxia, opisthotonus, recumbency.
❏ Death.

Note: (1) The progressive nature of the neurological signs means that repeat neurological examinations and assessment of cranial nerve function are important for diagnosis. (2) *Bradycardia* is an uncommon finding in the goat but occurs in the pituitary abscess syndrome and other space-occupying lesions of the brain because pressure on the hypothalamus causes increased vagal tone. Bradycardia may also occur in *severe milk fever, hypothermia, hypoglycaemia, botulism* and *trauma* to the head.

Laboratory findings

❏ CSF – elevated white cell count (mostly neutrophils), elevated protein level.
❏ Haematology – not diagnostic; fibrinogen and globulin often elevated.

Postmortem findings

❏ Pituitary abscess – generally evident grossly, occasionally only on histopathological examination.
❏ Generally a chronic infection elsewhere in the body.
❏ Histopathology shows coagulative and liquefactive necrosis of the pituitary gland, particularly the adenohypophysis with neutrophil and some mononuclear cell infiltration.
❏ Culture of abscess sample yields pure or mixed culture of aerobic bacteria.

Treatment

❏ None.

Oestrus ovis

Oestrus ovis, the sheep and goat nasal fly, deposits larvae around the nostrils. The larvae normally migrate to the nasal passages and then the frontal sinuses. Clinical signs are usually limited to panic when the flies are laying and a mucopurulent discharge when the larvae are in the nasal passages and sinuses. Larvae may rarely migrate via the ethmoid bones to the brain, producing clinical signs as for *Coenurus cerebralis*. Larvae may also occasionally enter the eye or nasolacrimal system, causing conjunctivitis.

Tumour

Brain neoplasms are very rare. There is a single report of a glioma.

Space-occupying lesions of the spinal cord.

Although more common in kids (qv), *spinal meningitis, abscessation* and *vertebral osteomyelitis* may occur in adult animals, producing varying degrees of paraparesis or tetraparesis. Cerebrospinal fluid (CSF) is variable, often showing an increased white cell count (neutrophils). Treatment should be based where possible on culture and sensitivity of the CSF or use long-term broad-spectrum antibiotic therapy.

Tumours, e.g. lymphosarcoma, meningioma and *Coenurus cerebralis* cysts (qv) may rarely act as space-occupying lesions of the spinal cord.

Cerebrospinal nematodiasis – aberrant spinal cord migration of any nematode – may occasionally cause neurological signs, generally referrable to spinal cord disease. CSF shows elevated white cells (mainly eosinophils and mononuclear cells) and protein levels. Treatment with ivermectin (Ivomec injection, Merial) and dexamethasone may be successful if combined with adequate supportive care.

Trauma

Trauma (qv) to the head and neck should always be considered, particularly in male goats running together or tethered animals.

Vestibular disease

Otitis media/interna

Otitis media/interna occur as sequelae to otitis externa or following rhinitis and pharyngitis; or via haematogenous spread.

Clinical signs

❑ Head tilt, circling towards side of affected ear, nystagmus with fast component directed away from the affected ear.
❑ Eye drop on the affected side.
❑ Facial paralysis.

Ear mite infection (psoroptic mange)

See Chapter 10.

Hepatic encephalopathy

Hepatic encephalopathy is uncommon; severe hepatic insufficiency may result in lethargy, depression and neurological signs such as behavioural changes, ataxia, tremors, fits, convulsions and coma.

Halothane-induced acute hepatic necrosis has been described as producing depression, lethargy, salivation, head pressing, chewing motions, icterus and recumbency.

Poisonings

A variety of drugs, plants and chemicals can be neurotoxic.

Lead

Aetiology

❏ Lead from old painted wood (check partitions, doors, etc.), car batteries, motor oil, etc.

Clinical signs

❏ Blindness (normal pupillary light reflexes), head pressing, ataxia.
❏ Abdominal pain, anorexia, weight loss.
❏ Diarrhoea, tenesmus.

Laboratory tests

❏ Blood lead estimation.
❏ Basophilic stippling of erythrocytes stained with Wright's stain.
❏ Kidney or liver lead levels: >4 ppm.
❏ CSF – acellular.

Postmortem findings

❏ Cerebral oedema.
❏ Mucoid enterocolitis.

Treatment

❏ **Sodium calciumedetate, 75 mg/kg, daily in four divided doses,** slowly **i.v. or s.c. (Sodium calciumedetate 250 mg/ml**, Animalcare) for 2 to 5 days. Dilute 1 ml in 4 ml glucose 5% or sodium chloride 0.9%.

Other heavy metals

Poisoning with other heavy metals such as *arsenic* and *mercury* may occasionally occur, giving neurological signs such as incoordination, blindness, muscle tremors and convulsions, together with abdominal pain and diarrhoea.

Plants

See Chapter 20. Plant poisoning is unlikely to produce nervous signs in goats in the UK. Rape (*Brassica rapus*) can produce blindness, head pressing and violent excitement. Bracken (*Pteridium aquilinum*), although unlikely to induce a thiamine deficiency under normal conditions where ruminal synthesis of thiamine is adequate, might exacerbate or precipitate cerebrocortical necrosis (qv). Oxalate poisoning, which can produce ataxia, muscle tremor, paralysis and death, might be produced by eating large amounts of rhubarb or common sorrel. Fool's parsley (*Aethusa cynapium*) can cause indigestion, panting and ataxia. Cherry laurel (*Prunus laurocerasus*) causes cyanide poisoning, with animals often being found dead. Less severe cases show dyspnoea, staggering gait, jerky movements and convulsions. Laburnum (*L. anagyroides*) and hemlock (*Corium maculatum*) contain nicotine-like alkaloids resulting in rapid respiration, salivation, excitement and muscle tremors followed by depression, incoordination, convulsions and death. Ragwort (*Senecio jacobaea*) produces an hepatic neurotoxicity.

Organophosphates

Aetiology

❏ Exposure to organophosphates, e.g. dips or drenches.

Clinical signs

❏ Abdominal pain, inappetence, incoordination, diarrhoea, muscular tremors, dyspnoea, paralysis, convulsions, coma and death.

Treatment.

❏ **Atropine, 0.6–1 mg/kg, 1–1.5 ml/kg (Atropine sulphate, C-Vet; Atrocare, Animalcare), one quarter i.v., the rest s.c. or i.m., every 4 to 6 hours for up to 24 hours.**

Rafoxanide

The flukicide rafoxanide has a much lower safety margin in goats (4 to 6 times) than sheep (20 times). Overdosage may cause degeneration and oedema of the retina, optic tract and related areas of the CNS, and death. Rafoxanide is no longer available in the UK, although it is available in Eire (**Flukex**, Univet).

Urea (hyperammonaemia)

Aetiology

❏ Overfeeding of urea in rations.

Clinical signs

❏ Abdominal pain, muscle tremor, ataxia, hyperaesthesia.
❏ Mydriasis, convulsions and death.

Treatment

❏ **Vinegar 0.5 to 1.0 l** orally, as an acidifying agent.

Epilepsy

A single case of partial epilepsy in a Nubian goat has been properly documented. However, the incidence of 'fits' is much higher. Because they are usually not fully investigated, the aetiologies of these fits are unknown. Most owners cull goats that have repetitive fits without resorting to medication. Kids which recover from disbudding meningoencephalitis may continue to have fits into adult life.

Further reading

General

Barlow, R.M. (1987) Differential diagnosis of nervous diseases of goats. *Goat Vet. Soc. J.*, **8**, 73–6.

Baxendell, S.A. (1984) Caprine nervous diseases. *Proc. Univ. Sydney, Post Grad. Comm. Vet. Sci.*, **73**, 333–42.

Brewer, B.D. (1983) Neurologic disease of sheep and goats. *Vet. Clin. North Am.: Large Animal Practice*, **5** (3), November 1983, 677–700.

Thompson, K.G. (1985) Nervous diseases of goats. *Proc. Course in Goat Husbandry and Medicine*, Massey University, November 1985, 152–61.

β-Mannosidosis

Kumar, K., Jones, M.Z., Cunningham, J.G., Kelly, J.A. and Lovell, K.L. (1986) Caprine β-mannosidosis: phenotypic features. *Vet. Rec.*, **118**, 325–7.

Caprine arthritis encephalitis

Adams, D.S., Klevjer-Anderson, P., Carlson, J.L., McGuire, T.C. and Gorham, J.R. (1983) Transmission and control of CAE virus. *Am. J. Vet. Res.*, **44** (9), 1670–75.

Dawson, M. (1987) Caprine arthritis encephalitis. *In Practice*, January 1987, 8–11.

Knight, A.P. and Jokinen, M.P. (1982) Caprine arthritis encephalitis. *Comp. Cont. Ed. Pract. Vet.*, **4** (6), S263–9.

Cerebrocortical necrosis

Baxendell, S.A. (1984) Cerebrocortical necrosis. *Proc. Univ. Sydney Post Grad. Comm. Vet. Sci.*, **73**, 503–7.

Smith, M.C. (1979) Polioencephalomalacia in goats. *J. Am. Vet. Med. Assoc.*, **174** (12), 1328–32.

Cerebrospinal fluid

Scott, P. (1993) Collection and interpretation of cerebrospinal fluid in ruminants. *In Practice*, **15** (6), 298–300.

Coenuriasis

Harwood, D.G. (1986) Metacestode disease in goats. *Goat Vet. Soc. J.*, **7** (2), 35–8.

Disbudding meningoencephalitis

Wright, H.J., Adams, D.S. and Trigo, F.J. (1983) Meningoencephalitis after hot iron disbudding of goat kids. *Vet. Med./Small Animal Clin.*, **78** (4), 599–601.

Ear Mites

Littlejohn, A.I. (1968) Psoroptic mange in the goat. *Vet. Rec.*, **82**, 148–55.

Williams, J.F. and Williams, S.F. (1978) Psoroptic ear mites in dairy goats. *J. Am. Vet. Med. Assoc.*, **173** (12), 1582–3.

Enzootic ataxia

Inglis, D.M., Gilmour, J.S. and Murray, I.S. (1986) A farm investigation into swayback in a herd of goats and the result of administration of copper needles. *Vet. Rec.*, **118**, 657–60.

Whitelaw, A. (1985) Copper deficiency in cattle and sheep. *In Practice*, May 1985, 98–100.

Hepatic encephalopathy

Morris, D.D. and Henry, M.M. (1991) Hepatic encephalopathy. *Comp. Cont. Ed. Pract. Vet.*, **13** (7), 1153–61.

Listeriosis

Harwood, D.G. (1988) Listeriosis in goats. *Goat Vet. Soc. J.*, **10** (1), 1–4.

Louping-ill

Reid, H. (1991) Louping-ill. *In Practice*, **13** (4), 157–60.

Meningitis

Jamison, J.M. and Prescott, J.F. (1987) Bacterial meningitis in large animals. Part I. *Comp. Cont. Ed. Pract. Vet.*, **9** (12), F399–406.
Jamison, J.M. and Prescott, J.F. (1988) Bacterial meningitis in large animals. Part II. *Comp. Cont. Ed. Pract. Vet.*, **10** (2), 225–31.

Metabolic and nutritional diseases

Andrews, A.H. (1985) Some metabolic conditions in the doe. *Goat Vet. Soc. J.*, **6** (2), 70–72.
Merrall, M. (1985) Nutritional and metabolic diseases. *Proc. Course in Goat Husbandry and Medicine*, Massey University, November 1985, 126–31.
Pinsent, J. and Cottom, D.S. (1987) Metabolic diseases of goats. *Goat Vet. Soc. J.*, **8** (1), 40–42.

Oestrus ovis

Dorchies, P., Duranton, C. and Jacquiet, P. (1998) Pathophysiology of *Oestrus ovis* infection in sheep and goats: a review. *Vet. Rec.*, **142**, 487–9.

Pituitary abscess syndrome

Perdrizet, J. and Dinsmore, P. (1986) *Comp. Cont. Ed. Pract. Vet.*, **8** (6), S311–18.

Scrapie

Collinge, J. and Palmer, M.S. (eds) (1997) Prion Diseases. Oxford University Press, Oxford.
Golmann, W., *et al.* (1996) Novel polymorphisms in the caprine PrP gene: a codon 142 mutation associated with scrapie incubation period. *J. Gen. Virol.*, **77**, 2885–91.
Kimberlin, R.H. (1981) Scrapie. *Brit. Vet. J.*, **134** (1), 105–112.

Sargison, N. (1995) Scrapie in sheep and goats. *In Practice*, **17** (10), 467–9.
Wood, J.L.N., Done, S.H., Pritchard, G.C. and Wooldridge, M.J.A. (1992) Natural scrapie in goats: case histories and clinical signs. *Vet. Rec.*, **131**, 66–8.
Wood, J.L.N. and Done, S.H. (1992) Natural scrapie in goats: neuropathology. *Vet. Rec.*, **131**, 93–6.

Tickborne diseases

Reid, H.W. (1986) Tick and tickborne diseases. *Goat Vet. Soc. J.*, **7** (2), 21–5.

Tumour

Marshall, C.L., Weinstock, D., Kramer, R.W. and Bagley, R.S. (1995) Glioma in a goat. *J. Am. Vet. Med. Assoc.*, **206** (10), 1572–4.

12 Diseases of the Mammary Gland

Mastitis

Mastitis is the inflammation of the mammary gland, regardless of cause, characterised by physiological, chemical and generally bacteriological changes in milk and by pathological changes in glandular tissue.

Investigation of mastitis

General clinical examination

❏ Assess severity of systemic infection, degree of pyrexia, etc.

Specific udder examination

❏ Visually and by palpation.
❏ Compare the two halves.
❏ Heat.
❏ Swelling.
❏ Lumps.
❏ Extent of fibrosis.
❏ Injuries to teats or body of udder.
❏ Superficial inguinal lymph nodes.

Milk sample examination

> In subclinical mastitis the milk may appear grossly normal.

❏ Use strip cup.
❏ Compare the two halves.
❏ Pus.
❏ Blood.

❑ Clots.
❑ Colour.

Laboratory tests

Somatic cell counts

> Somatic cell counts are useful as a herd test to monitor subclinical mastitis.

Unlike the bovine mammary gland, where milk is produced by merocrine secretion, that of the goat produces milk by apocrine secretion, which results in portions of cytoplasm from epithelial cells being pinched off and appearing in milk as DNA-free particles, similar in size to white blood cells. Intact epithelial cells from acini and ducts also appear in the milk.

There is poor correlation for goat milk between somatic cell counts obtained by particle counting machines (Coulter counters) and machines which count cell nuclei (Fossomatic counters) as the former cannot differentiate between particulate non-cellular debris and white blood cells. Counts from Fossomatic counters are themselves consistently higher than direct microscopic cell counts using Pyronin Y Methyl green stain.

Because goats are seasonal breeders, milk bulk tank somatic cell counts show a distinct seasonal variation, with the lowest in April and the highest in September or October. Counts begin to rise about 4 months after kidding and with the onset of oestrus cycles. As in cow's milk, mastitis due to bacterial infection causes a rise in the cell count of milk from the affected half, i.e. raised somatic cell counts are indicators of impaired udder health. However, as goats consistently have higher cell counts than cattle, particularly towards the end of lactation, results need careful interpretation. Variations in yield, feed intake and stage of lactation, as well as infection, are likely to affect cell counts.

At a cell count threshold of 1.5 million/ml, 80.5% of bacteriologically negative samples will be correctly classified, but 19.5% of negative samples will be diagnosed infected and only 41.4% of bacteriologically positive samples diagnosed. Lowering the threshold results in more false positive but fewer false negative results. At a 1 million/ml cell count threshold, 71.8% of bacteriologically negative samples are correctly classified, 28.2% of negative samples would be diagnosed infected and 56.5% of bacteriologically positive samples correctly identified.

California mastitis test and Whiteside test

The California mastitis test and the Whiteside test are likewise more suitable for excluding a diagnosis of mastitis than showing its presence. The California mastitis test is a simple semiquantitative test for determining the number of nucleated cells, measuring both neutrophils and epithelial cells. High scores can occur, in the absence of mastitis, when there are large numbers of epithelial cells present, such as towards the end of lactation or in systemically ill goats with low milk yield.

Bacteriology on a sterile milk sample

> In some types of mastitis excretion of bacteria is only intermittent, e.g. *Pseudomonas* spp. and chronic *Staph. aureus*.
>   Coagulase-positive *Staph. aureus* is the most common cause of caprine mastitis.

Collect a sample: clean teats thoroughly with 70% ethanol, discard foremilk, collect 20 ml of milk from each udder half in sterile containers; if not tested immediately store at 4°C (sample can be frozen for several weeks if necessary).

It is only necessary to use standard bacterial media, as *Mycoplasma* spp. are not implicated in mastitis in the UK. The bacteria present should be identified and antibiotic sensitivity tests carried out.

Coagulase positive *Staph. aureus* is the commonest cause of caprine mastitis, causing gangrenous, nongangrenous or subclinical mastitis.

Coagulase negative staphylococci are the most frequently isolated organisms, but are of uncertain significance and probably commensals rather than primary pathogens.

Environmental mastitis caused by organisms such as *E. coli*, *Pseudomonas* spp. and *Klebsiella* spp. is rare and most frequently seen as subclinical mastitis.

Many other bacteria, including *Streptococcus* spp. and *Pasteurella haemolytica* occasionally cause mastitis. *Yersinia pseudotuberculosis* has been isolated from the milk of an aborting goat. Fungi and yeasts such as *Candida albicans* are occasionally isolated.

Mycoplasma spp. have not been reported as causing mastitis in the UK, but they are an important problem in many other countries including a number of EU members. *Mycoplasma agalactiae* causes contagious agalactia; *Mycoplasma mycoides* subspecies *mycoides* is implicated in contagious pleuropneumonia and a variety of serious syndromes. *Mycoplasma putrefaciens* also causes agalactia.

Clinical mastitis

Peracute or gangrenous mastitis

Aetiology

❏ Commonly *Staph. aureus* infection following a slight injury to the teat at any stage of lactation: occasionally *E. coli*.

Clinical signs

❏ Marked pyrexia in early stages, often progressing to a toxaemia with subnormal temperature and death; may present as sudden death.
❏ Udder hard, hot, swollen and painful; minimal thin, bloody serous fluid from teat.
❏ Pain syndrome – teeth grinding, rapid pulse.

Prognosis

❏ Guarded; if the animal survives, the affected half becomes gangrenous, cold and clammy, turning blue through purple to black and eventually sloughing.

Treatment

❏ Economically, treatment is often not worthwhile. In a pet goat or where the goat is to be kept for breeding:
❏ Intensive intravenous antibiotic therapy.
   Ampicillin, 3 mg/kg (Penbritin Veterinary Injectable, Pfizer), every 8 hours.
   Oxytetracycline, 3–10 mg/kg (Alamycin, Norbrook; **Duphacycline**, Fort Dodge; **Engemycin**, Merial; **Oxytetrin**, Schering-Plough; **Terramycin**, Pfizer), every 12–24 hours.
   Fluoroquinalones, 1.25–2.5 mg/kg (Advocin, Pfizer; **Baytril**, Bayer; **Marbocyl**, Vetoquinol) every 24 hours.
❏ Non-steroidal anti-inflammatory drugs will help reduce the systemic and local udder temperature, decrease the production of inflammatory mediators and improve the clinical demeanour of the animal.
   Carprofen, 1.4 mg/kg, 1 ml/35 kg i.v. (Zenecarp Solution, C-Vet)
   Flunixin meglumine, 2 mg/kg, 2 ml/45 kg i.v. (Finadyne Solution, Schering-Plough)
   Ketoprofen, 3 mg/kg, 1 ml/33 kg i.v. (Ketofen, Merial)
   Meloxicam, 0.5 mg/kg, 1 ml/10 kg i.v. (Metacam 5 mg Solution, Boehringer Ingelheim), every 36–48 hours.

❏ Intravenous fluid therapy, **100–200 ml/kg** over 4–5 hours.
❏ Good nursing – rugs, heat and human company.
❏ As the udder sloughs and the teat is lost, milk may still be produced by the dorsal portion and *mastectomy* (see Chapter 23) may be necessary. Mastectomy can also be considered in male goats. Partial mastectomies under local or general anaesthetic may also be necessary to remove unsightly or necrotic tissue.
❏ As an alternative to mastectomy, infusions of **Lugol's iodine** or **acriflavine** or 60 ml of **10% formalin** under local anaesthetic can be used to dry up the affected half.

Acute mastitis

Aetiology

❏ A number of different bacteria.

Clinical signs

❏ Pyrexia, anorexia, lethargy.
❏ Udder hard, swollen and painful.
❏ Milk yield decreased; milk consistency changed.
❏ Milk often thin and watery with clots.

Prognosis

❏ Clinical recovery may result in subclinical disease or fibrosis and atrophy of the half.

Treatment

❏ Broad-spectrum antibiotics – parenteral and intramammary. *Staphylococcus aureus* is the most frequent cause of mastitis, so initial treatment should be aimed at this organism, which is frequently penicillin resistant. Use **cephalosporins, cloxacillin** or **amoxycillin/clavulinic acid preparations**. Better results are achieved by using parenteral and intramammary antibiotics together, as some drugs, e.g. cephalosporins, do not pass easily from blood to milk. Use a specific antibiotic once the results of laboratory tests are known.

At the present time, there are no intramammary preparations specifically licensed for goats available in the UK. Experimental work shows clearly that clearance times of antibiotic preparations from the mammary gland of goats may differ markedly from those from bovine mammary glands. In some cases, e.g. oxytetracycline, erythromycin, rapid elimination of the drug may occur to the extent that therapeutic efficiency may be compromised. With other preparations, e.g. amoxycillin trihydrate, potassium clavulanate, prednisolone (Synulox LC, Pfizer), a withholding time approximately double that for cows is required. With all preparations used outwith data sheet recommendations *a minimum 7-day withdrawal period* should be imposed for milk.

In addition, the nozzles of some intramammary preparations are too large to be inserted easily into goat teats, with the resultant risk of introducing infection or traumatising the teat. Long-acting preparations, e.g. **cephacetrite sodium** (**Vetimast**, Novartis) or **cefoperazone** (**Pathocef**, Pfizer), may thus be useful in that only a single tube need be inserted and prolonged action can be obtained within a 7-day withholding period.

It should be noted that when one half is treated, antibiotic may infuse into the milk in the other half.

Always thoroughly clean the teat with spirit before insertion of nozzles and use a teat dip after insertion.

❑ Oxytocin: **Oxytocin-S** (Intervet) (G), **20 U**, **2 ml i.m.** or **s.c.** initial dose, then **10 U**, **1 ml**, prior to each stripping out 2 or 3 times daily. Given immediately before the use of intramammary treatment, oxytocin causes contraction of the smooth muscle in udder ducts, maximising the stripping of the udder, removing infective and toxic material and allowing greater penetration of the intramammary infusion. Higher doses are given than those employed for milk letdown in normal goats.

❑ Supportive therapy, as for peracute mastitis, if necessary – intravenous fluids and non-steroidal anti-inflammatory drugs.

Mild clinical mastitis

Aetiology

❑ A number of different bacteria.

Clinical signs

❑ Only very mild or no systemic signs.
❑ Local udder reaction, possibly with slightly swollen half, small clots or pus in milk; milk often thinner than usual. Most milk samples presented for testing are from goats that are not clinically ill but where there are a few clots or crystals in the milk, poor keeping quality of milk, milk taint or curdling on boiling milk.

Terminal fibrosis and atrophy

The endpoint of most forms of mastitis is fibrosis and atrophy of the affected mammary tissue as healing takes place. Lesions may be confined to localised areas or may involve the greater part of the half. Fibrosis produces palpable induration and decreased milk yield. Contraction of the fibrous tissue produces visible and palpable atrophy.

Pockets of infection may remain and form abscesses.

Subclinical mastitis

Udder and milk secretions are clinically normal with subclinical mastitis, although fibrosis and atrophy may be present from a previous clinical infection. There is usually some reduction in milk yield which may be economically significant. There may also be a reduction in the levels of butterfat and no fat solids and a decreased keepability.

The true level of subclinical mastitis is unknown although surveys have suggested that between 4 and 6% of halves are affected with known pathogens.

Subclinical infections are much easier to treat when the goat is dry.

Dry-goat therapy

Dry-goat therapy with long-acting intramammary antibiotic treatments should be used whenever there has been clinical mastitis or evidence of subclinical mastitis during the lactation; many infections, e.g. *Staph. aureus*, are easier to treat during the dry period.

There are pros and cons to using dry-goat therapy routinely; there is danger of introducing infection when inserting tubes (especially with an inexperienced goatkeeper or goat with small teat orifice).

Always thoroughly clean the teat with spirit before insertion and use a teat dip after insertion.

Always use a separate tube for each half.

Drying off

An 8-week dry period before parturition as with cows is recommended. Many high yielding goats will still be giving substantial quantities of milk (4.5+ l daily) at this stage. Stop milking abruptly – in high yielders, the udder may become quite large until the pressure stops milk production, but within a few days the udder will shrink and become softer. Pressure of milk causes an inflammatory response so leucocytes collect in the udder helping to prevent infection. Reducing concentrates for a few days before drying off may help reduce milk production in very high yielders. Milking only once daily for a week before drying off will also help. *Never* partially milk out an udder as this increases the susceptibility to infection.

Teat dipping for a week after stopping milking will help prevent infection during drying off.

The milking machine and mastitis

The milking machine can affect the incidence of mastitis in three ways:

(1) Bacteria can be spread from goat to goat on contaminated liners.
(2) Teat-end damage allows bacteria to enter the udder. Teat-end damage can result from a number of factors, including vacuum levels being too high, defective pulsation and overmilking.
(3) Machine faults which lead to rapid fluctuations in vacuum will cause milk droplets to be driven back up against the teat-ends. Milk may penetrate the teat sphincter and enter the teat sinus, spreading disease if the milk contains pathogens.

Machine settings

Vacuum level: 37 kPa
Pulsation rate: 70–90 ppm
Pulsation ratio: 50 : 50

Preventing and controlling mastitis

❑ Keep goats in a clean, dry environment, on a well balanced diet.
❑ Goats are generally cleaner than cows, so it may not be necessary to wash udders before milking. However, udders should be washed if they are obviously dirty or if there is a problem with high bacterial cell counts in milk. Udder washing must avoid possible transfer of pathogens from goat to goat or from teat to teat:
■ use a disinfectant solution; washing with plain water will probably cause more problems than not washing at all.
■ use a spray system or wash and wipe with a single service paper towel soaked in disinfectant solution.
■ dry teats and udder thoroughly with separate disposable paper towel. Water running down the teats will drip into the bucket or be drawn into the liner during milking, carrying

bacteria into the milk. Wet udders during milking easily transmit infection.

❏ Routinely examine animals for mastitis at each milking – use a strip cup or filter in the long milk tube to detect milk clots. During milking the udders should be examined for cleanliness, teat lesions and teat orifice abnormalities and changes in the udder tissue.

❏ Use a postmilking teat disinfectant:
  ■ to remove mastitis bacteria which could be transmitted from goat to goat by the milker or milking machine;
  ■ to remove general bacteria from cut or sore teats (generally less of a problem in goats than cows).

The dip should be applied straight after milking has finished, whilst the teat canal is still open, so a small quantity of dip disinfects the epithelium of the teat canal. Unused dip should be discarded at the end of milking or as soon as it gets grossly contaminated.

❏ Treat mastitis cases promptly, using the full course of treatment. Treatment failures are usually due to:
  ■ using the wrong antibiotic;
  ■ waiting too long before treatment;
  ■ using too low a dosage;
  ■ stopping treatment too soon;
  ■ presence of microorganisms that have become resistant to treatment;
  ■ failure of treatment to reach walled off sites of infection;
  ■ chronic cases with poor recovery chances.

❏ Cull chronic or incurable cases.

❏ Use preventative treatment at drying off (dry-goat therapy) where necessary (but see above) – dry-goat treatments have at least twice the cure rates of treatments during lactation.

❏ Keep records.

❏ Maintain equipment in clean conditions; milking machines should be tested regularly.

'Hard udder'

'Hard udder' is indicated by a firm, swollen udder in freshly kidded goats (often first kidders), little milk production with poor milk letdown, and non-responsiveness to treatments for oedematous udders, e.g. diuretics. The milk appears normal with no evidence of bacterial mastitis. Increased milk production and softening of the udder occurs after about a week, but milk production remains suboptimal throughout the lactation because of the indurative changes in the udder tissue.

In the UK at least, the condition appears to be part of the CAE complex. All goats seen by the author with this condition have been CAE seropositive and since the widespread introduction of CAE control measures the incidence has fallen to zero.

Udder oedema

Occasionally, the normal physiological oedema of the udder which occurs prior to parturition is excessive, resulting in an udder which is hard and swollen. Unlike the 'hard udder' syndrome, milk production is not severely affected. In the UK, although some goats may need milking before kidding to ease the udder, it is extremely rare to have to resort to any further treatment. In contrast, the condition is reported to be common in British Alpines, particularly first kidders, in Australia, suggesting that some factor other than a normal physiological process is involved. In severe cases of oedema, hot compresses, liniments and frequent stripping may be necessary together with injections of a diuretic.

Frusemide, **5 ml i.m.** or **i.v.** (**Lasix 5% Solution**, Hoechst Roussel), every 12 hours for 3 days.

Trauma to the udder

Traumatic injury to the teats and udder associated with butting and being trodden on are common and may result in large painful swellings, possibly accompanied by mastitis. Any wounds should be carefully treated and antibiotic cover given to prevent the occurrence of mastitis.

Gangrenous mastitis commonly results from quite small abrasions near the teat tip.

Abscesses

Abscesses in the udder may arise from mastitic episodes or from penetrating lesions to the udder. Deep abscesses are not possible to treat; abscesses just below the skin of the udder can be satisfactorily drained.

Fibrous scar tissue

Fibrous lumps arise as a sequel to mastitis or trauma. Because they are an obvious fault in the show ring, owners resort to numerous methods to try to get rid of them. Topical applications of anti-inflammatory creams, herbal remedies, etc. will reduce the size of surface lumps, but the most successful treatment is cold laser treatment, initially twice weekly, then weekly.

Pustular dermatitis of the udder

See 'Staphylococcal dermatitis' (Chapter 10).

Fly bites

Biting flies may produce quite severe lesions, superficially resembling staphylococcal dermatitis on the udder. Topical creams and washes will ease the lesions.

Tumours

See Chapter 9.

Orf

See Chapter 9.

Maiden milkers

Many kids and goatlings from heavy milking strains show udder development and milk production particularly during the summer months. The vast majority of these animals do *not* require milking – milking stimulates production of more milk necessitating more regular milking, possibly predisposing to mastitis and acting as a nutritional drain on a growing animal. In well grown, well fed animals feed reduction may help control milk production. Milking is only necessary if the amount of milk makes the goat uncomfortable – the udder should be completely emptied as partial milking predisposes to infection; teats should be dipped after milking.

Empirically, treatment could be tried with drugs inhibiting prolactin secretion:

Cabergoline, 5 ug/kg, 0.1 ml/kg, orally (Galostop, Boehringer).

'Witch's milk'

Newborn kids occasionally show mammary development and milk production. No treatment is necessary.

Milking males (gynaecomastia)

Many males from high yielding families, particularly British Saanen and Saanen males, show mammary development and some degree of milk production during the summer months. For this reason, and to limit the risk of laminitis, the protein and energy levels of feed should be reduced during the summer. In most males, dietary management will control mammary development without resorting to milking. However, regular checks should be made as gangrenous mastitis is not an uncommon sequel in these animals. The fertility of males with mammary development is not affected.

Milk problems

Blood in the milk ('pink milk')

> 'Pink milk' is usually a sign of trauma rather than mastitis.

Haemorrhage into the udder from a damaged blood vessel occurs most commonly in first kidders in the first few days after kidding as the udder adapts to milk production and the stresses of regular milking. It may also occur at other times during lactation, particularly if the goat is milked by someone other than the regular attendant. The degree of haemorrhage determines whether the milk is coloured pink or there is merely a pink sediment after the milk has been allowed to stand. Culture of a sterile milk sample will confirm the absence of infection in these cases – bloody milk is not a common sign of mastitis.

Treatment is usually not necessary, the condition being self-limiting in a few days.

Milk leakage

Milk will sometimes leak from a teat, particularly at the junction between the teat and the udder. Some goats have milk-secreting tissue in the wall of the teat, and under pressure from milking, milk oozes through pores in the skin to the surface. The problem usually occurs shortly after lactation and first commencement of milking and, if pressure on the area can be avoided at milking, will often resolve itself. Cauterisation of the leaking area with a silver nitrate stick after each milking may help resolve the problem or suturing of severe leaks may be necessary. Milk may collect subcutaneously in the area rather than leaking out, forming a cyst which may interfere with milking.

Investigation of milk taint

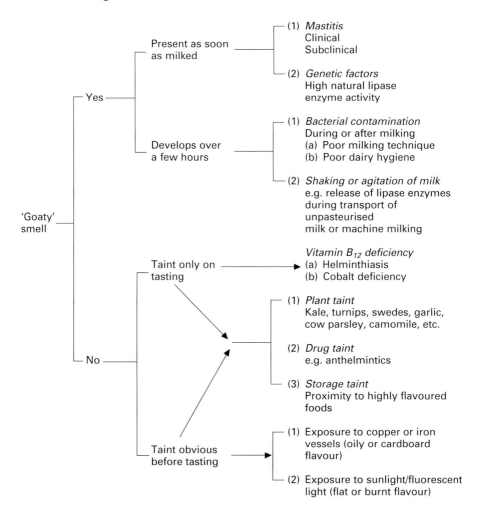

Figure 12.1   Identification of the cause of milk taint. [After Mews, A., 1987, *Goat Vet. Soc. J.*, **8** (1), 29–31.]

Initial assessment

- ❑ Individual or group of animals involved – generally an individual animal problem.
- ❑ Recent or persistent problem.
- ❑ Machine/hand milking – technique; relief milkers.
- ❑ Dairy hygiene and practice.
- ❑ Storage of milk.
- ❑ Type of taint:
  - ■ 'goaty' or not;
  - ■ obvious before tasting or only after tasting;
  - ■ present as soon as milked or develops over a few hours.

Herd problem

Consider:

- ❑ *Feed taint* – kale, turnips, swedes, garlic, cow parsley, camomile, etc. (see Chapter 20).
  Action – identify possible sources of taint, house animals and zero graze on hay rather than green plants.
- ❑ *Genetic factors* – certain goats have a high natural lipase enzyme activity causing release of fatty acids, particularly caproic acid.
  Action – identify particular families of goats involved.
- ❑ *Vitamin B$_{12}$ deficiency*
  - ■ Cobalt deficiency (see Chapter 8)
  - ■ Helminthiasis (see Chapter 13).
  Results in accumulation of branch chain and odd chain fatty acids and sweet sickly smell.
  Acion – worm animals and correct deficiency.
- ❑ *Mastitis* – widespread subclinical mastitis may present as a herd problem.
  Action – check milking technique, milking machine maintenance.
- ❑ *Poor milking technique* – bacterial contamination of milk.
- ❑ *Poor dairy hygiene* – bacterial contamination of milk, inadequate filtration, cooling, refrigeration and freezing of milk.
- ❑ *Agitation of milk* – releases free fatty acids, particularly caproic acid.
  Action – check pumps and length of milk lines, etc.
- ❑ *Oxidation*
  - ■ exposure to copper or iron (oily/cardboard flavour)
  - ■ exposure to sunlight or fluorescent light (flat/burnt flavour).
- ❑ *Storage taint* – milk readily picks up strong flavours from other foods, etc.

Individual goat problem

❏ Identify goat.
❏ One or both halves of udder involved? – unilateral generally means mastitis, bilateral may be mastitis.
❏ Examine udder for lumps, fibrosis, abscess, etc.
❏ If no bacteria isolated, consider other causes of taint as discussed under 'Herd problem'.

Self-sucking

Self-sucking is a quite common problem, which once started is very difficult to stop. A variety of preventative devices can be tried – udder bags, Elizabethan collars, noxious sprays such as Bitter Apple, teat tape (3 m), etc. – but many chronic suckers are culled.

Teat abnormalities

'Pea' in the teat

Occasionally a teat obstruction occurs preventing the flow of milk during milking. This is generally a crystal which is too big to pass through the teat orifice, but teat lumen granulomas also occur.

Crystals can usually be removed by manipulation and pressure; removal of a granuloma may require teat surgery.

Supernumerary and abnormal teats

Supernumerary and abnormal teats are inherited defects which result in disqualification in show animals. There is thus an ethical consideration before surgical interference is undertaken. All kids, male and female, should be checked for teat abnormalities at disbudding, but many abnormalities will not become apparent until later. Discrete, definite supernumerary teats can be removed at disbudding or later. Double teats and fishtail teats are best left intact.

Further reading

Machine milking

Edmondson, P. (1993) The milking machine and mastitis. *In Practice*, **15** (1), 12–17.

Lu, C.D., Potchoiba, M.J. and Loetz, E.R. (1991) Influence of vacuum level, pulsation ratio and rate on milking performance and udder health in dairy goats. *Small Ruminant Research*, **5**, 1–8.

Mottram, T.T., Smith, D.L.O. and Godwin, R.J. (1991) Analysis of parlour design parameters for goat milking. *Small Ruminant Research*, **6**, 1–13.

Roberts, J.R. (1989) The importance of correct maintenance of milking machines in goats. *Goat Vet. Soc. J.*, **10** (2), 89–93.

Mastectomy

Kerr, H.J. and Wallace, C.E. (1978) Mastectomy in a goat. *Vet. Med. Small Animal Clinician*, **73** (9), 1177–81.

Mastitis

Anderson, J.C. (1983) Mastitis in goats. *Goat Vet. Soc. J.*, **4** (1), 17–20.

Baxendell, S.A. (1984) Mastitis. *Proc. Univ. Sydney, Post Grad. Comm. Vet. Sci.*, **73**, 473–83.

Cripps, P. (1986) The prevention and control of mastitis in goats. *Goat Vet. Soc. J.*, **7** (2), 48–51.

Milk hygiene

Department of Agriculture and Fisheries for Scotland, Code of Practice (undated) *The Hygienic Control of Goats' Milk*. Department of Agriculture and Fisheries for Scotland, Edinburgh.

Ministry of Agriculture, Fisheries and Food, Code of Practice (undated) *The Hygienic Production of Goats' Milk*. MAFF Publications, Alnwick.

Milk taint

Baxendell, S.A. (1984) Goat milk taints. *Proc. Univ. Sydney Post Grad. Comm. Vet. Sci.*, **73**, 493–4.

Cousins, C.M. (1981) Milk hygiene and milk taints. *Goat Vet. Soc. J.*, **2** (1), 20–24.

Mews, A. (1987) Goat milk taints. *Goat Vet. Soc. J.*, **8** (1), 29–31.

Somatic cell counts

Francis, P.G. (undated) Somatic cell counts in sheep and goat milk. Issued by Chief Scientists' Group, MAFF, London.

Park, Y.W. (1991) Interrelationships between somatic cell counts, electrical conductivity, bacteria counts, percent fat and protein in goat milk. *Small Ruminant Research*, **5**, 367–75.

Udder conditions

Baxendell, S.A. (1984) Other udder conditions of goats. *Proc. Univ. Sydney Post. Grad. Comm. Vet. Sci.*, **73**, 484–9.

13 Diarrhoea

Diarrhoea may be produced by a number of pathogens, toxic substances and nutritional causes.

Initial assessment

The preliminary history should consider:

- ❏ Individual or group problem.
- ❏ Age of animal(s).
- ❏ Weaned or unweaned.
- ❏ Acute or chronic problem.
- ❏ Nutrition:
  - ■ basic diet
  - ■ change in diet
  - ■ level of concentrate feed (change in batch, excessive amount)
  - ■ possible mineral deficiencies.
- ❏ If unweaned kids consider:
  - ■ on dam or artificially reared
  - ■ whole milk or milk replacer
  - ■ ad lib or restricted feed
  - ■ bottle, bowl or machine fed
  - ■ type of milk powder, concentration fed and temperature
  - ■ one person or number of people responsible for feeding.
- ❏ Housing:
  - ■ individual or group
  - ■ deep litter or slats
  - ■ mixing of age groups.
- ❏ Grazing:
  - ■ zero grazed
  - ■ access to pasture
  - ■ pasture rotation.
- ❏ Access to toxic materials or plants.
- ❏ Preventative medications:
  - ■ clostridial vaccination
  - ■ anthelmintics (frequency, dose rate, accurate assessment of weight?, class of anthelmintic).

Clinical examination

❏ A full detailed clinical examination is essential to reach an accurate diagnosis.

❏ Diarrhoeic animals may be hypoproteinaemic with signs of oedema, e.g. bottle jaw, and/or anaemia (see Chapter 17).

❏ Examine mucous membranes.

❏ The diarrhoea may be a secondary problem, e.g. in severe toxaemias such as acute mastitis.

❏ Animals may be bright, afebrile and eager to feed or dull, lethargic, pyrexic and anorexic.

❏ Note type and consistency of faeces – colour, mucus, blood.

❏ Presence or absence of abdominal pain (see also Chapter 14).

❏ Signs of dehydration.

Laboratory investigation

❏ Fresh material is essential for diagnosis. Submission of a live, acutely ill animal may make a definitive diagnosis easier.

❏ A faeces sample (20 to 30 ml) should be collected early in the course of the disease. A faecal swab does not permit diagnosis of anything other than a bacterial infection.

❏ A complete range of samples for investigation from a live animal includes:
  ■ fresh faeces; air-dried smears of fresh faeces;
  ■ blood samples: EDTA, serum and air-dried blood films.

❏ At postmortem, freshly fixed sections from all levels of the small and large intestine and unopened loops of intestine.

❏ The antibody status of kids can be assessed by the use of the zinc sulphate turbidity test on serum.

Treatment

Specific treatments should be instigated where the cause of the diarrhoea is known. In other cases or before a laboratory diagnosis is reached, symptomatic treatments may be of value.

(1) Restrict food, particularly concentrates, for 24 hours, gradually increasing to the normal ration as the diarrhoea is controlled and correcting any obvious dietary excess.

Unweaned kids should be taken off milk for 24 hours and fed water or elctrolyte replacer. Reduced quantities of normal strength milk should be offered subsequently.

Note: feeding milk replacers at less than the recommended concentration is likely to exacerbate the diarrhoea as the milk will not clot properly.

(2)   *Fluid therapy* to replace fluid loss and correct the electrolyte balance.

❑   Oral rehydration therapy with electrolyte solutions (**Lectade**, Pfizer; **Life-Aid**, Norbrook), **250–500 ml** every 6 hours. Healthy diarrhoeic kids will generally drink from a bottle.

❑   Intravenous balanced electrolyte solutions, **20–120 ml/kg**, given over a period of 4 to 5 hours, depending on the degree of dehydration.

The amount of replacement fluid required can be estimated from the percentage fluid loss based on body weight (see Table 13.1).

Table 13.1   Fluid loss and associated clinical signs of diarrhoea.

Percentage fluid loss based on body weight	Clinical signs
0–5	Mild, barely detectable, increased thirst
5–10	Moderate, mouth dry, skin remains erect when pinched
10	Severe, body cold, eyes shrunken, comatose

A dehydrated kid requires a weight of fluid equal to the estimated loss due to dehydration, plus a weight of fluid equal to 10% of body weight for daily maintenance. For practical purposes, 1 kg = 1 l of fluid.

Thus, a 5-kg kid with 5% fluid loss requires:

5% of 5 kg to replace lost fluid = 0.25 kg
plus 10% of 5 kg for maintenance = 0.50 kg
Total fluid required is 0.75 kg = 0.75 l = 750 ml

Additional bicarbonate is required to combat acidosis in cases of severe diarrhoea, i.e. 150 to 650 mg sodium bicarbonate depending on the degree of dehydration (1 teaspoonful = 5 g).

(3)   Use non-specific treatments such as kaolin, chalk, bismuth, etc.

Light kaolin/pectin, 1–2 ml/kg (**Kaopectate**, Pharmacia & Upjohn) every 8 hours.

Calcium chloride, aluminium hydroxide, light kaolin, magnesium chloride, potassium acetate, sodium acetate, sodium chloride, 1–2 ml/kg (**Stat**, Intervet) every 8 hours.

(4) Reduce intestinal motility:

Loperamide hydrochloride, 100–200 µg/kg, 0.5–1 ml/kg orally (Immodium syrup, Janssen-Cilag), every 8 or 12 hours or 1–2 capsules/20 kg orally (Immodium capsules, Janssen-Cilag), dissolving contents in small amount of water, every 8 to 12 hours.

(5) Use oral or parenteral antibiotics if a bacterial cause is strongly suspected or confirmed, but do not use them indiscriminately. Some antibiotics may prolong the diarrhoea by delaying regeneration of the intestinal mucosa. In ruminating animals, antibiotic therapy may have deleterious effects on the rumen micoflora. Parenteral antibiotics are essential if the kid is septicaemic.

(6) Use spasmolytics to relieve pain and intestinal spasm:

Metamizole, hyoscine butylbromide, 0.5–2 ml (Buscopan Compositum, Boehringer Ingelheim).

(7) Use non-steroidal anti-inflammatory drugs for analgesia and to limit the cytokine cascade following release of endotoxin:

Flunixin meglumine, 2 mg/kg, 0.2 ml/4.5 kg (Finadyne, Schering-Plough).

(8) Once antibiotic treatment has ceased, re-establishment of a beneficial intestinal flora can be aided by the use of live yoghurt, or probiotics or ground up fresh faecal pellets from an adult goat.

Birth to 4 weeks

Dietary scour

> Nutritional mismanagement is the major cause of diarrhoea in kids under 4 weeks.

The majority of cases of diarrhoea in artificially reared kids between 2 and 12 weeks of age are related to nutrition; either directly through sudden changes in concentration or type of milk replacer, changing between goat's milk and milk replacer, overfeeding or varying the temperature at which the milk is fed, or indirectly through dirty utensils or contamination of feed. Correction of feeding practices and symptomatic treatment will result in the rapid resolution of uncomplicated nutritional diarrhoea, but where secondary infection is involved the treatment may need to be more prolonged. Nutritional scours may also predispose to or coexist with bloat, colic and mesen-teric torsion (see Chapter 15), all of which are potentially life threat-ening.

In older kids and adults, overfeeding of concentrates without adequate roughage either through bad management or stealing food (see Chapters 14 and 15) will cause diarrhoea. Similarly, overgrazing on lush grass, excessive feeding of roots, e.g. mangolds, or kale, excess fruit or bread or mouldy hay will all cause digestive upsets.

The role of infectious agents in diarrhoea in young kids

> The role of infectious agents in diarrhoea of young kids is unclear.

In kids under 4 weeks, the specific aetiology of the diarrhoea will often remain unknown. Viruses, such as rotavirus and coronovirus, are commonly isolated from diarrhoeic kids but are also identified in non-diarrhoeic kids. Enterogenic *E. coli* can also be isolated from both diarrhoeic and non-diarrhoeic kids. In contrast, the identification of *Cryptosporidium* spp. is always significant.

E. coli

Coliform bacteria are commensals of the alimentary tract and can readily be identified on faecal culture. Enterotoxigenic *E. coli* (ETEC) are significant as a cause of diarrhoea in newborn kids and may complicate infections caused by cryptosporidia, rotavirus and cor-onavirus in kids up to 2 to 3 weeks of age. Other strains of *E. coli* cause septicaemia and chronic arthritis.

Aetiology

❑ Enterotoxigenic *E. coli* produce an enterotoxin which causes the release of electrolytes and water from the cells lining the small intestine, resulting in diarrhoea. The enterotoxin is non-antigenic, but ETEC have the antigenic K99 pilus which enables the bacteria to adhere to the intestinal epithelium.

Clinical signs

❑ Acute, profuse, watery diarrhoea in very young kids.
❑ Dehydration and death.

Laboratory diagnosis

❑ Isolation of the organism on faecal culture.
❑ Detection of the K99 antigen by isolation on special media and slide testing for the antigen with specific antisera.
❑ Immunofluorescence of frozen sections of small intestine.

Treatment

❑ Antibiotics – orally or parenterally.
❑ General supportive therapy (qv).

Salmonella

Salmonellosis causes *peracute septicaemia* and sudden death in neonatal kids and an *acute diarrhoea* in kids and older goats, often following stress, and *abortion* in later gestation (see Chapter 2).

Outbreaks of diarrhoea and abortion may occur concurrently.

Aetiology

❑ *Salmonella typhimurium* and *S. dublin* are most common, but several other serotypes have been associated with the disease.

Transmission

❑ Infection is most often acquired from other goats which are excreting the organism and are either clinical or preclinical cases of the disease or symptomless carriers. However, other sources of infection may occasionally be significant.
❑ Infection from food and water.
❑ Infection from other domestic animals or man.
❑ Infection from wild animals or birds.

Clinical signs

❑ Lethargy, pyrexia.
❑ Diarrhoea, often profusely watery and yellow ± dysentery.
❑ Abdominal pain.
❑ Dehydration.
❑ Death in severe cases.
❑ Sudden death in very young kids.

Postmortem findings

❑ Enteritis, abomasitis, septicaemia, enlarged mesenteric lymph nodes.

Laboratory diagnosis

❑ Culture of faeces – rectal swabs or faeces using selective media.
❑ Isolation of organism from mesenteric lymph nodes, hepatic lymph nodes, heart blood, spleen, lungs, etc.
❑ The organism may be excreted in milk.

Treatment

❑ Antibiotics – orally or parenterally.
❑ General supportive therapy (qv).

Clostridium perfringens types **B** and **C**

Clostridium perfringens types B and C cause an acute harmorrhagic enteritis of kids under 3 weeks of age.

Aetiology

❑ Clostridia produce beta toxin in the small intestine causing local necrosis with resultant haemorrhagic diarrhoea.

Clinical signs

❑ Acute, profuse haemorrhagic diarrhoea.
❑ Abdominal pain.
❑ Death.

Postmortem findings

❑ Severe harmorrhagic enteritis affecting part or most of the ileum. The mucosa is congested and dark red and large deep ulcers are often present.

Laboratory investigation
Confirmation of the disease at postmortem is generally only possible in a freshly dead animal as beta toxin is very unstable.

❑ Collect 20 to 30 ml of intestine contents, to which 2 to 3 drops of chloroform have been added, in a universal container and submit to the laboratory.
❑ Gram-stained impression smears from the small intestine show gram-positive rods.
❑ Beta toxin can be demonstrated using mice protection tests with specific antisera or by an ELISA test.
❑ *Clostridium perfringens* is a normal inhabitant of the intestine and its isolation at postmortem is *not* necessarily significant.

Prevention

❏ Vaccination of the dam in late gestation to confer protection on the kids via the colostrum (see *Clostridium perfringens* type D in 'Colic in kids', Chapter 14).

Treatment

❏ Administration of **clostridial antitoxins** (**Lambisan**, Hoechst Roussel).
❏ General supportive therapy (see 'Treatment' section, this chapter).

Campylobacter

Campylobacter spp. have occasionally been isolated from diarrhoeic kids and are a potential zoonotic hazard.

Viral diarrhoea

Rotavirus, coronavirus and adenovirus have been reported to cause diarrhoea in kids. Mixed infections with enterotoxigenic *E. coli* or *Cryptosporidia* may occur. Other viruses such as a herpes virus have also been implicated in diarrhoea in goats, but the clinical significance of these isolates is unclear.

Rotavirus is the most common enteric virus of goats.

Aetiology

❏ Rotavirus infects and destroys the epithelial cells of villi in the small intestine, producing malabsorption and diarrhoea.

Clinical signs

❏ Acute, profuse watery diarrhoea, dehydration and death.
❏ Many kids will carry inapparent infections.

Laboratory investigation

❏ Demonstration of viral particles in faeces by electron microscopy.
❏ Demonstration of viral antigen in faeces by an ELISA test.
❏ Immunofluorescence on frozen intestinal section.

Cryptosporidium

Aetiology

❏ *Cryptosporidium parvum* is a small protozoan parasite related to enteric coccidia which parasitise the distal small intestine, caecum and colon, reducing the mucosal surface area, resulting in malabsorption and deficiencies in mucosal enzymes, particularly lactose. The life cycle is direct and closely resembles that of other Eimerian coccidia, although it is as short as 3 or 4 days, so environmental contamination can reach high levels very rapidly.

Transmission

❏ *Cryptosporidium* lacks host specificity so one domestic species may spread infection to another.
❏ Purchased infected animals will introduce the disease into a herd.
❏ Mice and rats may act as a reservoir of infection.
❏ Infective oocysts are highly resistant and will persist in paddocks or in pens for over a year.
❏ Oocysts sporulate in the intestine and are immediately infective when passed in the faeces, so rapid transmission occurs.
❏ Kids are usually infected within the first week of life and are fairly resistant by 4 weeks of age.

Clinical signs

❏ Watery diarrhoea in kids 1 to 4 weeks of age.
❏ Dehydration.
❏ Anorexia.
❏ High morbidity.
❏ Mortality may be high because of dehydration.

Postmortem examination

❏ Postmortem lesions resemble those due to other causes of diarrhoea.

Laboratory investigation

> The isolation of *Cryptosporidium* is always significant.

❏ Faecal smears air dried, fixed in methanol and stained with Giemsa will show the oocysts as blue circular structures with reddish granules.
❏ Oocysts can be concentrated by flotation in saturated salt or sugar solutions and examined by phase contrast microscopy or after staining.
❏ *Cryptosporidium* can be demonstrated in histological sections of

small and large intestines provided the postmortem material is very fresh.
❑ Fluorescent antibody on faecal smears; ELISA for faecal antigen/oocysts.

Treatment

❑ No specific therapy exists – anticoccidial drugs and antibiotics do not influence the course of the infections.
❑ Symptomatic treatment, including correction of dehydration (qv).

Control

❑ Improve hygiene – regular weekly cleaning of pens with high pressure water; allow to dry thoroughly before restocking.
❑ Reduce infection – separate kids at birth and feed colostrum from bottle; house kids in small groups, or individually, away from adult herd; immediately isolate any kid with diarrhoea.

Prevention

❑ Once the disease is established on a premises, only steam or hot water cleaning of pens is likely to destroy the infective oocysts.

Public health considerations

Cryptosporidium is potentially zoonotic, causing no or only mild disease in adults, but possibly severe disease in children or the immuno-suppressed.

Strongyloides papillosus

Strongyloidosis is a relatively common infection, occasionally producing diarrhoea in suckling kids. Kids are initially infected via the dam's milk so feeding of pooled milk or milk replacer will reduce the number of larvae transmitted. Subsequently, infection is by ingestion or skin penetration and heavy infections may result in a localised dermatitis (see Chapter 10).

Diagnosis

❑ Faecal examination for typical embryonated eggs.

Treatment

❑ Any broad-spectrum anthelmintics.

From 4 to 12 weeks

Gastrointestinal parasitism

Gastrointestinal parasitism is the major differential diagnosis in older kids or adult goats showing diarrhoea, unthriftiness, poor growth rates, anaemia or hypoproteinaemia.

Investigation of suspected gastrointestinal parasitism

❏ History.
❏ Clinical examination – any of the following may indicate worm infestation, particularly in the kid or young goat, but all ages are potentially susceptible as only limited protective immune response develops with age:
  ■ reduced growth rate/weight loss (see Chapter 8)
  ■ reduced fibre growth
  ■ reduced milk production
  ■ diarrhoea
  ■ anaemia (see Chapter 17)
  ■ sudden death (see Chapter 18).

Note: (1) Subclinical levels of infection may cause significant losses in production (weight gain, milk production, etc.) without other overt clinical signs. (2) Combinations of clinical signs may be seen as animals are usually parasitised by more than one species.

As in sheep, the main species involved in producing scouring are *Ostertagia* spp. and *Trichostrongylus* spp. *Haemonchus contortus* infection causes severe anaemia, oedema and lethargy.

Clinical signs and history may be diagnostic; if not, laboratory diagnosis is necessary.

Laboratory diagnosis

Faecal egg counts

Kids
Generally good correlation between egg counts, worm burden and disease:

500 to 2000 eggs/g faeces = subclinical infection
>2000 eggs/g faeces   = clinical infection

One to two weeks after treating with anthelmintics counts should approach zero. If not, suspect anthelmintic resistance or drenching procedure.

Confusion may occur if kids are given anthelmintic treatment shortly before a faecal sample is taken as clinical signs may persist due to chronic intestinal damage even though egg counts are low.

Adults

❑ Correlation less exact and counts may be misleading:
- depressed egg production as a result of partial host immunity: worm burden and therefore damage greater than count suggests.
- worm burden required to produce clinical disease depends on other factors such as nutrition and milk production level.
- larvae may produce disease before egg production.
- diurnal and seasonal variations in egg production occur.

Note: significant worm burdens can develop in deep litter systems given suitable conditions of temperature and humidity.

Postmortem examination

❑ Identify various worms present – goats are infected with the same parasites that affect sheep and also some of the parasites that affect cattle:

Abomasum: *Haemonchus contortus, Ostertagia* spp., *Trichostrongylus axei*

Small intestine: *Trichostrongylus* spp., *Nematodirus* spp., *Bunostomum trigonocephalum, Cooperia curticei, Strongyloides papillosus*

Large intestine: *Oesophagostomum columbianum, Chabertia ovina, Trichuris ovis.*

❑ Estimate number of worms present – significance of numbers depends on other factors such as overall herd health, clinical signs, etc. As a rough guide:

Trichostrongylus colubriformis	4000	=	subclinical infection
	8000	=	diarrhoea in young goats
	20 000	=	death in young goats
Haemonchus contortus	500	=	subclinical infection
	1000	=	anaemia in young goats
	2500	=	death in young goats.

Plasma pepsinogen levels

❑ Levels >3 U may indicate severe ostertagiasis.

Haematology

❏ Anaemia and hypoproteinaemia are consistent with *haemonchosis* and *trichostrongylosis*

Treatment and control

> Goats do not develop immunity to nematodes.
> Control is necessary at all ages.

Adult goats are susceptible to infection with gastrointestinal nematodes and often have levels of infection high enough to cause clinical or subclinical disease. Newly kidded goats, kids and debilitated animals are most susceptible and control is most important in these groups.

No single control system is suitable for all goat systems, but all rely on a combination of the following:

❏ Avoid infection.
  - *Extensive husbandry* allows goats to follow their preferred browsing habits, without close cropping of grass.
  - *Rotation of grazing*: adopt a 3-year rotation of paddocks, growing crops such as kale or lucerne and sharing grazing with horses or cattle (but not sheep).
  - *Zero grazing*, the only financially practical solution for large milking herds because the minimum milk withholding time for anthelmintics is 7 days. Only very low levels of infection, if any, develop in deep litter systems.
❏ Limit infection by grazing management, together with minimal anthelmintic treatment.
  - *Maintain safe pasture*, particularly for kids. Safe pasture is pasture not grazed in the second half of the previous year or pasture ungrazed until mid-July when overwintered larvae have died off.
  - *Kid early, indoors*, to prevent the periparturient rise in faecal egg counts.
  - *Delay turnout* until overwintered larvae on pasture have died off in mid-July.
  - If safe pasture is available in the spring, worm in the spring at kidding time, worm again in June and move onto clean pasture, avoiding the midsummer rise in infection.
  - If no safe pasture is available in the spring, worm in the spring at kidding time, then worm again in June and move to safe pasture.

■ If no safe pasture is available in the spring or later in the year, worm in the spring at kidding time, then worm every 3 weeks from spring to autumn.

Preventing the spread of anthelmintic resistance

> Only three groups of anthelmintics are available.

Anthelmintic resistance is forever.

Anthelmintic resistance has been reported in all the major gastro-intestinal nematodes of sheep and goats, in particular *Haemonchus*, *Ostertagia* and *Trichostrongylus*, but also *Nematodirus* and *Cooperia* spp. Resistance has occurred in all three groups of anthelmintics (see Table 13.2). Most studies in the UK have looked at Angora and cashmere goats. The situation in dairy goats is largely unknown.

Table 13.2 Groups of broad-spectrum anthelmintics.

Group 1	Benzimidazoles	Probenzimidazoles
	Albendazole	Netobimin
	Fenbendazole	Febantel
	Mebendazole	Thiophanate
	Oxfendazole	
Group 2	Imidazothiazoles/tetrahydropyrimidines	
	Levamisole	
	Morantel	
	Pyrantel	
Group 3	Avermectins	Milbemycin
	Abamectin	Moxidectin
	Doramectin	
	Eprinomectin	
	Ivomectin	

Administer the correct dose

Dose rates for sheep cannot be directly extrapolated to goats. Higher dose rates are often required in goats.

Benzimidazoles and probenzimidazoles: 1.5–2 times sheep dose rate; Albendazole, febantel, fenbendazole, oxfendazole, **7.5 mg/kg orally**; mebendazole, **22.5 mg/kg**; netobimin, **11.25 mg/kg orally**.

Levamisole: 1.5 times sheep dose rate, 12 mg/kg orally (do not exceed this rate as levamisole is toxic in goats at dose rates approaching 20 mg/kg; do not use injectable preparations).

Avermectins: use sheep dose rate; 200 µg/kg, **10 mg/50 kg, 1 ml/ 50 kg s.c.**

Estimation of the weight of goats is often very imprecise and many goats are underdosed. Underdosing increases the rate of selection for anthelmintic resistance by exposing nematodes to sublethal concentrations of anthelmintic. Wherever possible goats should be weighed, e.g. while at shows, in cattle markets, or weigh bands can be used (see Appendix 1). Groups of goats should be dosed at the rate for the largest in the group.

Drenching equipment should be well maintained and correctly calibrated.

The use of topical anthelmintics ('pour-ons') in goats is not well documented and there is very little data available concerning efficacy and drug dosages. The avermectin, eprinomectin is potentially a very useful anthelmintic in milking goats:

Eprinomectin, 'pour-on', 0.5 mg/kg (Eprinex, Merial).

Because of its low milk to plasma ratio (< 0.2), eprinomectin has a nil milk withdrawal period in cattle, although further research is required on the pharmokinetics and optimum drug dosage in goats and there are no reported milk residue studies. Eprinomectin has been shown to have a high activity against gastrointestinal nematodes in goats when applied topically at 0.5 mg/kg body weight, with 99 to 100% efficacy demonstrated against adult strongyles of *Haemonchus contortus* and *Ostertagia circumcincta* and 98% efficacy demonstrated against *Trichostrongylus colubriformis*.

Use the minimum number of treatments

Increasing the frequency of treating with anthelmintics increases selection pressure and leads to increased prevalence of resistant genotypes. Establishing an effective control programme on each holding prevents unnecessary dosing.

Rotate type of anthelmintic group used annually

Annual (slow) rotation between anthelmintic groups minimises the development of both single and multiple resistance. Prolonged use of a single drug family increases the selection pressure for the development of resistance to that family. Rapid alternation of drug families exposes a single generation of nematodes to two different drugs and may lead to selection of individuals with dual resistance.

The only anthelmintics licensed for use in goats in the UK are the avermectin **ivermectin,** 200 µg/kg, **2.5 ml/10 kg orally (Oramec Drench**, Merial) and the probenzimidazole **thiophanate, 9 kg/tonne feed** as single dose or **2.8 kg/tonne feed (Nemafax 14**, Merial) daily for 5 days. Ivermectin is not suitable for milking goats as the withholding time for milk is 14 days if treated during lactation and 28 days if treatment occurs before lactation commences. Nemafax is an in-feed medication, unsuitable for treating individuals or small groups of goats. However, Nemafax, with a milk withhold time of 3 days and a meat withhold time of 7 days, is the only anthelmintic in the UK with a milk withhold time of less than 7 days. There are no products licensed for goats in the levamisole group.

In this specific instance, it is essential, on scientific and welfare grounds, to ignore the 'cascade system' and rotate anthelmintic groups annually as recommended, using suitable products.

Avoid introducing resistant worms

Wherever possible, a history of anthelmintic treatments and possible resistance should be obtained for goats entering a new holding. All goats should be treated with effective anthelmintics from two different families on arrival, then held on concrete for at least 24 hours before being allowed on pasture. As most resistance in the UK is to the benzimidazoles, the other two groups should be used.

Fibre goats are most likely to carry resistant genotypes and should not be grazed with dairy goats unless the effectiveness of anthelmintic treatment has been established.

Establish an optimum worm control strategy for each holding

Detection of resistant nematodes Faecal egg count reduction test – groups of goats are marked, faecal sampled, weighed and then dosed according to live weight with the drug(s) under investigation. The same animals are then resampled 10 days later and the percentage reduction in faecal egg count is calculated. Efficacies < 90% are indicative of the presence of resistant strains.

In vitro tests – a number of different *in vitro* tests can be used to determine resistance, including the *egg hatch test* which determines the ability of eggs to hatch in different concentrations of anthelmintic and the *larval development test*.

If resistance is diagnosed

❏ Stop using the group of anthelmintics to which resistance has been diagnosed.
❏ Alternate annually between the remaining two anthelmintic groups.
❏ Check annually to ensure that these groups are still effective.
❏ Minimise anthelmintic use by strategic control methods.

Cestode infection

Moniezia spp. commonly affect goats and proglottids can be detected in faeces, but clinical, or even subclinical, infection is unlikely to be attributed to tapeworms unless very large numbers are present in kids. Heavy infestation in kids may produce poor growth rates, a pot-bellied appearance and constipation. Complete occlusion of the intestinal lumen produces colic (see Chapter 14).

Benzimidazole drugs (see Table 13.2) **albendazole, 10 mg/kg, febantel, 7.4 mg/kg, fenbendazole, 15 mg/kg** and **oxfendazole, 10 mg/kg** are effective against *Moniezia* spp. at higher doses than required for nematode control.

Praziquantel, 5 mg/kg, 1 ml/10 kg s.c. or **1 tablet/10 kg orally (Droncit**, Bayer) is effective but not licensed for food-producing animals in the UK. Some goats are irritated by the injection.

Coccidiosis

> Coccidiosis is the most important cause of diarrhoea in housed kids > 4 weeks.

Aetiology

❑ Coccidia are protozoan parasites: goats are affected by 12 species of *Eimeria* which are all specific for the goat except *E. caprovina* which is transmissible between sheep and goats. Related protozoa such as *Isospora, Sarcocystis* and *Toxoplasma* do not generally multiply in the intestinal tract of the ruminant. The coccidial species of cattle, poultry or domestic pets do not cause coccidiosis in the goat.

Transmission

❑ All goats are infected with coccidia.
❑ It is probable that all kids are infected during their first few weeks of life and that management standards determine whether or not the levels of infection are sufficient to cause clinical signs of the disease. Kids become infected by ingestion of food, bedding and water contaminated with sporulated oocysts.
❑ Oocysts are ingested by the kid, rapidly undergo maturation and multiply. The cycling of a single oocyst could result in 1 to 2 million oocysts being passed 3 to 4 weeks later.
❑ Infection can occur indoors in intensive rearing situations or at pasture when the grass is sufficiently short for ingestion of oocysts lying on the soil surface.
❑ Oocysts are resistant to low temperature and will overwinter on pasture or indoors to provide a source of infection the following spring.

Epidemiology

❑ Kids become infected in the first few weeks of life, with the highest incidence of clinical disease between 4 and 7 weeks of age. After this, faecal oocyst excretion decreases as the kids acquire immunity to coccidia.

❑ Stress factors such as weaning, transport, changes in diet and adverse weather conditions can also predispose to the development of clinical disease possibly by producing a relaxation of immunity.

Clinical signs

❑ Depression.
❑ Anorexia.
❑ Weight loss.
❑ Diarrhoea, possibly with blood and/or mucus.
❑ Dehydration.
❑ Death.

In severely infected kids massive release of meronts and merozoites from the intestinal cells can produce sudden onset colic, shock and collapse or kids may be found dead with no signs of diarrhoea.

Recovered kids may show illthrift with a reduced growth rate and poor fibre production.

Diagnosis

The diagnosis of clinical coccidiosis must be based on the history, observation of clinical signs, postmortem findings, faecal oocyst counts and oocyst speciation. Diagnosis based on the number of oocysts in faecal samples poses a number of problems:

❑ All kids are infected with coccidia.

❑ A severe challenge and the subsequent asexual reproductions can result in considerable damage to the intestine and clinical signs in the prepatent phase before the sexual cycle occurs with release of oocysts in the faeces. In very heavy infections the damage to the intestinal mucosa may not leave enough epithelial cells in the villi for the sexual cycle to occur.

❑ The intestines may be so damaged by the infection that clinical signs, i.e. diarrhoea, persist after the peak of oocyst production.

❑ Normal kids may have 1000 to 1 000 000 oocysts/g faeces; clinically ill kids may have 100 to 10 000 000 oocysts/g faeces.

❑ Identification of the species of coccidia present may be helpful. The predominant species in the faeces of the normal goat are *E. arloingi* and *E. hirci*. The most pathogenic species which predominate in kids which are clinically ill are *E. ninakohlyakimovae*, *E. caprina* and *E. christenseni*.

Postmortem findings

❑ Gross postmortem finds are often limited.
❑ Haemorrhage or mucoid enteritis may be obvious in severe infections, but in less severe infections there is generally little haemorrhage into the intestine.
❑ Small white pinpoint lesions may be present on the mucosal surface of the intestine. Smears taken from these areas show the presence of meronts, gametocytes and oocysts.

Control

> Improved hygiene is the cornerstone of coccidiosis control.
>   Helminthiasis can occur concurrently with coccidiosis in kids at grass.

The environment

❑ Avoid overcrowding.
❑ Provide clean, dry, well strawed pens for each batch of kids.
❑ Do not mix kids of different age groups.
❑ Raise food and water containers above the floor to avoid faecal contamination.
❑ Clean deep litter pens every 3 weeks.
❑ Slatted floors rather than deep litter may help reduce the oocyst level in some husbandry systems.

The doe

❑ Feeding a coccidiostat to the does in late pregnancy will reduce oocyst output and thus contamination of the environment, but enough oocysts will remain to infect the kids in intensive housing conditions and the coccidia can rapidly multiply in the non-immune kid.

The kid

❑ Prophylactic medication may have some success in controlling coccidiosis by reducing the challenge to the kids and allowing them to develop immunity by exposure to a low number of oocysts. However, drug treatment in a contaminated environment will only have a temporary effect. Most drugs are coccidiostats with only a limited coccidiocidal effect.

Treatment

❏ *Coccidiostats* – most anticoccidial drugs are coccidiostats that arrest development of one or more stages in the coccidial life cycle by interfering with cell development but do not totally eliminate the organism. Most drugs act early in the life cycle. Diclazuril has a coccidiocidal effect on the asexual or sexual stages of the development cycle of the parasite, dependent on the coccidia species. No anticoccidial drugs are specifically licensed for goats in the UK.

 Sulphadimidine, 200 mg/kg, 6 ml/10 kg initial dose, then **100 mg/kg, 3 ml/10 kg s.c.** or **i.v.** (preferred) (**Bimadine 33 1/3**, Bimeda; **Intradine**, Norbrook; **Sulfoxine 333**, Vetoquinol; **Vesadin**, Merial), daily for up to 5 days total.

 Sulphadimidine, 200 mg/kg initial dose, then **100 mg/kg orally** (**Bimadine Oral Powder**, Bimeda), daily for 5 days total.

 Note: sulphadimidine injectable solutions can be given orally in milk or water as an alternative to powder.

 Sulphamethoxypyridazine, 20 mg/kg, 1 ml/12.5 kg s.c. (**Bimalong**, Bimeda; **Midicel**, Pharmacia & Upjohn; **Sulfapyrine LA**, Vetoquinol), daily for 3 days.

 Decoquinate, 100 g/tonne feed or **1 mg/kg** (**Deccox, Deccox prescription**, Merial), for 28 days.

 Diclazuril 1 mg/kg, 1 ml/2.5 kg orally [**Vecoxan**, Janssen] as a single dose.

 Amprolium, 5–10 mg/kg orally, daily for 3–5 days and **Toltrazuril, 20 mg/kg orally** (**Baycox**, Bayer), once every 3–4 weeks have been used successfully to control coccidiosis in kids but are only licensed for use in poultry in the UK.

❏ *Supportive therapy* – fluids, analgesics, intravenous corticosteroids – is essential in severe cases.

Prevention

In feed

 Decoquinate, 100 g/tonne feed or **1 mg/kg** (**Deccox, Deccox prescription**, Merial), for 28 days to kids.

 Decoquinate, 50 g/tonne feed or **0.5 mg/kg** (**Deccox, Deccox prescription**, Merial), for 28 days to does.

Monensin is now classified as a growth promoter in the UK and cannot be used in the control of coccidiosis in goats. Other growth promoters such as **Lasalocid** and **Salinomycin** are also prohibited. Conversely, monesin is approved for use in non-lactating goats in the USA.

In milk
> **Sulphadimidine, 200 mg/kg** initially, then **100 mg/kg** for a further 2–4 days every 3 weeks will reduce the level of environmental contamination of oocysts as 3 weeks is close to the prepatent period for many goat *Eimeria*. Sulphadimidine can be given as oral powder or the injectable solution can be added to milk.
>
> **Toltrazuril, 20 mg/kg** (**Baycox**, Bayer), every 3–4 weeks (only licensed for poultry in the UK).

Orally
> **Diclazuril 1 mg/kg, 1 ml/2.5 kg orally** [**Vecoxan**, Janssen] at about 4–6 weeks of age. Under conditions of high infection pressure, a second treatment can be given about 3 weeks after the first dosing.

Clostridium perfringens type D (enterotoxaemia, pulpy kidney disease)

See Chapter 15.

Salmonella

See Chapter 2 and this chapter.

Giardiasis

Aetiology

❏ A protozoan parasite, *Giardia.*

Transmission

❏ Faecal contamination of water, food or environment by an infected animal.

Clinical signs

❏ Chronic but sometimes intermittent watery diarrhoea.

Laboratory investigation

❏ Demonstration of motile flagellates in wet faecal smears stained with Giemsa to show the flagellae, pear-shaped central bodies and binucleate appearance.
❏ Cysts can be concentrated by flotation in zinc sulphate.

Treatment
- **Fenbendazole, 7.5 mg/kg orally** (**Panacur**, Hoechst Roussel), for 3 days.
- **Metronidazole, 20 mg/kg, 0.5 ml/10 kg orally** or **s.c.** (**Torgyl Forte Solution**, Merial), daily. (*Note:* metronidazole is banned from use in food-producing animals in the EU.)

Public health considerations
Giardia is a possible zoonosis by direct contact with sick animals or through faecal contamination.

Yersiniosis

Aetiology
- *Yersinia enterocolitica* and *Y. pseudotuberculosis*, gram-negative coccobacilli.

Clinical signs
- *Yersinia pseudotuberculosis* is reported to cause abortion and post-parturient deaths, liver abscesses and granuloma formation and acute and chronic mastitis.
- Both *Y. pseudotuberculosis* and *Y. enterocolitica* cause diarrhoea, with *Y. enterocolitica* being more frequently implicated. All ages can be affected, but generally kids between 1 and 6 months.
- Diarrhoea is watery and non-haemorrhagic.
- Mortality is high and some kids may present as sudden deaths.
- A more chronic illness with dehydration and weight loss may occur.

Treatment
- **Tetracyclines** will control outbreaks of diarrhoea and abortion.

Public health considerations
Affected animals and faeces are a potential hazard for humans and *Y. enterocolitica* has been isolated from goats' milk.

Nutritional factors

See 'Abortion', Chapter 2.

Campylobacter jejuni

See 'Abortion', Chapter 2.

Toxic agents causing diarrhoea

Poisonous plants

Poisonous plants may be eaten direct or in hay. Plants reported to cause diarrhoea include aconite, bluebell, box, buckthorn, dog's mercury, irises, rhododendron, spurges and wild arum.

Mycotoxins

Mycotoxins are fungal toxins found in mouldy conserved fodder or badly dried cereals.

Poisonous minerals

- ❏ Copper (footbaths, sprays, etc.); see Chapter 14.
- ❏ Basic slag, nitrogenous or other types of *fertiliser* from recently top-dressed pasture.
- ❏ Industrial waste – fluorides, arsenicals, barium, chromium, mercury, zinc and selenium.
- ❏ Fruit sprays.
- ❏ Teart pastures – molybdenum.
- ❏ Lead – access to old paint or batteries (qv).

Drugs

Drugs include sulphonamides, carbon tetrachloride, copper sulphate and warfarin.

Over 12 weeks

- ❏ Parasitic gastroenteritis (qv).
- ❏ Coccidiosis (qv).
- ❏ *Clostridium perfringens* type D (see Chapter 15).
- ❏ Salmonella (qv).
- ❏ Nutritional factors (qv).
- ❏ Toxic agents (qv).
- ❏ Liver disease (see Chapter 14) – hepatic disease and bile duct obstruction lead to a decrease in the level of bile salts in the alimentary tract. This together with general liver distension causes gastrointestinal disturbances of anorexia and constipation, with attacks of diarrhoea.
- ❏ Copper deficiency (see Chapter 5) – results in anaemia, illthrift, poor coat, infertility and diarrhoea in growing and adult goats.

❏ Johne's disease (see Chapter 8) – diarrhoea is an uncommon finding in Johne's disease in goats but may occur terminally.

Further reading

General

Blackwell, R.E. (1983) Enteritis and diarrhoea. *Vet. Clin. North Am.: Large Animal Practice*, **5** (3), November 1983, 557–70.

Thompson, K.G. (1985) Enteric diseases of goats. *Proc. Course in Goat Husbandry and Medicine*, Massey University, November 1985, 78–85.

Coccidiosis

Gregory, M. and Norton, C. (1986) Anticoccidials. *In Practice*, January 1986, 33–5.

Gregory, M. and Norton, C. (1986) Caprine coccidiosis. *Goat Vet. Soc. J.*, **7** (2), 32–4.

Howe, P.A. (1984) Coccidiosis. *Proc. Univ. Sydney Post Grad. Comm. Vet. Sci.*, **73**, 468–72.

Lloyd, S. (1987) Endoparasitic disease in goats. *Goat Vet. Soc. J.*, **8** (1), 32–9.

Van Veen, T.W.S. (1986) Coccidiosis in ruminants. *Comp. Cont. Ed. Pract. Vet.*, **8** (10), F52–8.

Cryptosporidiosis/giardiasis

Angus, K.W. (1987) Cryptosporidiosis in domestic animals and humans. *In Practice*, March 1987, 47–9.

Kirkpatrick, C.E. (1989) Giardiasis in large animals. *Comp. Cont. Ed. Pract. Vet.*, **II** (1), 80–84.

Lloyd, S. (1986) Parasitic zoonoses. *Goat Vet. Soc. J.*, **7** (2), 39–44.

Gastrointestinal parasites

Baldock, C. (1984) Helminthiasis in goats. *Proc. Univ. Sydney Post Grad. Comm. Vet. Sci.*, **73**, 450–67.

Coles, G.C. (1992) Anthelmintic resistance in nematodes of goats. *Goat Vet. Soc. J.*, **13** (2), 48–54.

Coles, G.C. and Roush, R.T. (1992) Slowing the spread of anthelmintic resistant nematodes of sheep and goats in the United Kingdom. *Vet. Rec.*, **130**, 505–9.

Jackson, F. (1991) Anthelmintic resistance in goats. *Goat Vet. Soc. J.*, **12** (1), 1–6.

Lloyd, S. (1982) Control of parasites in goats. *Goat Vet. Soc. J.*, **3** (1), 2–6.

Lloyd, S. (1987) Endoparasitic disease in goats. *Goat Vet. Soc. J.*, **8** (1), 32–9.

14 Colic

Initial assessment

❏ Feeding history – overfeeding, change in diet, mouldy feed, etc.
❏ General physical examination – to determine whether the problem is related to a specific alimentary condition, associated with a more general disease, or not connected with the alimentary tract at all (e.g. urolithiasis).
❏ Specific examination of the digestive system:
  ■ visual inspection: abdominal contour from behind, abdominal distension;
  ■ palpation of the left abdominal wall and rumen: filling of the rumen;
  ■ percussion: tympanitic sounds, pain;
  ■ auscultation: rumen mobility, sounds of left-sided abomasal displacement.

Further investigations

❏ Passage of a stomach tube allows release of accumulated gas and the collection of a sample of ruminal fluid. A simple gag to facilitate stomach tubing can be made by drilling a hole in a piece of wood.
❏ *Trocharisation* of the left paralumber fossa releases accumulated gas.
❏ *Abdominocentesis* – in adults, use an 18 or 20 gauge needle at the lowest point of the ventral abdomen, 2 to 4 cm to right of midline to avoid rumen. Aseptically prepare area, use local anaesthetic and possibly sedation in nervous animals.

Examination of rumen contents

❏ Measure pH with indicator papers: pH 4.5 to 5.0 suggests a moderate degree of abnormality; <4.5 suggests severe rumen acidosis and requires emergency treatment.
❏ Methylene blue reduction test measures the redox potential of the ruminal fluid and reflects the level of activity of aerobic rumen microflora; 20 ml of ruminal fluid is added to 1 ml of 0.03%

methylene blue solution in a test tube and the time required for the methylene blue to decolorise is measured. The faster the decolorisation the more active the microflora – microfloral inactivity will give results of 15 minutes or longer and severe rumen acidosis >5 minutes. A normal goat with a high concentrate ration will have a time of 1 to 3 minutes and a goat on an all hay diet 3 to 6 minutes.

Clinical signs of colic

❑ Lethargic, depessed, reluctant to move or frequently gets up and down.
❑ Bleating.
❑ Pawing ground with front feet, shifting of weight between feet.
❑ Teeth grinding.
❑ Tachypnoea, shallow respirations.
❑ Tachycardia.
❑ Tenesmus.
❑ Arched back.
❑ Tucked up at abdomen, staring at abdomen, kicking at abdomen (uncommon).

Goats rarely roll. Clinical signs may be continuous or spasmodic.

COLIC IN ADULT GOATS

Diarrhoea/enteritis

See Chapter 13.

Indigestion (ruminal atony)

Aetiology

❑ Minor degrees of dietary mismanagement, particularly inadequate protein and energy with a high fibre diet, mouldy or frosted feeds, a moderate overfeeding of concentrates or insufficient water, produce various degrees of ruminal impaction and atony.
❑ Oral dosing with antibiotics or sulphonamides (due to destruction of the normal ruminal flora).
❑ Lack of exercise.
❑ Oral dosing with linseed oil produces a foul-tasting cud which is often spat out and normal chewing of the cud ceases.

Clinical signs

❏ Reduced appetite or complete anorexia.
❏ Reduced milk yield.
❏ Constipation with small amounts of faeces or occasionally diarrhoea.
❏ Generally a firm, pliable rumen palpable on the left side but occasionally moderate degrees of tympany as ruminal atony becomes established.
❏ No signs or only weak signs of rumination.
❏ Often few signs of abdominal pain, although occasionally typical spasmodic colic signs such as pawing the ground with the front feet, looking at the abdomen, frequent getting up and down and grinding of teeth.

Treatment

❏ Many mildly affected animals will recover spontaneously. In other cases, symptomatic treatment should be adopted.
❏ Use **Epsom Salts (200 g)** in **300 ml water** as a drench on the first day, then 100, 75 and 50 g on successive days if necessary.
❏ Give **vegetable oil (30 ml)** in about **100 ml liquid paraffin** as a drench.
❏ Rehydration if necessary.
❏ Relief of pain where present.
❏ In animals with a recurrent problem, *bran mashes* two or three times weekly may help prevent impaction – mix four handfuls of bran scalded with sufficient boiling water to make a crumbly mash and leave to stand for 10 minutes.
❏ Feed on browsings, leaves and branches, to encourage the resumption of cudding.
❏ Re-establish ruminal microflora with yoghurt, probiotics or by drenching fresh rumen contents or ground-up faeces.

Note: abomasal impaction may occur in animals with poor rumination. The abomasum is palpable in the low right abdomen. Treat as for ruminal atony.

Acute impaction of the rumen (acidosis)

Aetiology

❏ Excess ingestion of high energy feeds such as barley, wheat, dairy cake, etc. results in a rapid fermentation of the carbohydrate in the feed with the formation of large quantities of lactic acid decreasing the rumen pH. As the pH falls, rumen motility decreases and the normal rumen microflora are destroyed and replaced by lactobacilli and streptococci. The lactic acid produces a severe rumenitis with necrosis of the mucous membrane, and lactic acid and the toxic products from the degeneration of the rumen bacteria are absorbed, causing a toxaemia. The ruminal contents are hypertonic to plasma, so fluids are lost into the alimentary tract resulting in diarrhoea and dehydration.

❏ Certain feeds which are acidic in their own right, e.g. mangolds, apples, rhubarb, etc., may produce acidosis if they are suddenly fed in large quantities.

❏ Secondary infection by fungi or bacteria such as *Fusibacterium necrophorum* may lead to a more prolonged rumenitis after the animal has survived the acute disease.

Clinical signs

❏ Lethargy.
❏ Anorexia.
❏ Abdominal pain – grinding of teeth, kicking at abdomen.
❏ Subnormal temperature.
❏ Fast, weak pulse.
❏ Ruminal movements absent.
❏ Diarrhoea.
❏ Death.
❏ Laminitis (see Chapter 6) may develop in animals that have recovered due to changes in the corium of the feet.

Treatment

❏ Mild cases can be treated as for indigestion (qv).
❏ Drenching with 100 g sodium bicarbonate will help reduce the acidosis (but overdosing may lead to alkalosis); alternatively, 15 ml milk of magnesia is a good antacid that will not convert to metabolic alkalosis if excess is given. Repeated in 3 to 4 hours if necessary.
❏ Dehydration should be corrected with parenteral administration of 3 to 5 l of isotonic fluids (Ringer's solution, **0.9% saline**). *Note:* avoid lactic acid solutions, such as Hartmann's.
❏ Metabolic acidosis can be corrected with intravenous **sodium bicarbonate**, given over 1 to 3 hours. To estimate bicarbonate deficit:

Severity of clinical signs	% Dehydration	Base deficit (mmol/l)
Mild	5	5
Moderate	8	10
Severe	10	15

(body weight in kg) × 0.5 × base deficit = mmol bicarbonate required, where 0.5 is the extracellular fluid volume (ECFV). Thus, a 50-kg goat that is 10% dehydrated will have a base deficit of 15 mmol/l and will need:

    50 × 0.5 × 15 = 375 mmol bicarbonate

    1 ml of 1.26% sodium bicarbonate = 0.15 mmol bicarbonate

    1 ml of 4.2% sodium bicarbonate = 0.50 mmol bicarbonate

    1 ml of 8.4% sodium bicarbonate = 1.00 mmol bicarbonate

The goat will require 750 ml of 4.2% sodium bicarbonate. If sodium bicarbonate solutions are not available, sodium bicarbonate can be added to 0.9% saline:

    1 g sodium bicarbonate = 12 mmol bicarbonate.

The 50-kg goat with 10% dehydration needs 31.25 g sodium bicarbonate.

❑ **Thiamine, 10 mg/kg i.v. or i.m., 1 ml/10 kg (Vitamin B$_1$**, Bimeda) daily for 3 days may help prevent cerebrocortical necrosis. Multi-vitamin preparations can be used if thiamine is not available, but must be given according to the thiamine content (usually 10 or 35 mg/ml).

❑ **Procaine benzylpenicillin, 10 mg/kg i.m. (Duphapen**, Fort Dodge; **Norocillin**, Norbrook) every 12 hours for as long as 10 to 14 days will help eliminate or prevent anaerobic bacterial rumenitis.

❑ Surgical – rumenotomy should be performed in serious cases, the rumen completely emptied and washed out and the contents replaced by hay, water and preferably rumen contents from a normal goat.

❑ The re-establishment of the normal rumenal microflora should be assisted by dosing with yoghurt, probiotics, ground-up faecal pellets, etc.

Ruminal tympany

Primary ruminal tympany (frothy bloat)

See Chapter 15.

Secondary ruminal tympany ('choke')

See Chapter 15.

Enterotoxaemia (*Clostridium perfringens* type D, pulpy kidney disease)

Aetiology

❑ *Clostridium perfringens* type D produces epsilon toxin in the small intestine. Rapid proliferation of the organism in response to dietary changes such as overgrowing lush pasture or overfeeding cereals results in toxin being absorbed into the bloodstream and damage to blood vessels in the brain, lungs and heart.

Transmission

❑ *Clostridium perfringens* is present in the intestine of normal sheep and goats and has also been isolated from soil.

Clinical signs

❑ Peracute – sudden death or terminal shocked condition with convulsions.
❑ Acute:
  ■ diarrhoea, initially yellow–green and soft, later watery with mucous, blood and shreds of intestinal mucosa;
  ■ sternal and later lateral recumbency;
  ■ severe abdominal pain: pitiful intermittent cry of pain;
  ■ shock: cold extremities;
  ■ paddling movements and throwing back of head prior to death.
❑ A chronic form has been described in adult goats showing periodic bouts of severe diarrhoea and wasting which responds to vaccination.

Postmortem findings

❑ Pericardial fluid that clots on exposure to air.
❑ Petechial or ecchymotic haemorrhages on the epicardium, endocardium, diaphragm, small intestine serosa and abdominal muscles.
❑ Mucosa of small intestine inflamed.
❑ 'Pulpy kidneys' may or may not be present.
❑ Symmetrical areas of haemorrhage, oedema and liquefaction in the brain, particularly the basal ganglia; focal symmetrical encephalomalacia (see Chapter 11).

Laboratory investigation

❑ Confirmation of the disease even at postmortem is generally difficult and only possible in a freshly dead animal.

❏ Collect 20 to 30 ml of intestine contents to which 2 to 3 drops of chloroform have been added in a universal container and submit to the laboratory.
❏ *Clostridium perfringens* type D is a normal inhabitant of the gut and may be found, with its toxin, in healthy animals.
❏ Gram-stained impression smears from the small intestine show gram-positive rods.
❏ Epsilon toxin can be demonstrated using mice protection tests with specific antisera or by an ELISA test.
❏ Urine collected from the bladder may contain glucose.

Treatment

❏ *Clostridium perfringens* **type D antitoxin**, adults at least **12.5 ml**, kids **5 ml**, s.c. or **i.m.** (**Lambisan**, Hoechst Roussel).
❏ Pain relief with:
   Flunixin meglumine, 2 mg/kg, 2 ml/45 kg i.v. (**Finayne Solution**, Schering-Plough).
   Carprofen, 1.4 mg/kg, 1 ml/35 kg i.v. (**Zenecarp Solution**, Pfizer).
❏ Supportive therapy – intravenous balanced electrolyte solutions, **120 ml/kg** over 4 to 5 hours (not glucose saline as hyperglycaemia occurs terminally), warmth and company.

Prevention

❏ Avoid digestive disturbances – overeating of concentrates, high concentrate diet with insufficient fibre, excessive grazing of lush grass, etc. – and make any feed changes gradually.
❏ Vaccination with a multivalent clostridial vaccine will give some protection against enterotoxaemia, *Cl. perfringens* types B and C and tetanus. However, protective thresholds have not been established for goats and the antibody response to vaccination is often unclear. The immunity produced in goats appears less satisfactory than that produced in sheep. It has been postulated that vaccination may give adequate protection against absorbed epsilon toxin but not against clostridial-induced damage to the intestinal mucosa. However, recent work has shown that vaccination with epsilon toxoid can definitely protect against enterotoxaemia so the reason for reported failures of routine vaccination is still unclear. There is some evidence that 4 in 1 vaccines give better protection than 7 or 8 in 1 vaccines. However, any vaccine used should contain toxoids of *Cl. perfringens* types B, C and D and *Cl. tetani* [**Lambivac**, Hoechst Roussel (G); **Quadrivexin**, Schering-Plough]. A 2 in 1 vaccine giving protection against enterotoxaemia and

tetanus is also available (**Pulpy Kidney and Tetanus Vaccine**, Schering-Plough). Other clostridial diseases are extremely rare in the UK. A 5 in 1 vaccine (**Heptavac**, Hoechst Roussel) should only be used if *Cl. novyi* or *chauvoei* infections have been confirmed in a herd (see Chapter 18). The use of combined clostridial and pasteurella vaccines is not recommended.

> Primary course: **2 ml s.c.** (**Lambivac**, Hoechst Roussel) (G), two doses 4 to 6 weeks apart. This interval of 4 to 6 weeks is important and should not be reduced.
>
> Booster: every 6 months; 4 to 6 weeks before kidding.
>
> Kids: primary course starting at 3 to 4 weeks of age for kids from unvaccinated dams and 8 weeks of age for kids from vaccinated dams.

The length of persistence of maternally derived antibodies and their effect on vaccination is not clear. The age of immunological maturity in kids is likewise not well documented. The recommended site for injection is the lateral side of the neck. Sterile swellings commonly occur as a reaction to vaccination and may range in size from small nodules to several centimetres in diameter.

Note: although generally considered a major disease of goats in the UK, difficulties in confirming the diagnosis mean that the true incidence is unknown. Any 'sudden death' is usually attributed by goatkeepers to enterotoxaemia so that other causes of sudden death, e.g. bacterial septicaemia or mesenteric torsion, are underdiagnosed. Even the finding of epsilon toxin in intestinal contents does *not* prove conclusively that death was caused by *Cl. perfringens* type D and *histological examination of the brain is essential for diagnosis.*

Abomasal ulceration

Aetiology

❑ Abomasal ulceration is poorly documented but probably due to a high concentrate/low roughage diet, particularly in early lactation. Ulceration may be a sequel to chronic acidosis and rumen stasis.

Clinical signs

❑ Many goats with superficial abomasal ulceration show no apparent illness or only occasionally become inappetent. However, deeper ulceration will lead to more severe clinical signs.

❑ Changes in the abomasal tone and motility will in turn affect the motility of the rumen and reticulum.

❑ Perforation with omental adhesion which seals the perforation produces low grade intermittent pain, with grinding of teeth, intermittent pyrexia, reduced ruminoreticular movement, weight loss, reduced milk yield, marked inappetence and intermittent diarrhoea.
❑ Perforation without the defect being sealed may result in an acute diffuse peritonitis and death.
❑ Severe haemorrhage may occur and produce displacement (see below) with adhesions to the left side of the abdomen.

Treatment

❑ Symptomatic; correct the diet.
❑ **Metaclopramide, 0.5–1.0 mg/kg, 5–10 ml/50 kg i.v.** initially, then **i.m. (Emequell,** Pfizer) twice daily (maximum two doses by i.m. injection) to restore abomasal tone and encourage gastric emptying.
❑ Broad-spectrum antibiotics.

Left-sided displacement of the abomasum

See Chapter 15.

Urolithiasis

Urolithiasis is a metabolic disease of male goats, particularly castrates of any age and male kids but occasionally entire males of any age, characterised by the formation of calculi within the urinary tract and urethral blockage. The calculi are generally phosphatic, but oxalates and silicates sometimes occur. In the UK, urolithiasis is virtually always associated with concentrate feeding.

Aetiology

Anatomy

❑ Male animals affected; females can pass calculi easily through their shorter, wider urethra.
❑ Castration arrests penile development so the urethra remains narrow.
❑ Mature animals have a larger urethra than immature animals. *Young castrated animals are at greatest risk.*

Urinary phosphorus excretion

❏ High levels of urinary phosphorus increase the likelihood of the formation of insoluble phosphates and urinary calculi.

❏ Factors which increase urinary phosphorus excretion predispose to calculi formation.

❏ Urinary phosphorus excretion is normally very low in ruminants as any excess phosphorus absorbed is secreted back into the digestive system via the saliva and excreted in the faeces. However, a number of factors may lead to increased urinary phosphorus:

   ■ *High levels of dietary phosphorus:* at a certain level the salivary phosphorus recycling system becomes saturated and urinary phosphorus excretion occurs.

   ■ *Low levels of dietary calcium (low calcium : phosphorus ratio):* a high calcium : phosphorus ratio in the diet reduces the incidence of calculi formation by decreasing the absorption of phosphorus from the gut, thus reducing urinary phosphate levels. Conversely, rations low in calcium increase phosphorus intake.

   ■ *Low fibre diet:* goats on high grain/low fibre diets secrete much lower amounts of saliva than animals on high roughage diets, thus decreasing the amount of phosphorus excreted in the faeces.

   ■ *Low urine output:* any reduction in voluntary water intake will lead to decreased urine volume and increase the likelihood of calculi formation. Feeding concentrates instead of roughages significantly reduces the urine volume.

   ■ *Dietary magnesium levels:* some research has suggested that high magnesium levels *per se* do not cause urolithiasis and may in fact reduce the incidence of calculi formation by reducing urinary phosphorus excretion.

   ■ *Genotypic predisposition:* in sheep, individual differences in phosphorus metabolism have been shown to have a genetic basis – phosphorus is excreted mainly in the faeces by some sheep and in the urine by others. It is probable that there is a similar situation in goats – a familial tendency to calculi formation has been shown in Saanen males. There are definite breed differences in sheep – it is not known if the same applies to goats.

   ■ *Alkaline urine pH:* phosphate calculi form more readily in alkaline urine.

Oxalate-containing plants

❏ Calcium oxalate crystals may form in animals fed on oxalate-containing plants such as sugar beet tops.

❏ This has led to a widespread misconception among goatkeepers that sugar beet *pulp* should not be fed to male goats – there is no scientific evidence to support this theory.

Clinical signs

❏ Anorexia, lethargy.
❏ Signs of abdominal pain – grinding of teeth, looking at abdomen, kicking at abdomen.
❏ Reluctant to walk; stands with legs stretched out.
❏ Strains to urinate; may dribble urine before complete blockage occurs; small calculi may collect on preputial hairs.
❏ Palpation of the abdomen is resented; tight bladder may be palpable in kids.
❏ Rupture of the urethra results in infiltration of urine into the perineal subcutaneous tissues; bladder rupture results in urine accumulation in the scrotum or intra-abdominally.

Diagnosis

❏ Clinical signs. *Note:* initial signs may be mild, i.e. lethargy, inappetence, slight straining – careful examination may be required over 1 or 2 hours.
❏ Examination of the urethral process, palpation of urethra. Angoras can be sat on their rump or laid on their back with front and back legs tied tightly together so that the penis can be exteriorised and held with a swab or cotton wool; larger dairy goats will require sedation with Xylazine.
❏ A provisional diagnosis of urolithiasis is supported by greatly increased levels of blood urea nitrogen (BUN) and creatinine concentrations (up to 10-fold increase or more). Normal level of BUN in the goat is 3.6 to 7.5 mmol/l and creatinine 53 to 124 µmol/l. In cases of urolithiasis, BUN concentrations may be greater than 40 mmol/l.
❏ Plain and contrast radiography will help determine the extent of urethral obstruction, the location of calculi, the numbers of calculi present or if there is urethral rupture.
❏ A distended bladder is identifiable by ultrasonography in the standing goat, using a 5-MHz sector or linear probe head in contact with the inguinal region. Ultrasonography can also readily identify the presence of free urine in the abdomen, following bladder rupture. Urine may leak through the distended bladder wall, without rupture of the bladder, so that free urine in the abdomen may be present even in the presence of a distended bladder.
❏ In cases of bladder rupture, urine can be collected by abdomino-

centesis. Urine can be identified by its smell and urine dipsticks can be used for further analysis.

Treatment

❏ The penis should be exteriorised (see 'Diagnosis') and the urethral process examined – this is the most common site of blockage. Sedation with Xylazine may provide sufficient muscle relaxation to allow a stone to be passed. In most cases, the urethral process will require removing with scissors. If only the urethral process is blocked, urine flow will occur within 5 minutes.

❏ Complete catheterisation to the bladder is anatomically impossible – catheters will not pass the ischial arch as they enter a diverticulum of the urethra – but retrograde catheterisation from the bladder to the penis is possible following surgery.

❏ Where further stones are present or the blockage is not at the urethral process, surgery will be necessary to locate and remove the obstruction. The surgical treatment of obstructive urolithiasis is discussed fully in Chapter 23.

General management for all male goats

❏ Ensure adequate water intake:
- Clean water should always be available; change twice daily.
- Give warm water in cold weather.
- Check the height and suitability of any automatic drinkers and check that the goats know how to use them.

❏ Feed palatable fodder – *good* hay, pea straw, etc.

❏ Feed dried grass products, e.g. lucerne, instead of concentrates – lucerne has the added advantage of being high in calcium.

❏ Do not feed buffers, e.g. $NaHCO_3$.

❏ Feed a well balanced diet with 2:1 Ca:P ration – add calcium as calcium chloride to adjust ration where necessary.

❏ Do not add P to concentrate diets.

Additional control measures in problem herds/flocks

Control

❏ Control in the UK is generally directed towards prevention of phosphatic calculi forming, but it is sensible to have the calculi analysed after each episode and to measure the urine pH before beginning control measures.

❏ Increase the salt (NaCl) content of the ration – an increase to 4% will

be required to alter water intake. Up to 9% NaCl can be fed before decreasing palatability.
❏ Add urine pH modifiers, e.g. NH_4Cl (2% of concentrate ration), fishmeal, citrus pulp, maize gluten.
❏ Give **10 g ammonium chloride** dissolved in 40 ml water by mouth daily.
❏ Ammonium chloride can be fed at 40 mg/kg daily in feed, but is not very palatable and will need disguising in molassed food.
❏ Give **3 mg/kg ascorbic acid**, orally or s.c. daily.
❏ Aim to stabilise urine pH around 5.5 to 6.0.

Liver disease

A general increase in the size of the liver or specific parenchymal changes may result in abdominal pain, either a localised pain detectable by palpation or more generalised pain with changes in posture and unwillingness to move. Other clinical signs of liver disease include oedema, ascites, hepatic encephalopathy (see Chapter 11), photosensitivity (see Chapter 10), anorexia, constipation, diarrhoea (see Chapter 13), jaundice (qv), or weight loss (see Chapter 8).

Diagnosis

❏ *Biochemistry* – aspartate transaminase (AST), gamma glutamyltransferase (GGT), glutamate dehydrogenase (GLDH), sorbitol dehydrogenase (SDH), albumin, globulin; serum protein electrophoresis. The biochemical profile shows whether there is significant liver disease and gives some indication of the type of liver pathology present.
■ *Primary hepatocellular disease*
Damage to hepatocytes gives an increase in serum of specific hepatocyte enzymes. In goats these are GLDH and SDH. In the absence of damage to the bile duct system, GGT remains low.
– Severe anaemia: haemorrhage, haemolytic disease, haemonchosis.
– Copper poisoning (qv).
– Shock.
– Congestive cardiac failure.
– Bacteraemia: liver abscess, salmonellosis.
■ *Cholangiohepatitis*
Damage to the biliary system and the hepatocytes results in elevated serum GLDH *and* GGT.
– Fascioliasis (qv).
– Bacterial cholangitis.

- Pyrrolizidine alkaloid poisoning (qv).
- Primary neoplasia.
- Metastatic neoplasia.
- Aflatoxicosis.

■ *Hepatic cirrhosis*
Persistent liver damage and fibrosis from whatever cause results in a decrease in the functional liver mass. Early or moderate fibrosis is difficult to detect biochemically but when severe will result in decreased serum albumin and increased globulin; GGT and GLDH may be moderately elevated.
Note: jaundice is an uncommon sign in the goat even with severe hepatocellular damage but may occur:
- in haemolytic disease where there is excess production of bilirubin, e.g. copper toxicity, leptospirosis, eperythrozoonosis and poisoning by brassicas or onions.
- following bile duct obstruction, e.g. fascioliasis.

With haemolytic disease, most of the bilirubin is indirect as it has not been conjugated by the hepatocytes; in cholestatic diseases more of the bilirubin will be direct.

Urine bilirubin may not be elevated in haemolytic disease because unconjugated bilirubin is bound to serum protein and will not be filtered by the kidney. Conjugated bilirubin in obstructive cholestasis is water soluble and may be detected in urine.

Urine urobilinogen may be increased in haemolytic jaundice because of increased production but is absent in obstructive cholestasis because no bilirubin is converted into urobilinogen in the intestine.

❏ *Liver biopsy* – use a transthoracic approach via the right ninth intercostal space.
■ Primary hepatocellar disease: necrosis of hepatocytes, cirrhosis, fatty changes, biliary hyperplasia.
■ Bile duct obstruction: plugs of bile in canaliculi, biliary cirrhosis, etc.

Toxic minerals

Copper poisoning

Goats are relatively more resistant to copper poisoning than sheep, but poisoning may occur from high copper mineral licks, eating pig rations containing high levels of copper, drinking footbaths, or dosing with copper sulphate. Calf milk replacers containing high copper levels have also been implicated. Low dietary levels of zinc and molybdenum, which are copper antagonists, may increase copper intake even when dietary copper levels are not obviously high. Copper accumulates in the liver until maximum hepatic levels are reached, when copper is released into the bloodstream, causing an acute intravascular haemolysis.

Clinical signs

- ❏ Often sudden death.
- ❏ Dull, lethargic, pyrexic.
- ❏ Severe abdominal pain.
- ❏ Mucoid diarrhoea.
- ❏ Haemoglobinuria/anaemia if goat survives long enough.
- ❏ Jaundice.

Laboratory findings

- ❏ Heinz body anaemia.
- ❏ Elevated liver enzyme.
- ❏ Marked bilirubinaemia.

Postmortem findings

- ❏ Liver enlarged, friable, icteric.
- ❏ Entire carcase may be jaundiced.
- ❏ Kidneys dark green/black.

Diagnosis

- ❏ Liver, kidney and faecal copper levels markedly elevated.

Treatment

- ❏ **Ammonium tetrathiomolybdate** either **1.7 mg/kg i.v.** or **3.4 mg/kg s.c.** in three doses on alternate days.

Lead poisoning

See Chapter 11.

Fertiliser ingestion

See Chapter 13.

Post kidding problems

Metritis

See Chapter 4.

Retained kid

See Chapter 4.

Peritonitis

Peritonitis from whatever cause produces abdominal pain, ileus, pyrexia and possibly abdominal distension. Most infections occur post kidding, following a uterine tear, as a sequel to metritis or following caesarian section, but peritonitis may also occur as a sequel to rumenitis, after trocharisation of the rumen or other abdominal catastrophe.

Cystitis

Cystitis occurs sporadically, particularly in does. Some does will merely show frequent urination with small amounts of urine being passed, but acute cases will show moderate abdominal pain and occasionally systemic illness.

Cystitis rarely occurs as a sequel to kidding, even when there is infection of the posterior reproductive tract. Stricture of the cervix and vagina, caused by fibrosis following trauma at kidding, has been associated with blockage of the urethra and ureter, obstructing urine flow and leading to cystitis and pyelonephritis. *Pyelonephritis* occurs infrequently in goats, much less frequently than in cattle, possibly because there is a lower incidence of uterine infections postpartum.

Most urinary tract infections involve *Corynebacterium renale*, which is susceptible to procaine penicillin. This is the drug of choice in treating cystitis and pyelonephritis as it is cheap and secreted unchanged by the kidney:

Procaine penicillin, 10 mg/kg i.m. (Duphapen, Fort Dodge; **Norocillin**, Norbrook) daily.

Transabdominal ultrasonography of the standing goat with a 5-MHz sector scanner will identify the bladder and allow an assessment of bladder distension and the thickness of the bladder wall.

Note: (1) Many does will urinate frequently when nervous; (2) it is sometimes difficult to distinguish between the end result of hydro-metra (see Chapter 1), i.e. 'cloudburst', and cystitis. In most cloud-bursts the fluid is rapidly released with sudden decrease in abdominal size and wetting of flanks and perineum, but occasionally the fluid is released slowly over a few days with intermittent straining and pass-ing of small amounts of fluid.

Leiomyoma

Although tumours of the reproductive and urinary systems are uncommon, leiomyomas have been reported as a cause of abdominal straining and urinary tenesmus in goats. Leiomyomas are benign smooth-muscle tumours which arise from the cervix, uterus or vagina. Large tumours may produce sufficient mass in the pelvic inlet to activate the pelvic reflex, as occurs during second-stage labour, or may obstruct the urethra, resulting in a distended bladder. Intravaginal tumours can be detected by digital or speculum examination of the vagina. Intra-abdominal tumours can be detected by ultrasonography, using a 5-MHz sector scanner.

Plant poisoning

See Chapter 20.

COLIC IN KIDS

Any colic signs in kids should be treated as a potential emergency and the owner encouraged to seek veterinary help if the signs persist. Kids regularly die after quite short periods of abdominal pain.

Diarrhoea

See Chapter 13.

Abomasal bloat

See Chapter 15. Abomasal bloat is common in artificially reared kids and is a significant cause of death between 4 and 12 weeks of age.

Mesenteric torsion

Mesenteric torsion leads to infarction of the abomasum, intestine or caecum. Torsion should be considered in cases of bloat that do not respond to treatment.

Aetiology

❏   The aetiology of the condition is poorly understood, but it occurs most commonly in artificially reared kids, probably after an excessive feed of milk in a short time. Torsions occasionally occur in older animals, but the predisposing factors in these cases are not known.

Clinical signs

❏   As for bloat, with severe abdominal pain, distended abdomen and intermittent piercing screams; the kid may throw itself about.
❏   Kids are often found dead.

Postmortem findings

❏   The affected portion of the alimentary tract is enlarged, dark red and filled with gas or blood-stained fluid.
❏   Careful examination reveals a twist in the mesentery.

Treatment

❏   Surgical intervention to correct the torsion may be effective if the condition is diagnosed early. Supportive therapy with intravenous fluids is essential to combat shock, together with analgesics such as **flunixin meglumine (Finadyne**, Schering-Plough).

Note: other abdominal catastrophes such as *intussusception* and *caecal torsion* will also produce signs of severe colic.

Coccidiosis

In heavy coccidial infections, intense colic and shock can be produced by the damage to the intestinal cells during release of meronts and merozoites so that kids may be found collapsed or dead.

Ruminal bloat

See Chapter 15.

Clostridium perfringens type D (enterotoxaemia)

Enterotoxaemia is a potential problem in all ages of goat as the causative agent is present in most herds (see earlier this chapter).

Urolithiasis

Urolithiasis (see earlier this chapter) should be considered as a cause of colic in older male kids.

Visceral cysticercosis

Infection with large numbers of *Cysticercus tenuicollis*, the metacestode of the canine tapeworm *Taenia hydatigena*, occasionally causes acute disease in kids under 6 months because of damage to the liver parenchyma. Clinical signs include depression, anorexia, pyrexia, weight loss, abdominal discomfort and occasionally death due to acute haemorrhage.

Plant poisoning

See Chapter 20.

Further reading

Acute impaction of the rumen

Braun, U., Rihs, T. and Schefer, U. (1992) Ruminal lactic acidosis in sheep and goats. *Vet. Rec.*, 18 April, 343–9.
Michell, R. (1990) Ruminant acidosis. *In Practice*, November 1990, 245–9.
Underwood, W.J. (1992) Rumen lactic acidosis. Part I. Epidemiology and pathophysiology. *Comp. Cont. Ed. Pract. Vet.*, **14** (8), 1127–33.
Underwood, W.J. (1992) Rumen lactic acidosis. Part II. Clinical signs, diagnosis, treatment and prevention. *Comp. Cont. Ed. Pract. Vet.*, **14** (9), 1265–70.

Enterotoxaemia

Baxendell S.A. (1984) Enterotoxaemia of goats. *Proc. Univ. Sydney Post. Grad. Comm. Vet. Sci.*, **73**, 557–60.
Blackwell, T.F. and Butler, D.G. (1992) Clinical signs, treatment, and post-mortem lesions in dairy goats with enterotoxaemia; 13 cases (1979–1982). *J. Am. Vet. Med. Assoc.*, **200** (2), 214–17.

Uzal, F.A. and Kelly, W.R. (1998) Protection of goats against experimental enterotoxaemia by vaccination with *Clostridium perfringens* type D epsilon toxoid. *Vet. Rec.*, **142**, 722–5.

Leiomyoma

Cockcroft, P.D. and McInnes, E.F. (1998) Abdominal straining in a goat with a leiomyoma of the cervix, *Vet. Rec.*, **142**, 171.
Scott, P. (1998) Ultrasonography of the ovine urinary tract. *UK Vet*, **3** (6), 67–73.

Liver disease

Ellinson, R.S. (1985) Some aspects of clinical pathology in goats. *Proc. Course in Goat Husbandry and Medicine*, Massey University, November 1985, 105–122.
Pearson, E.G. (1981) Differential diagnosis of icterus in large animals. *Calif. Vet.*, **2**, 25–31.
Pearson, E.G. and Craig, A.M. (1980) The diagnosis of liver disease in equine and food animals. *Mod. Vet. Pract.*, **61** (3), 233–7.

Urolithiasis

Baxendell, S.A. (1984) Urethral calculi in goats. *Proc. Univ. Sydney Post. Grad. Comm. Vet. Sci.*, **73**, 495–7.
Cuddeford, D. (1988) Ruminant urolithiasis: cause and prevention. *Goat Vet. Soc. J.*, **10** (1), 10–14.
Oehme, F.W. and Tillman, H. (1965) Diagnosis and treatment of ruminal urolithiasis. *J. Am. Vet. Med. Assoc.*, **147**, 1331–9.

15 Abdominal Distension

Abnormal distension must be distinguished from normal anatomical changes. Goats carry their fat deposits intra-abdominally rather than subcutaneously, so *overweight goats* may appear to have abdominal distension. *Pygmy goats* are achondroplastic dwarfs with relatively large abdomens, when compared to other breeds. In older goats of some breeds, particularly British Toggenburgs, the abdominal muscles may drop ventrolaterally in late pregnancy so that subsequently the abdomen remains permanently lower than normal. Many causes of abdominal distension will produce some degree of abdominal pain (see Chapter 14). Tables 15.1 and 15.2 list the causes of abdominal distension in adults and kids, respectively.

Initial assessment

❑ Age and sex, pregnant or non-pregnant.
❑ Sudden or slow onset of abdominal distension.
❑ Feeding history – type of feed, change in diet, age at weaning, kid feeding regime.
❑ Routine medication, including worming.
❑ General physical examination – most cases of abdominal distension will involve the alimentary tract or pregnant goats.
❑ Specific examination of the digestive system:
  ■ visual inspection: abdominal contour from behind, position of distension;
  ■ palpation of left abdominal wall and rumen: filling of rumen;
  ■ percussion: tympanitic sounds, pain;
  ■ auscultation: rumen mobility.

Further investigations

❑ Abdominocentesis, trocharisation, passage of stomach tube (see Chapter 14).
❑ Ultrasonography in the standing goat, using a 5-MHz sector transducer, to determine presence or absence of live fetuses.

Table 15.1 Abdominal distension in adult goats.

	Distension
Normal goats	
Abdominal fat	Bilateral
Dropped stomach	Bilateral
Pygmy goats	Bilateral
Ruminal distension	
Primary ruminal tympany (frothy bloat)	Left paralumbar fossa initially, then entire left side, then also right ventral abdomen
Secondary ruminal tympany (choke)	As primary tympany
Impacted rumen	Low left
Abomasal distension	
Abomasal impaction	Right ventral
Left-sided displacement	
Reproductive	
Pregnancy	Bilateral, particularly low right
False pregnancy (hydrometra)	Bilateral
Hyrops uteri (hydroallantois, hydramnios)	Bilateral
Ovarian tumour	Bilateral
Ventral hernia	Low right
Ascites	
Chronic liver congestion	Bilateral
Fascioliasis	Bilateral
Cardiac failure	Bilateral
Abdominal tumour	Bilateral
Ruptured bladder (urolithiasis)	Bilateral ventral

ADULT GOATS

Ruminal distension

Primary ruminal tympany (frothy bloat)

Aetiology

❏ Grazing lush pastures, particularly clover or lucerne in the spring; sudden introduction of grass clippings or excessive vegetable waste, etc. produces a rumen filled with gas or frothy material.

Clinical signs

❏ Depression.
❏ Abdominal pain – teeth grinding, shifting of weight on the feet, kicking at the abdomen.

- ❏ Abdominal distension – more obvious in the left flank, but the whole of the abdomen is enlarged.
- ❏ Dyspnoea – mouth breathing, extension of the head, protrusion of the tongue.

Treatment

- ❏ First-aid treatment by owner – drench with 100 to 200 ml of any non-toxic vegetable or mineral oil or with a proprietary bloat drench; or with 8 to 10 ml medical turpentine in 100 ml liquid paraffin. In an emergency 10 ml washing-up liquid will suffice. Massage the abdomen to spread the oil.

  Stand the goat with the front feet raised, tie a 30-cm stick through the mouth like a bridle and smear honey or treacle on the back of the tongue to promote continual chewing. Gentle exercise may encourage eructation.

  Trocharise the rumen on the left side with a 14- or 16-g 38- or 50-mm needle.
- ❏ Veterinary treatment continues the treatment started by the owner with release of gas by means of a stomach tube or trocharisation with a needle or sheep trocar and cannula. Oil or bloat remedy can be introduced directly into the rumen through a cannula.
- ❏ Increase the fibre in the diet by feeding hay before a return to feeding legumes or grazing.

Prevention

- ❏ Allow only limited access to grazing.
- ❏ Avoid any sudden introduction of fermentable material to the diet.
- ❏ Provide sufficient fibre in the diet in the form of hay.
- ❏ Smearing vegetable oil on the coat before grazing will promote a regular intake of oil by licking so preventing gas buildup.

Secondary ruminal tympany ('choke')

Aetiology

- ❏ A physical obstruction to eructation causes a build up of gas in the rumen, e.g. *oesophageal obstruction* caused by a foreign body such as a piece of apple or rootcrop or a tumour at the region of the thoracic inlet, e.g. thymoma (see Chapter 9).
- ❏ Spasm of the reticuloruminal musculature in *tetanus* and interference with oesophageal groove functions in cases of *diaphragmatic hernia* may also lead to chronic ruminal tympany.

❏ A degree of ruminal tympany may be observed in diseases such as *listeriosis* because of pharyngeal paralysis.

Treatment

❏ First-aid treatment by the owner as for primary tympany – small amounts of oil may help lubricate an obstruction.
❏ Veterinary treatment – trocharisation to relieve the build up of gas.
❏ Administration of an antispasmolytic drug will aid relaxation of oesophageal musculature around a foreign body.
  Metamizole, Hyoscine butylbromide, 5 ml i.v. (Buscopan Compositum, Boehringer Ingelheim).
❏ Consider oesophagostomy where the foreign body is palpable in the neck if conservative methods are unsuccessful.

Rumen impaction

Rumen impaction is uncommon in the UK, unless goats are fed high fibre, low energy diets. The distension is in the lower left ventral abdomen, where the rumen is palpably hard. Affected animals are lethargic and inappetent, with decreased milk yield. Some animals have mild bloat. Daily dosing with 100 to 200 ml non-toxic mineral or vegetable oil may soften the impaction, but many goats will require a rumenotomy.

Abomasal distension

Abomasal impaction

Abomasal impaction is uncommon in the UK, as diets do not generally predispose to the condition, which is the result of high fibre, low digestible feeds, particularly during pregnancy. There is progressive lower right ventral abdominal distension and the abomasum may be palpably hard and doughy. Affected animals lose weight and pass soft, fibrous, smelly faeces. Treatment with 100 to 200 ml non-toxic mineral or vegetable oil daily, coupled with an improved, less fibrous diet will resolve early cases. Severe impactions have a more problematical outcome.

Left-sided displacement of the abomasum

Aetiology

❏ Left-sided displacement of the abomasum is poorly documented in the goat, but is probably related to high levels of concentrate feeding in late pregnancy. During pregnancy the abomasum is pushed under the rumen by the expanding uterus. After parturition the rumen resumes its normal position, trapping the abomasum.

Clinical signs

- ❏ Selective anorexia – refuses concentrates but eats hay.
- ❏ Reduced ruminal contractions; rarely cuds.
- ❏ Initial constipation, then diarrhoea.
- ❏ Secondary ketosis – smell of ketones on breath, positive Rothera's reaction to milk.
- ❏ Auscultation of the left flank reveals abnormal sounds – high pitched metallic tinkling and ringing sounds which may be spontaneous or can be elicited.

Treatment

- ❏ A spontaneous cure may occur with exercise and access to browsings.
- ❏ Conservative treatment with starvation and rolling.
- ❏ Surgical replacement and anchorage.
- ❏ After spontaneous cure or surgery, concentrate feeding should be reintroduced very gradually over a period of 2 or 3 weeks.

Other causes of abomasal distension

Apart from abomasal impaction and left-sided displacement, there are virtually no reports of abomasal problems in goats. In sheep, abomasal enlargement has variously been caused by abomasal emptying defects, inadequate rumination caused by conditions such as teeth problems, vagus indigestion and adenomata of the abomasal mucosa.

Distension related to pregnancy and the reproductive tract

Normal pregnancy, false pregnancy (*hydrometra*) and *hydrops uteri* (*hydrallantois* and *hydramnios*) all cause abdominal distension (see Chapter 1). *Ovarian tumours* can produce large amounts of intra-abdominal fluid.

Ventral hernia

Rupture of the ventral abdominal muscles occasionally occurs following trauma or abdominal distension, resulting in abdominal swelling and dropping of the udder. Most cases occur in late pregnancy when increasing intra-abdominal pressure weakens the muscle and tendinous support of the abdominal wall, particularly the external and internal abdominal oblique muscles. Manual or surgical intervention at parturition is usually necessary. The hernia can be corrected surgically after kidding.

Ascites

Ascites is uncommon in goats but may arise in *fascioliasis* (see Chapter 8) as a result of blood loss and decreased hepatic synthesis of albumin and occasionally from *chronic liver congestion* or *right-sided cardiac failure*.

Abdominal tumours

Both *intestinal* and *ovarian adenocarcinomas* have been associated with accumulation of large amounts of intra-abdominal fluid.

Ruptured bladder (urolithiasis)

A blocked urethra as a result of urolithiasis in male goats will lead to rupture of the urinary bladder and collection of urine in the ventral abdomen (see Chapter 14).

KIDS FROM BIRTH TO 1 WEEK OLD

Prematurity

Many premature kids have a flaccid, slightly distended abdomen. There may be additional evidence of abortions or stillbirths within the herd.

Congenital abnormalities

Alimentary tract defects – **atresia ani**, **atresia coli** and **atresia recti** – occur occasionally in kids, leading to increasing abdominal distension, with no production of faeces, decreasing appetite and lethargy. **Pyloric stenosis** produces a more rapid abdominal distension than lower alimentary tract blockages.

Kidney defect or *heart defect* could produce ascites, with slowly increasing abdominal distension.

High alimentary tract obstruction

Rarely, *pyloric obstructions*, e.g. with milk curd, or *abomasal torsion* occur in very young kids.

OLDER KIDS

Abomasal bloat

Abomasal bloat is common in artificially reared kids and is a significant cause of death in kids between 4 and 12 weeks of age. It should be distinguished from other causes of abdominal distension (Table 15.2).

Aetiology

❑ It is poorly understood, but probably related to the rapid ingestion of large quantities of milk, leading to excessive fermentation and rapid distension of the abdomen with gas and fluid. Proliferation of microorganisms that release an excessive quantity of gas has also been postulated.

Clinical signs

❑ Abdominal distension with drum-like tension on left and right sides.
❑ Colicky pain – grinding of teeth, yawning, constant stretching of the back.
❑ Diarrhoea.
❑ Shock.
❑ Death.

The condition may present as a 'sudden death' (Chapter 18) with the kid being found dead in the morning. All cases of bloat even if mild should be treated seriously and the kid checked at regular intervals.

Treatment

❑ Mild cases may respond to administration of a drench of a table-spoonful of vegetable oil or a proprietary bloat drench. Linseed oil is recommended in many older goat books but is not suitable as a

Table 15.2   Abdominal distension in kids.

	Onset of distension
Birth to 1 week	
Prematurity	Present at birth
Congenital abnormalities	
Alimentary tract defect	Generally slow
Kidney defect	Slow
Heart defect	Slow
High alimentary tract obstruction	
Pyloric obstruction	Sudden
Abomasal torsion	Sudden
Older kids	
Abomasal bloat	Sudden
Ruminal bloat	Sudden
Mesenteric torsion (intestinal bloat)	Sudden
'Pot belly'	
Inadequate nutrition	Slow
Gastrointestinal parasitism	Slow

drench as it may cause cessation of rumination since the regurgitation of stomach contents containing the oil is offensive in the mouth.

More severe cases will require veterinary attention:

❑ Release pressure by trocharising the abdomen on the left side with a 16- or 18-g needle.
❑ Relieve spasm and pain
    Metamisole, Hyoscine, 0.5–2 ml i.v. or i.m. (**Buscopan Compositum**, Boehringer Ingelheim).
❑ Help restore abomasal tone and promote emptying
    Metaclopramide, 0.5–1.0 mg/kg, 0.5–1 ml/5 kg i.v. (**Emequell**, Pfizer).
❑ Administer broad-spectrum antibiotics intramuscularly or intravenously.
❑ Fluid therapy for shocked kid.

Prevention

❑ Regular feeding with milk at the correct temperature and concentration.
❑ Consider feeding whole goats' milk in problem herds – but this is more expensive and there is the danger of CAE spread.
❑ Kids fed from bowls rather than bottles are possibly more prone to

bloat (due to more rapid intake of milk?); consider bottle feeding or a multisuckling system in these herds – but this is more time consuming.
❏ Early wean any kid which has repeat episodes of bloat.

Ruminal bloat

Ruminal bloat may occur in kids during weaning.

Aetiology

❏ Sudden dilation of the abomasum by rapid intake of milk causes inhibition of forestomach motility.
❏ Failure of the oesophageal groove closure reflex allows milk to leak into rumen, leading to excessive fermentation.
❏ Secondary to ruminal stasis and/or diarrhoea.
❏ Secondary to oesophageal obstruction (choke).

Clinical signs and treatment
As for abomasal bloat.

Prevention

❏ Correct feeding technique – establish a routine to ensure oesophageal groove closure at feeding; smaller feeds more frequently.
❏ If the bloat is repetitive, wean the kid completely as early as possible.

Constipation

Constipation seems to be quite common in artificially reared kids in certain herds, presumably as a result of management practices.

Aetiology

❏ Excess of concentrates with insufficient water intake (?), as a sequel to *abomasal impaction*(?)

Clinical signs

❏ Depressed.
❏ Frequent unsuccessful attempts to defaecate.
❏ Low grade abdominal pain – stretching, yawning.
❏ Unwilling to feed or take milk.

Treatment

❑ Drench with a tablespoonful (15 ml) of liquid paraffin with about 2 teaspoonfuls (10 ml) of vegetable oil or proprietary colic drench containing turpentine oil and polymethylisoloxone (**Gaseous Fluid**, Day, Son & Hewitt).

Mesenteric torsion

See Chapter 14.

'Pot belly'

Poorly thriving kids will assume a 'pot bellied' appearance, coupled with poor growth rate. This is generally due to too early weaning, inadequate nutrition or gastrointestinal parasitism.

16 Respiratory Disease

Respiratory disease in goats is generally poorly researched worldwide. There is a paucity of information on the aetiology and frequency of respiratory disease in the UK, but it would appear to be relatively common, ranging from sudden death from peracute pneumonia to slight but persistent coughs and nasal discharges (Table 16.1).

Initial assessment

The preliminary history should consider:

❏ Individual or herd/flock problem.
❏ Possible exposure to infected animals – shows, brought-in stock, etc.
❏ Feeding, e.g. dusty hay; root crops, etc.
❏ Housing – ventilation, building design.
❏ Vaccination.
❏ Overall level of coughing/sneezing in the building.

Normal respiratory rate: adult 15 to 30/minute
                          kid 20 to 40/minute.

Clinical examination

> Clinical signs of respiratory distress may arise from many conditions not directly related to the respiratory tract.

❏ A thorough clinical examination should be made – temperature, pulse, respiratory rate, auscultation of the lungs – to localise lesions to the upper and lower respiratory tract.
❏ Many clinical conditions not directly involving the respiratory tract can result in hyperpnoea and tachypnoea, e.g. bloat, anaemia, pain, hyperthermia and acidosis. Hypocalcaemia may present as an apparently excited pyrexic and pneumonic goat.

Table 16.1   Differential diagnosis of respiratory diseases.

❏   *Nasal discharge*
    Bilateral
        Rhinitis
            viral
            bacterial
            fungal
            mycoplasmal   } unlikely, UK
        Pneumonia (see cough)
        Dusty conditions

    Unilateral
        Sinusitis – *oestrus ovis* (rarely reported)
        Nasal tumour
        Foreign body

❏   *Cough*
    Pneumonia
        bacterial
        inhalation (drench, force feeding, dip, rhododendron poisoning)
        parasitic
        fungal (unlikely, UK)
    Allergic bronchitis
    Congestive cardiac failure
    Oesophageal obstruction
    Lymph node enlargement – lymphosarcoma, caseous lymphadenitis
    Tuberculosis

❏   *Dyspnoea*
    Primary respiratory disease
        bacterial pneumonia
        inhalation pneumonia
        chronic interstitial pneumonia (CAE)
        mycoplasma
        pulmonary adenomatosis
        lung/nasal tumours
        tracheal collapse
    Heat stroke
    Poisoning
        cyanide (*Prunus* family)
        nitrite/nitrate
        urea
        salt
        organophosphorus
    Anaemia
    Cardiac disease – congenital, acquired
    Bloat
    Selenium/vitamin E deficiency
    Hypocalcaemia
    Terminal stages of many disease conditions
    Trauma – thoracic injuries, diaphragmatic hernia

Infectious respiratory disease

> Respiratory disease may have a multifactorial aetiology.

Aetiology

Although several organisms known to produce severe respiratory disease in goats are absent from the UK, including the mycoplasma responsible for contagious caprine pleuropneumonia (CCPP) and peste des petits ruminants virus (PPRV), a number of infectious agents have been isolated from clinical cases or experimentally shown to produce disease in goats in the UK.

Bacteria

Pasteurella

Pasteurella haemolytica and *P. multocida* have been isolated from pneumonic lungs of goats. *Pasteurella haemolytica* serotypes A1, A2 and A6 are the most common isolates in the UK. The disease may be precipitated by stress, e.g. transport, etc. *Pasteurella trehalosi* appears to have no role in caprine respiratory disease.

Clinical signs

❑ The disease syndrome of 'pasteurellosis' may involve other aetiological agents such as viruses or other bacteria and a wide variety of clinical signs ranging from occasional coughing to sudden death, but often an acute pneumonia, particularly in kids.
❑ Lethargic, anorexic, pyrexic.
❑ Tachypnoea, hyperpnoea, dyspnoea.
❑ Abnormal lung sounds – rales, rhonchi, noisy expiration.

Postmortem findings

❑ Exudative bronchopneumonia.
❑ Extensive consolidation of the lung.
❑ Fibrinous pleurisy.

Diagnosis

> Identification of *P. haemolytica* from a swab does not prove the goat has pasteurellosis.

❏ *Pasteurella haemolytica* may be isolated from a nasal or naso-pharyngeal swab as an incidental finding and does *not* indicate that the goat has pasteurellosis.

❏ Postmortem confirmation depends on bacteriology and histology of lung lesions.

❏ *Pasteurella multocida* has been shown to produce an atrophic rhinitis with nose bleeding, sneezing and nasal turbinate atrophy.

Mycoplasma

> Mycoplasma are increasingly reported from cases of respiratory disease in the UK.

Mycoplasma ovipneumoniae and *M. arginini* have been isolated from goats and may act as a predisposing agent for *Pasteurella* infection. *Mycoplasma capricolum, M. conjunctivae* and *Acholeplasma oculi* have also been isolated from animals in the UK. Their role in respiratory disease is uncertain and they are discussed more fully in Chapter 19.

Outwith the UK, severe respiratory disease is produced by a number of mycoplasma, e.g. *M. capripneumoniae* (F38 species), *M. mycoides* subspecies *capri, M. mycoides* subspecies *mycoides* (large colony type).

Other bacteria

Corynebacterium pyogenes, Staphylococcal spp., *Streptococcal* spp., *Haemophilius* spp. and *Klebsiella pneumoniae* among others have been isolated from infected goats. Goats are also susceptible to infection with *Mycobacterium bovis, M. tuberculosis* and *M. avium* (see Chapter 8).

Viruses

> The role of viruses in the aetiology of respiratory disease is unknown.

Several viruses have been isolated from or shown serologically to be present in association with clinical disease.

Herpes

Infectious bovine rhinotracheitis (IBR, BHV-1) virus has been isolated from goats with respiratory and ocular disease, although the goat may not be a natural host for the virus.

Caprine herpes virus type 1 (BHV-6) which causes vulvovaginitis and infertility in New Zealand and Australia does not appear to cause respiratory disease, but strains of caprine herpes virus in the USA have caused severe systemic illness including dyspnoea in kids.

Parainfluenza

A role for parainfluenza virus (PI3) in respiratory disease in goats has been suggested, possibly as a predisposing agent for pasteurellosis.

Respiratory syncytial virus

Although respiratory syncytial virus (RSV) has been isolated from goats in the UK its role in respiratory disease is unclear. In the USA, RSV has been associated with nasolacrimal discharge, pyrexia and coughing.

Caprine arthritis encephalitis

See Chapter 6. Some goats infected with CAE develop a progressive intestinal pneumonia characterised by a chronic cough and weight loss. Pneumonia may occasionally be the major presenting sign.

Pulmonary adenomatosis (jaagsiekte)

Pulmonary adenomatosis (jaagsiekte) is a disease of sheep which has been transmitted experimentally to goats. There is a chronic progressive pneumonia with adenomatosis lesions of the lung alveoli.

Laboratory investigation of infectious respiratory disease

- ❑ Bacteriology – isolation of bacteria from nasal swabs does not confirm an organism as being responsible for disease, merely that it is present in the nasal passages; nasopharyngeal swabs are more useful.
- ❑ Virology – nasopharyngeal swabs can be used for virological examination.
- ❑ Paired serum samples 10 to 14 days apart may be of value.
- ❑ Postmortem examination – histopathology; bacteriology/virology, etc.

Treatment of infectious respiratory diseases

- ❑ Isolate affected animal(s) and carefully observe other animals for early signs of disease.

❏ Provide a warm, draught-free environment.
❏ Use antibiotics to control bacterial pneumonias or prevent secondary bacterial infection. [Do not use **tilmicosin** (**Micotil**, Elanco), as this drug is associated with a high death rate in goats.]
❏ Use non-steroidal anti-inflammatory drugs to reduce pulmonary congestion and pyrexia:

> **Flunixin meglumine, 2 mg/kg, 2 ml/45 kg i.v. or i.m. (Finadyne Solution,** Schering-Plough).
> **Carprofen, 1.4 mg/kg, 1 ml/35 kg i.v. or s.c. (Zenecarp Solution,** C-Vet).
> **Ketoprofen, 3 mg/kg, 1 ml/33 kg i.v. or i.m. (Ketofen,** Merial).
> **Meloxicam, 0.5 mg/kg, 1 ml/10 kg i.v. or s.c. (Metacam 5 mg Solution,** Boehringer Ingelheim).

Control of infectious respiratory diseases

❏ Strong, well-nourished kids will be less susceptible to respiratory infection.
❏ Avoid mixing different age groups in one air space.
❏ Operate an 'all-in-all-out' policy for batches of kids.
❏ Ensure a well ventilated draught-free environment.
❏ *Pasteurella* vaccination – ideally *Pasteurella* vaccines should contain *P. haemolytica* serotypes A1, A2 and A6 and all serotypes of *P. multocida*, but no vaccine available in the UK meets these requirements. The cattle vaccine **Pastobov** (Merial) has been used in goats. Pastobov contains serotype A1, but some cross immunity to other types, including A6, can be expected, but not to *P. multocida*. The vaccine also stimulates development of antileucotoxin antibodies.

> Primary course, 2 ml, two injections at 3- to 4-week intervals.
> Booster dose – 2ml annually.
> The vaccination can be given at the same time as clostridial vaccination but at a separate site.

> It is not recommended to use combined clostridial and pasteurella vaccines.

❏ Vaccination against respiratory viruses – at present there is no convincing evidence that vaccination against respiratory viruses, such as RSV or PI3, is useful in controlling respiratory disease in goats.

Parasites

Dictyocaulus filaria

❑ The lungworm *Dictyocaulus filaria* infects both sheep and goats.
❑ Direct life cycle with larvae being passed in faeces.
❑ Found in the trachea and bronchi.
❑ Not often a major pathogen; respiratory signs most likely in the south of England during late summer/autumn following larval buildup on pasture during the summer.

Epidemiology

❑ Larvae overwinter on pasture.
❑ Carrier sheep perpetuate the infection.

Clinical signs

❑ Coughing, tachypnoea, naso-ocular discharge.
❑ Inappetence, weight loss.
❑ Secondary infection may result in pyrexia and dyspnoea but severe clinical parasitic bronchitis is rare.

Diagnosis

❑ Larvae in faeces after a Baerman or $ZnSO_4$ flotation.

Treatment

❑ **Levamisole 12.5 mg/kg, orally.**
❑ **Mebendazole 22.5 mg/kg; Febental, Fenbendazole, Oxfendazole, 7.5 mg/kg, orally.**
❑ **Ivermectin 10 mg/50 kg, 12.5 ml/50 kg** orally [**Oramec**, Merial] G.
❑ **Abamectin, Doramectin, Ivermectin, Moxidectin, 10 mg/50 kg, 1 ml/50 kg sc.**

> Do not use injectable levamisole in goats with possible lung worm infection.

Muellerius capillaris

❑ The lungworm *Muellerius capillaris* infects both sheep and goats; goats are more susceptible to disease.
❑ Indirect life cycle, with slugs and snails ingesting the larvae and acting as intermediate hosts.

❏ Found in the alveolar ducts, small bronchioles, subpleural connective tissue and lung parenchyma.

Epidemiology

❏ Goats are infected during their first summer on pasture by eating intermediate hosts on herbage. Level of infection increases with age so that clinical disease is generally seen in adult goats over 3 years old.

Clinical signs

❏ Variable, ranging from mild cough to severe chronic cough and dyspnoea.

Diagnosis

❏ Larvae in faeces after Baerman or $ZnSO_4$ flotation.

Treatment

❏ **Fenbendazole**, **30 mg/kg** in single dose or **15 mg/kg** daily for 3 to 5 days orally.
❏ **Abamectin, doramectin, ivermectin, moxidectin, 10 mg/50 kg, 1 ml/50 kg s.c.**
❏ Immature worms may not be eliminated by treatment, which should therefore be repeated after about 3 weeks.
❏ Levamisole, particularly in injectable form, may produce a hypersensitivity reaction in the lungs due to the death of large numbers of *M. capillaris* and should thus be used with extreme caution in any animals suspected of having a heavy worm burden.

Protostrongylus rufescens

❏ The lungworm *Protostrongylus rufescens* has not been reported as pathogenic in the UK but reported as leading to secondary pneumonia and pleuritis in the USA.
❏ Found in the bronchioles.

Hydatid cysts

❏ A proportion of hydatid cysts reach the lungs and may produce respiratory signs, particularly if a secondary pasteurellosis occurs.

Airway obstruction

Foreign bodies in the trachea or the oesophagus [see "Secondary ruminal tympany ('choke')", Chapter 15] can result in coughing and signs of respiratory distress. *Lymph node enlargement* in the neck can impede air flow (may be caused by caseous lymphadenitis). *Tracheal collapse* has been recorded. *Tumour* – thymomas or thymic involvement in multi-centric lymphosarcoma may affect the respiratory or cardiovascular systems.

Inhalation pneumonia

Inhalation pneumonia may follow drenching, stomach tubing, etc. or *rhododendron poisoning* (see Chapter 20) where vomiting results in inhalation of rumen contents.

Trauma

Injury to the throat from drenching guns or barbed plant material can result in cellulitis, pharyngitis and respiratory signs. Trauma can also result from penetrating thoracic wounds, fractured ribs, etc., and *diaphragmatic hernia*.

Heat stress

Goats being transported, confined in buildings or attending agricultural shows in hot weather will often show heat stress – excessive panting, increased heart rate, excessive thirst, etc. Severe cases progress to respiratory and circulatory collapse, convulsions, coma and death.

Allergic alveolitis

Exposure to dusty conditions or feed may result in an allergic alveolitis with a chronic non-productive cough.

Treatment

❏ Remove from cause, damp hay.
❏ **Clenbuterol, 0.8 mcg/kg, 1.25 ml/50 kg**, slow **i.v.** or **i.m.** (**Ventipulmin**, Boehringer Ingelheim)
            2.5 g/50 kg orally (Ventipulmin granules, Boehringer Ingelheim) in feed twice daily.

Neoplasia

Primary and secondary lung tumours are very rare. *Enzootic intranasal tumours* have been described in goats, with a serosanguinous nasal exudate, stertorous breathing and dyspnoea.

Other conditions producing respiratory signs as part of a clinical syndrome

❏ *Hypocalcaemia* (see Chapter 11) may present as an apparently excited, pyrexic and pneumonic goat. When in doubt give calcium and magnesium.
❏ *Poisoning:*
  ■ nitrites/nitrates
  ■ urea
  ■ organophosphorus.
❏ *Bloat* (see Chapter 14).
❏ *Anaemia* (see Chapter 17).
❏ *Selenium/vitamin E deficiency* (see Chapter 7) – kids with white muscle disease may show dyspnoea, coughing and abnormal respiratory sounds.

Further reading

General

Harwood, D.G. (1989) Goat respiratory disease. *Goat Vet. Soc. J.*, **10** (2), 94–8.
Martin, W.B. (1983) Respiratory diseases induced in small ruminants by viruses and mycoplasma. *Rev. Sci. Tech. Off. Int. Epizool.*, **2** (2), 311–34.
McSporran, K.D. (1985) Pneumonia. *Proc. Course in Goat Husbandry and Medicine*, Massey University, November 1985, 123–5.
Robinson, R.A. (1983) Respiratory disease of sheep and goats. *Vet. Clin. North Am.: Large Animal Practice*, **5** (3), November 1983, 539–56.

Lungworms

Lloyd, S. (1982) Control of parasites in goats. *Goat Vet. Soc. J.*, **3** (1), 2–6.

Mycoplasma

Jones, G.E. (1983) Mycoplasmas of sheep and goats. *Vet. Rec.*, **113**, 619–20.
MacOwan, K.J. (1984) Mycoplasmosis of sheep and goats. *Goat Vet. Soc. J.*, **5** (2), 21–4.

17 Anaemia

Initial assessment

The preliminary history should consider:

❑ Individual or flock/herd problem.
❑ Grazing – haemonchosis and fascioliasis common in certain areas; access to poisonous plants.
❑ Feeding – brassicas, onions, cow colostrum to kids.
❑ Trauma – accidents, fights or dog attacks, obstetric trauma.
❑ Anthelmintic treatment.

Clinical examination

Individual animals should be examined for signs of:

❑ Trauma/lacerations – may be internal haemorrhage without obvious external signs.
❑ External parasite infestations, e.g. sucking lice.
❑ Diarrhoea.
❑ Haemoglobinuria.
❑ Oedema – bottle jaw, ascites, ventral abdominal oedema.
❑ Many anaemic animals are also *hypoproteinaemic.*
❑ The mucous membranes should be carefully examined – pale or cyanotic or jaundiced.
❑ Cardiac rhythm may be altered with severe anaemia.
❑ Jaundice (but see below).

Jaundice

> Jaundice is uncommon in goats and always has a poor prognosis.

Jaundice is an uncommon sign in the goat even with severe hepato-cellular damage. However, it may occur (1) in *haemolytic diseases*, e.g. copper toxicity, leptospirosis, eperythrozoonosis and poisoning by brassicas or onions where indirect (unconjugated) bilirubin levels are elevated, or (2) following *bile duct obstruction* in fascioliasis or tumours where direct (conjugated) bilirubin levels are raised. In some cases of liver dysfunction, e.g. hepatitis or photosensitisation, both direct and indirect bilirubin levels may be elevated.

Laboratory investigation

Blood samples

❏ EDTA, serum, fixed smears. For normal haematological values, see Appendix 1.
❏ Normcytic anaemia – infection, carcinomas, protein deficiency, cobalt deficiency, plant poisoning, acute fascioliasis.
❏ Macrocytic anaemia – haemonchosis, recovery from trauma, eperythrozoonosis, subacute/chronic fascioliasis.
❏ Microcytic anaemia – copper deficiency, chronic blood loss.
❏ Examination of smears may show parasitised red blood cells (eperythrozoonosis) or abnormal shaped cells (poikilocytosis) associated with formation of a different type of haemoglobin (HbC).

Table 17.1 shows laboratory findings with different causes of anaemia and suggests possible aetiology.

Faecal sample

❏ Egg counts for haemonchosis and trichostrongylosis (see Chapter 13).
❏ Egg counts for *Fasciola* if in 'fluke' area.
Use sedimentation technique.

Treatment

> Avoid stress by handling patient as little as possible.

A healthy goat can cope with an acute loss of up to 25% of its red cell mass and up to 50% over 24 hours. With chronic blood loss, a PCV as low as 9% can be tolerated without overt signs of clinical disease, provided the goat is not stressed or exerted or is not suffering from another concurrent disease.

Table 17.1   Anaemia. (After Bennett, 1983)

Cause of anaemia	PCV	Haemoglobin	Hypoproteinaemia	Bilirubin	Possible aetiology
Blood loss	Low	Low	Yes	Normal	Haemonchosis Trichostrongylosis Coccidiosis Lice Trauma
Haemolytic anaemia	Low	Low	No	High	Rape, kale or onion poisoning Copper poisoning Leptospirosis Eperythrozoonosis
Hepatic disease	Low or normal	Low or normal	Yes	High	Pyrrolizidine alkaloid poisoning
Hepatic disease + blood loss	Low	Low	Yes	High	Fascioliasis
Aplastic anaemia	Low	Low	No	High	Chronic inflammatory disease Protein deficiency Copper deficiency Cobalt deficiency
Protein loss	High or normal	High or normal	Yes	Normal	Coccidiosis Johne's disease Salmonellosis Trichostrongylosis

❏ Specific therapy for particular disease.
❏ Supportive therapy to correct anaemia and hypoproteinaemia.
  ■ Avoid stress: better to leave untreated than severely stress patient.
  ■ Fluid replacement:
      Lactated Ringer's (Hartmann's) solution, 20–80 ml/kg slowly **i.v. (Aquapharm No. 11**, Animalcare; **Isolec**, Ivex), depending on severity of blood loss.
  ■ Multivitamin/mineral preparations, **5 ml i.m.** or slow **i.v.** (**Vitatrace**, Vetoquinol; **Haemo 15**, Arnolds) every 48 hours.
  ■ High protein diet.
  ■ *Blood transfusion* is probably only indicated in shocked animals following severe acute blood loss.
      Donor: CAE seronegative; take **10 ml/kg** into collection bottle with 50–100 ml of 4% sodium citrate per 400 ml of blood.

> Recipient: give **10–20 ml/kg i.v.** into jugular or cephalic vein or more rapidly in kids **intraperitoneally**.
>
> Avoid repeat transfusions; use adrenaline if transfusion reaction occurs. An immediate improvement should be evident following intravenous transfusion and within 12 to 14 hours of peritoneal administration.

- Hypertonic saline has been used to resuscitate animals in haemorrhagic/hypervolaemic shock, by rapid plasma volume expansion and associated increase in systemic arterial pressure and cardiac output.

  > **Hypertonic saline (7.2%, 2400 mOsm/l), 5 ml/kg** rapidly **i.v.** (in < 7 minutes).

  Immediately after infusion animals will often drink large amounts of warm water to which oral electrolytes can be added if appropriate. Treatment with hypertonic saline should be followed by full replacement of fluid deficits using isotonic solutions.

Helminthiasis

Haemonchosis

> Haemonchosis may present as sudden death.

(See gastrointestinal parasitism, Chapter 13.) A sudden hot spell can produce rapid development of larvae on pasture and sudden development of disease in kids or even adults in the spring or summer. Severe anaemia and hypoproteinaemia may be produced very rapidly, before loss of condition is observed, and a kid may be found dead.

Chronic haemonchosis occurs in cooler years, with ingestion of low to moderate numbers of larvae, leading to prolonged chronic blood loss and anaemia.

Note: Suspect resistance to anthelmintics or underdosing (*weigh* animals) where goats have been regularly wormed.

Diagnosis

- ❏ Anaemia/hypoproteinaemia.
- ❏ Abomasal contents reddish/black with 'barber pole' worms in large numbers.
- ❏ Faecal egg counts.

Trichostrongylosis

(See gastrointestinal parasitism, Chapter 13.) In trichostrongylosis, anaemia is generally present as part of a clinical syndrome involving diarrhoea, weight loss, unthriftiness and hypoproteinaemia.

Diagnosis

❏ Anaemia/hypoproteinaemia.
❏ Egg counts.

Fascioliasis

See Chapter 8. Generally, fascioliasis is a chronic condition in goats, resulting in hypoproteinaemia and anaemia.

Diagnosis

❏ Anaemia/hypoproteinaemia.
❏ Faecal egg counts.
❏ Postmortem findings.

Protozoal causes

Coccidiosis

See Chapter 13. Haemorrhage in the intestine caused by coccidiosis may result in anaemia and hypoproteinaemia.

Diagnosis

❏ History.
❏ Clinical signs.
❏ Faecal occyst counts.
❏ Postmortem findings.

Eperythrozoonosis

As *Eperythrozoon ovis* occurs in the UK and may infect goats, it should be considered as a remote possible cause of anaemia.

Babasiosis and anaplasmosis

Babasiosis and anaplasmosis infect goats outwith the UK.

Sarcocystosis

See Chapter 2.

Bacterial causes

Leptospirosis

Goats do not appear to act as primary reservoirs of leptospiras, infection occurring spasmodically from contact with the organism in their environment or from carrier animals of other species.

Infection is generally poorly documented worldwide, with the serovar *pomona* the most common reported. Serological surveys in New Zealand have shown the serovars *bratislava* and *ballum* and *copenhagi* to predominate, followed by *pomona, hardjo, tarassovi* and *australis*, but despite serological evidence of widespread exposure to leptospira species there has been little evidence of active infection. No serological surveys of goats in the UK have been carried out.

Most animals exposed to leptospira do not develop clinical disease, but, outwith the UK, sporadic reports of acute disease have been recorded. Severely affected animals are pyrexic and dyspnoeic, with anaemia, haemoglobinuria and occasionally jaundice as a result of intravascular haemolysis. In goats, abortion is reported to occur only following septicaemia in acute infections, although in sheep the serovars *hardjo, pomona, ballum* and *bratislava* have been implicated in late term abortions, stillbirths and the birth of weak lambs in the UK without other clinical signs of disease. *Hardjo* infection in sheep has been shown to produce an agalactia similar to that seen in cows, with soft udders, return to milk in 3 to 4 days and starvation of lambs if not hand reared. *Hardjo* has also been recovered from the brains of young lambs showing meningitis.

Plant poisoning

See Chapter 20.

Bracken (*Pteridium aquilinum*)

Goats seem less susceptible to bracken poisoning than sheep, but prolonged grazing of the plant may result in an acute haemorrhagic syndrome or blood loss due to tumours in the bladder or intestine.

Pyrrolizidine alkaloids

Pyrrolizidine alkaloids, e.g. found in *ragwort* (qv), result in haemor-rhages following liver damage.

Brassicas

Prolonged feeding of kale and other brassicas such as rape, cabbage, Brussels sprouts and swede tops in large quantities results in haemolytic anaemia as a result of the conversion of S-methyl cysteine sulphoxide (SMCO) to dimethyl disulphide that destroys red blood cells.

Clinical signs

❏ Lethargy, inappetence, depressed milk yield.
❏ Anaemia, haemoglobinuria, jaundice.
❏ Pyrexia, tachypnoea.
❏ Diarrhoea.
❏ Death usually occurs in 24 to 48 hours.

Treatment

❏ Remove brassica from diet.
❏ Treat anaemia.

Onions

Onions can be fed over long periods without signs of poisoning but in large amounts produce haemolytic anaemia.

External parasites

Sucking lice

See Chapter 10.

Keds

Keds can also affect goats and produce anaemia.

Trauma

Chronic blood loss from internal or external wounds will result in anaemia.

Cow colostrum

Feeding bovine colostrum to kids may produce a haemolytic syndrome similar to that seen in lambs. Affected kids have severe anaemia and sometimes jaundice. The PCV declines to below normal by 7 days after birth and below 10% within 2 weeks, when clinical signs will be noticed. Initial signs are lethargy and failure to feed, progressing to collapse and death.

Laboratory findings

❏   Direct Coombs test demonstrates bovine IgG on erythrocytes.

Postmortem findings

❏   Extreme pallor, very watery blood; creamy appearance to bone marrow.

Treatment

❏   Blood transfusion (qv), corticosteroids, antibiotics and supportive therapy. Treat any other kids which have received the same batch of colostrum.

Mineral deficiencies

Copper deficiency

See Chapter 5. Copper deficiency may occur alone or in combination with cobalt deficiency. Anaemia occurs as a result of poor iron absorption, with a resultant deficiency in haemoglobin synthesis and microcytic, hypochromic anaemia.

Cobalt deficiency

See Chapter 8. Cobalt deficiency results initially in normocytic, normochromic anaemia, often with haemoglobin and erythrocyte levels within the normal range because of haemoconcentration. Later there may be marked poikilocytosis and macrocytic anaemia with polychromasia.

Mineral poisoning

Copper poisoning

See chapter 14. Copper poisoning results in an acute haemolytic crisis which occurs with sudden release of copper into the bloodstream when maximum hepatic levels are exceeded.

Protein deficiency

Primary protein deficiency due to malnutrition and secondary protein deficiency due to disease, e.g. Johne's disease, may both result in anaemia.

Chronic disease

Chronic disease states such as Johne's disease (qv or alimentary tumours) may result in anaemia through blood loss or secondary protein deficiencies.

Congenital disease

Myelofibrosis is an inherited lethal disease of Pygmy goats in California. Kids are normal at birth but become weak and inactive as early as 2 weeks of age as a progressive profound anaemia, neutropaenia and thrombocytopaenia become established because of a primary bone marrow dysfunction. There is no treatment and kids are usually euthanised.

Further reading

Bennett, D.G. (1983) Anaemia and hypoproteinaemia. *Vet. Clin. North Am.: Large Animal Practice*, **5** (3), November 1983, 511–24.

18 Sudden Death

> Genuine sudden death is rare in animals inspected regularly.

Initial assessment

The preliminary history may play a major role in deciding the cause of death. Consider:

- Individual or group of animals involved.
- Recent introduction or movement of animal(s) involved.
- Age of animal, pregnant/non-pregnant, stage of lactation.
- Feeding – recent changes, access to feed, etc., artificial rearing of kids, milk or milk replacer.
- Vaccination.
- Known disease status.
- Signs of ill health.
- Weather.
- Season of year.

Examination of carcase

- Position of body – possibility of trauma or electrocution.
- Signs of struggling? – terminal convulsions.
- Condition of body:
  - emaciated/good condition
  - bloat
  - discharges from orifices.

Postmortem examination

> Postmortem examination is only of use if carried out very shortly after death.

A thorough, prompt postmortem examination should be carried out. Delay will result in decomposition and reduce the chances of a successful outcome. Some causes of sudden death, e.g. some poisons, hypomagnesaemia, produce no obvious postmortem changes.

Sudden death in kids

Non-infectious causes

> Trauma and abdominal catastrophe are the most common causes of sudden death in kids.

Kids regularly die after short periods of abdominal pain or as a result of trauma, e.g. strangulation in haynets. Other causes are listed below:

❏ Hypothermia/hypoglycaemia – see Chapter 5.
❏ Abomasal bloat ⎫
❏ Ruminal bloat ⎬ – see Chapter 15.
❏ Mesenteric torsion ⎭
❏ Disbudding meningoencephalitis – see Chapter 11.
❏ Trauma.
❏ Anaphylactic shock – it is commonly believed that goats are more likely than other species to suffer anaphylactic shock following repeated injections, particularly of procaine penicillin but also local anaesthetics and occasionally clostridial vaccines.
❏ Plant poisoning – see Chapter 20. Plant poisons may produce no obvious pathological changes, so that evidence of consumption or leaves in the forestomachs may provide vital information.
❏ Chemical poisoning – uncommon
   ■ Copper poisoning (see Chapter 14).
   ■ Arsenic, lead (qv) and other metal poisonings produce acute or chronic illness, but occasionally present as sudden death.
   ■ Organophosphorus insecticides produce no obvious gross lesions at postmortem.
❏ White muscle disease – see Chapter 7.

Infectious causes

❏ Septicaemia, e.g. *Pasteurella*, streptococci.
❏ Coccidiosis – see Chapter 13.
❏ Enterotoxaemia (*Clostridium perfringens* type D) – see Chapter 15.
❏ Listeriosis – see Chapter 11.

❑ Pasteurellosis – see Chapter 16.
❑ Haemonchosis – see Chapter 13.
❑ Salmonellosis – see Chapter 13.

Sudden death in adult goats

Non-infectious causes

❑ Ruminal bloat – see Chapter 14.
❑ Acidosis (ruminal impaction) – see Chapter 14.
❑ Trauma.
❑ Cold stress – Angoras and Cashmere goats shorn in inclement weather without adequate shelter or nutrition.
❑ Anaphylactic shock – see 'Sudden death in kids'.
❑ Plant poisoning – see 'Sudden death in kids'.
❑ Chemical poisoning – see 'Sudden death in kids'.
❑ Hypomagnesaemia – see Chapter 11.
❑ Transit tetany – see Chapter 11.

Infections causes

❑ Gangrenous mastitis – see Chapter 12.
❑ Enterotoxaemia (*Clostridium perfringens* type D) – see Chapter 15.
❑ Listeriosis – see Chapter 11.
❑ Pasteurellosis – see Chapter 16.
❑ Haemonchosis – see Chapter 13.
❑ Acute fascioliasis – see Chapter 8.
❑ Anthrax ⎫
❑ Black leg ⎪
❑ Malignant oedema ⎬ (see below).
❑ Black disease ⎪
❑ Botulism ⎭

Anthrax

Anthrax is rare. The peracute form may produce death in 1 to 2 hours. Acute cases may show pyrexia, tremor, dyspnoea and mucosal congestion. After death, dark unclotted blood discharges from the nostrils, mouth, anus and vulva. The carcase undergoes rapid decomposition and there is absence of rigor mortis.

If anthrax is suspected, the carcase should not be opened until the disease has been proved absent. If a postmortem has been carried out inadvertently there will be evidence of widespread haemorrhage and a grossly enlarged spleen.

Diagnosis

❏ Blood smears from an ear vein should be air dried, fixed with heat and stained with polychrome methylene blue to show *Bacillus anthracis* rods with purple staining reaction of capsule.

Black leg

Black leg is also rare. Goats appear less susceptible than sheep.

Aetiology

❏ Acute infection by *Clostridium chauvoei* spores which enter by skin wounds or via the vulva and vagina at kidding or occasionally via the intestines and settle in muscle masses of the hindquarters, shoulder or lumbar areas. Bruising in these areas provides the anaerobic environment suitable for germination of spores.

Clinical signs

❏ Generally goat is found dead, often in a characteristic position with the affected limb stuck out stiffly and gas and oedema at the affected site.
❏ Decomposition and bloating occur rapidly and there may be blood from the nostrils and anus.

Malignant oedema

Malignant oedema is characterised by acute anaerobic wound infection caused by *Clostridium septicum* or other clostridial organisms. Goats appear less susceptible than sheep, but the disease may occur following fighting and head butting in males ('swelled head' or 'big head').

Clinical signs

❏ Death occurs within 12 to 24 hours of first appearance of clinical signs; affected areas are swollen with emphysema, erythema and extensive frothy exudate from the wound.

Note: multivalent clostridial vaccines should be used as a herd preventative whenever black leg or malignant oedema have been diagnosed in a herd (**Heptavac**, Hoechst Roussel).

Black disease (infectious necrotic hepatitis)

Black disease is rare. It causes acute toxaemia by combined infection with the liver fluke, *Fasciola hepatica* (qv), and *Clostridium novyi* (*Cl.*

oedematiens). Animals are generally found dead with blood-stained froth from the nostrils. Decomposition occurs rapidly. Postmortem shows dark subcutaneous tissue, blood-stained fluid in body cavities and a dark liver with scattered necrotic areas. In fluke areas, routine clostridial vaccination should include *Clostridium novyi* (**Heptavac**, Hoechst Roussel).

Botulism

Ingestion of botulism toxin, produced by *Clostridium botulinum*, in food has occasionally been reported to cause an acute onset of paralysis or sudden death.

Further reading

King, J.M. (1983) Sudden death in sheep and goats. *Vet. Clin. North Am.: Large Animal Practice*, **5** (3), November 1983, 701–10.

19   Eye Disease

Infectious keratoconjunctivitis

Infectious keratoconjunctivitis ('pink eye' or contagious ophthalmia) is an acute contagious disease characterised by inflammation of the conjunctiva and cornea in one or both eyes.

Aetiology

- ❏ The causal agents of the disease are still unclear; it is probable that several agents are involved.
- ❏ Predisposing factors include dusty hay, wind, bright sunlight and dust; overcrowding; long grass; flies.

Mycoplasma

There is strong evidence that *Mycoplasma conjunctivae* is a major causal agent of keratoconjunctivitis in the UK. *Ureaplasma, M. ovipneumoniae, M. arginini* and *Acholeplasma oculi* have also been isolated from keratoconjunctivitis in sheep and goats, but their role in natural disease remains debatable. Predisposing factors such as wind or dust probably play an important part.

Chlamydia

Chlamydia psittaci produces keratoconjunctivitis in both sheep and goats. There may be abortions (see Chapter 2) occurring in the same herd/flock and polyarthritis in kids (see Chapter 7).

Rickettsia

Colesiota (Rickettsia) conjunctivae is reportedly a common cause of keratoconjunctivitis in sheep and possibly goats outwith the UK, although in goats only a mild conjunctivitis is produced. It is probable that many cases attributed to this organism were in fact produced by *Mycoplasma* spp.

Bacteria

Bacteria probably act as secondary invaders where the primary damage is produced by smaller organisms, increasing the severity of the condition. *Branhamella ovis* is commonly isolated from sheep with affected eyes. *Moraxella* spp. may also be involved.

Listeria monocytogenes (see Chapter 11) may also cause keratoconjunctivitis as part of a syndrome involving neurological signs and/or abortion. Individual goats occasionally only show the ocular lesions – conjunctivitis, nystagmus, hypopyon and endophthalmitis.

Viruses

Infections bovine rhinotracheitis (IBR) can cause a mucopurulent conjunctivitis in goats.

Transmission

❑ Flies and lice are possible vectors for the disease.
❑ Carrier goats exist for *Mycoplasma* spp. and *C. psittaci* and can thus introduce the disease into a new herd; carriers continue the disease within a herd and as immunity is poor individual goats may suffer repeated infection.
❑ Contact at shows will facilitate spread between herds.
❑ Close contact at feeding or even at grass will spread the disease within a herd.
❑ Cross infection occurs between sheep and goats.

Clinical signs

❑ This is a herd/flock problem as it is very infectious; Angoras may be more severely affected than dairy breeds; older goats may be more severely affected, following previous exposure.
❑ Conjunctivitis with marked hyperaemia, excessive lacrimation and blepharospasm so animals stand with affected eyes closed.

Note: cobalt deficiency ('pine') (see Chapter 8) and *iodine toxicity* (see Chapter 5) can produce excessive lacrimation which might be confused with keratoconjunctivitis.

❑ Later corneal opacity and vascularisation; corneal ulceration in severe cases with a purulent ocular discharge and possible rupture of the anterior chamber of the eye.
❑ Vision is affected in severe cases so animals may have difficulty feeding and lose condition.
❑ Cloudiness of the cornea may persist for several weeks.

Diagnosis

- ❏ Clinical signs as herd/flock outbreak.
- ❏ Swab *early* cases – vigorously swab conjunctivae and cornea:
  - ■ submit dry or in Stuart's medium for bacteriology;
  - ■ place in mycoplasma transport medium;
  - ■ place in chlamydia transport medium.
- ❏ Scrapings of everted conjunctiva can be placed on a slide, fixed in methanol and stained with Giemsa or examined using fluorescent antibody techniques for *Mycoplasma* or *Chlamydia*.
- ❏ Blood samples for *Chlamydia* serology.

Treatment

- ❏ Topical **tetracycline ointments** daily for 5 to 6 days, together with **long-acting tetracycline injections intramuscularly**, are generally effective if started early in the course of the disease.
- ❏ Long-acting tetracycline injections can be used prophylactically in the rest of the herd.

Note: treatment will not eliminate the organism in all cases, so carrier animals will remain to perpetuate the infection.

- ❏ Severely affected animals should be penned separately in dark surroundings with easy access to food and water.
- ❏ With severe corneal ulceration, third eyelid flaps can be used to protect the cornea.

Foreign bodies

Foreign bodies, such as seeds, shavings, etc., will result in severe conjunctivitis and possible corneal ulceration if untreated. Foreign bodies may lodge behind the third eyelid and will need careful removal, with the goat securely held. Sedation and/or the use of a topical anaesthetic such as 0.5% proparacaine (Ophthaine, Squibb) is advisable. After removal of the foreign body, treatment is as for infectious keratoconjunctivitis.

Trauma

The cornea of goats is commonly traumatised, often by stalks of hay or straw; overlarge tags on the ears of Angora kids may irritate the eye and the eye will also be damaged when entropion is present. Treatment involves correcting or removing the cause of the trauma, then treating the resultant conjunctivitis or corneal damage.

Entropion

Entropion has been reported as an occasional congenital condition in all breeds of dairy goats and Angoras, but is uncommon in the UK. Because it is an hereditable defect, possible carriers, especially male goats, should be identified wherever possible. Surgical correction of the defect can be simply carried out using similar techniques to those used in the dog. Alternatively, the lower eyelid can be everted with skin sutures or by the subconjunctival injection of liquid paraffin or long-acting penicillin – the initial bleb produces immediate reversal of the entropion, followed by a degree of fibrosis which often prevents recurrence. Acquired entropion can arise following trauma and scar formation.

Secondary bacterial infection may occur where chronic irritation of the cornea has been present for some time and should be treated with topical ophthalmic antibiotic ointments.

Photosensitisation

Photosensitisation (see Chapter 10) from whatever cause will affect the head, resulting in swelling of unpigmented skin of the muzzle, drooping ears, swollen eyelids and ocular lesions, i.e. conjunctivitis, keratitis, excessive lacrimation, corneal oedema, blepharospasm and photophobia.

Affected animals should be removed from exposure to sunlight and any possible photosensitising substance.

Blindness

Blindness is an uncommon presenting sign in goats, usually occurring in conjunction with other neurological signs (see Chapter 11) or severe keratoconjunctivitis. The following conditions should be considered in apparently blind goats:

❏ Keratoconjunctivitis.
❏ Cerebrocortical necrosis.
❏ Pregnancy toxaemia.
❏ Pituitary abscess syndrome.
❏ Cerebral abscess.

❏   Coenurosis cerebralis (gid).
❏   Caprine arthritis encephalitis virus.
❏   Listeriosis.
❏   Poisoning:
  ■   lead,
  ■   plant, e.g. rape,
  ■   rafoxanide.
❏   Focal symmetrical encephalomalacia.
❏   Scrapie.
❏   Louping ill.

Further reading

General

Baxendell, S.A. (1984) Caprine ophthalmology. *Proc. Univ. Sydney Post Grad. Comm. Vet. Sci.*, **73**, 235–7.

Moore, C.P. and Whitley, R.D. (1984) Ophthalmic diseases of small domestic ruminants. *Vet. Clin. North Am.: Large Animal Practice*, **6** (3), November 1984, 641–65.

Wyman, M. (1983) Eye disease of sheep and goats. *Vet. Clin. North Am.: Large Animal Practice*, **5** (3), November 1983, 657–76.

Keratoconjunctivitis

Greig, A. (1990) Keratoconjunctivitis. *Goat Vet. Soc. J.*, **11** (1), 7–8.

Hosie, B.O. (1989) Infectious keratoconjunctivitis in sheep and goats. *Vet. Annu.*, **29**, 93–7.

Mycoplasma

Jones, G.E. (1983) Mycoplasma of sheep and goats. *Vet. Rec.*, **113**, 619–20.

MacOwan, K.J. (1984) Mycoplasmoses of sheep and goats. *Goat Vet. Soc. J.*, **5** (2), 21–4.

20 Plant Poisoning

> Goats frequently consume small amounts of
> potentially harmful plants with no apparent ill effect.

Goats, being of an inquisitive nature and of browsing habit, commonly consume small quantities of poisonous plants without ill effect, particularly when the rumen is full of other foodstuffs, and there are very few well documented cases of plant poisoning occurring in goats in the UK. The rumen provides a significant protection from plant poisons for the goat compared to monogastric animals. Thus, moderate levels of oxalates, as found in sugar beet tops or rhubarb, can be metabolised in the rumen, and glycosidic steroidal alkaloids as found in solanaceous plants such as green potatoes and tomatoes can be safely hydrolysed. Most cases of poisoning are caused by garden shrubs, in particular rhododendrons, azaleas and laurels. It seems safest to assume that all evergreen shrubs are poisonous and to keep goats and such plants well separated.

Many plants cause an *immediate poisoning*, e.g. yew, rhododendron. Some plants cause *delayed poisoning* as well as immediate poisoning, e.g. ragwort, St. John's wort, etc. Some plants are equally toxic when fed dry in hay, e.g. ragwort. Some plants are harmless when fresh but poisonous when dry and wilted, e.g. leaves of the *Prunus* family.

In addition to the plants listed in Table 20.1, British Goat Society publications list the following as being dangerous to goats, at least under certain circumstances:

Mayweed, old man's beard or traveller's joy, charlock, bryony, woody nightshade or bittersweet, deadly nightshade, honeysuckle, fool's parsley, buttercup, anemone, lesser celandine, bulbs and their leaves, e.g. daffodil, tulip, aconite, etc., walnut and spindle berry.

Some of the plants listed, e.g. walnut, are generally safe when eaten in small amounts, but large quantities should not be given to stall-fed goats.

Table 20.1 Clinical signs of plant poisoning. (Adapted from Spratling, 1980)

Diarrhoea	*Photosensitisation*	*Vomiting*
Hemlock	Ragwort	Rhododendron
Oak (young leaves)	St. John's wort	Azalea
Wild arum	Buckwheat	Pieris
Castor seed (in foodstuffs)	Bog asphodel	Black nightshade
Foxglove		*Gladiolus* corms
Water dropwort	*Sudden death*	
Box		*Goitre and stillbirth*
Potato (green)	Yew	
Rhododendron	Laurel	Brassica spp.
Linseed	Linseed	Linseed
Blue–green algae	Foxglove	Some clovers
	Water dropwort	
Haemorrhage	Blue–green algae	*Oestrus*
Bracken	*Frothy bloat*	Some clovers
Nervous signs	Legumes, e.g. rapidly growing lucerne	*Stomatitis*
Ragwort		Giant hogweed
Horsetails	*Anaemia*	Cuckoo pint
Hemlock	Rape	
Water dropwort	Kale	*Discoloured urine*
Potato		
Black nightshade	*Constipation*	Haematuria
Male fern		Bracken
Rhododendron	Oak (acorns and old leaves)	Oak
Laburnum	Ragwort	Haemaglobinuria
Rape	Linseed	Rape
Rhubarb		Kale
Common sorrel		Cabbage
Sugar beet tops		Brussels sprouts
Prunus family		
Blue–green algae		

Public health considerations

The excretion in milk of toxins from poisonous plants (Table 20.2) is unlikely in the UK, at least at high enough levels to provide a human health hazard. However, certain plant toxins, e.g. bracken toxins, and carcinogens and pyrrolizidine alkaloids are known to be excreted in goats' milk and the possibility of affecting humans should always be considered, particularly as a particular goat's milk may be consumed by a limited number of people over a long period.

Table 20.2   Plant toxins excreted through milk.

Pyrrolizidine alkaloids	Glucosinolates
Senecio (ragwort)	*Amoracia* (horseradish)
Crotalaria	*Brassica* (cabbage, broccoli, etc.)
Heliotropium	*Nasturtium* (watercress)
Echium	*Raphanus* (radish)
Symphytum (comfrey)	
Cynoglossum (hound's tongue)	Quinolizidine alkaloids
	Lupinus
Piperidine alkaloids	
Conium (hemlock)	

Treatment of plant poisoning

Advice to owners

- ❏ Separate the goat from the plant – it may be possible to actually remove the plant material from the goat's mouth.
- ❏ Keep the goat walking slowly so that it does not settle and start cudding.
- ❏ Give large quantities of strong tea (do not attempt to dose a vomiting animal). The tannic acid in the tea will precipitate many alkaloids and salts of heavy metals and will also have a useful stimulant effect. Strong coffee will also have a stimulant effect.

Note: poisoning by acorns is due to their high tannic acid content – tea should not be given in cases of acorn poisoning.

- ❏ Large doses (500 ml) of liquid paraffin are also commonly used as a first-aid remedy.
- ❏ Treat shock.
- ❏ If possible, identify the source of poisoning.
- ❏ Give demulcents, e.g. a mixture of eggs, sugar and milk, to soothe and relieve irritation of the stomach linings.

Veterinary treatment

- ❏ In most cases there is no specific antidote to the toxic principle involved in the poisoning, and first aid should be continued together with symptomatic treatment, e.g. spasmolytics, intravenous fluids, oral laxatives, B vitamins and antibiotics if there is a danger of inhaling vomit.
- ❏ **Etamiphylline camsylate, 20 mg/kg, 1 ml/7 kg (Millophylline,** Arnolds), can be used as a cardiac and respiratory stimulant.

❏ Rumenotomy should be considered to remove plant material, particularly if this can be done before clinical signs of poisoning have developed.

Specific plant poisoning

> Vomiting in goats is almost always due to plant poisoning.

Rhododendron (rhododendron, azalea, kalma, pieris species)

Aetiology

❏ Rhododendron is the most common plant poison of goats in the UK, from browsing on the living shrubs and eating discarded prunings.
❏ Toxic principle is an andromedotoxin together with a glucoside arbutin.

Clinical signs
Clinical signs appear about 6 hours after ingestion of leaves.

❏ Lethargy, anorexia.
❏ Salivation, repeated swallowing.
❏ Abdominal pain.
❏ Vomiting.
❏ Ruminal bloat.
❏ Recumbency and death.
❏ Inhalation pneumonia may occur secondarily to the vomiting.

Postmortem findings

❏ No characteristic lesions.

Treatment

❏ Symptomatic and supportive therapy.
❏ Spasmolytics, B vitamins, antibiotics, analgesics.

Oxalates

Aetiology

❏ Ingestion of plants containing oxalic acid or its salts, e.g. sugar beet tops, mangold tops, rhubarb leaves, docks (*Rumex* spp.) and wood sorrel (*Oxalis acetosella*).

❏ Goats can detoxify large amounts of ingested oxalates, so poisoning is only likely to arise if large amounts are eaten over a short period. Oxalates combine with blood calcium to produce insoluble calcium oxalate and severe *hypocalcaemia*.

Note:

> The feeding of dried sugar beet to male goats does *not* lead to urolithiasis.

(1) In castrated male goats, the urethra may become blocked by calcium oxalate crystals – this association of sugar beet tops with urolithiasis has led to the common misconception among goatkeepers that sugar beet pulp should not be fed to male goats.

(2) *Ethylene glycol* (*antifreeze*) poisoning results in increased salivation, ataxia, staggering, seizures, recumbency and death. Metabolites of ethylene glycol, e.g. glycolic acid formed by the liver, are responsible for metabolic acidosis and hyperosmolality. Glycolic acid is excreted or further converted to oxalic acid with formation of oxalate crystals and signs of oxalate poisoning.

Clinical signs

❏ Depression, inappetence.
❏ Muscular tremors, ataxia, staggering.
❏ Dyspnoea.
❏ Paralysis, recumbency and death.
❏ May present as sudden death.

Postmortem findings

❏ Calcium oxalate crystals in kidneys and urinary tract.
❏ Hyperaemia of the lungs; scattered haemorrhages.

Confirmation of diagnosis

❏ Oxalate can be detected in kidneys and rumen contents.

Treatment

❏ **Calcium borogluconate 20%, 80–100 ml**, slowly **i.v.** or **s.c.** or half by each route.
❏ Provided treatment is early and kidney damage has not occurred there is rapid response to treatment.

Diagnosis

❑ Ethylene glycol in rumen contents.
❑ Glycolic acid in urine serum or ocular fluid.

Photosensitisation

See Chapter 10.

Prunus family (cyanide)

Aetiology

❑ The leaves of the *Prunus* family, e.g. cherry, laurel, peach, plum, contain a cyanogenic glycoside amygdalin which is converted into hydrogen cyanide in crushed and wilted plants. Thus dried leaves are more dangerous than fresh leaves.

Clinical signs

❑ Sudden death.
❑ Dyspnoea.
❑ Muscular tremors, dilated pupils, ataxia, convulsions.
❑ Mucous membranes bright red.

Postmortem findings

❑ Blood bright red.
❑ Bitter almond smell of rumen contents.

Confirmation of diagnosis

❑ Cyanide estimation on rumen contents or blood (preserve with 1% sodium fluoride).

Treatment

❑ Rumenotomy.
❑ **1% sodium nitrite, 25 mg/kg i.v.** – induces formation of methaemoglobin to which hydrocyanic acid is preferentially bound; followed by **25% sodium thiosulphate, 600 mg/kg i.v.** – combines with hydrocyanic acid to form non-toxic thiocyanate; then **sodium thiosulphate, 30 g orally** every hour to prevent further absorption of cyanide.

Nitrites/nitrates

Aetiology

❏ Nitrates occur in many plants, e.g. mangolds, sugar beet tops and rape. When excess accumulation of nitrate occurs, the plant may be toxic to ruminants. Poisoning is uncommon in the UK but in the USA and Australia may be caused by consumption of weed species which accumulate nitrite.

❏ In the rumen, nitrates are converted to nitrite, which is absorbed and combines with haemoglobin in the blood to form methaemoglobin, preventing the uptake of oxygen and resulting in *hypoxia*.

Clinical signs

❏ Depression.
❏ Abdominal pain, diarrhoea.
❏ Dyspnoea, convulsions, tachycardia.
❏ Ataxia, incoordination, coma and death.

Postmortem findings

❏ Chocolate-coloured blood, petechiation of mucous membranes.

Confirmation of diagnosis

❏ Diphenylamine test on clear body fluids (urine, serum, CSF, aqueous humour).
❏ Nitrite estimation in blood or urine.
❏ Methaemoglobin estimation (stabilise sample in pH 6.6 phosphate buffer).

Treatment

❏ **Adrenaline 20 µg/kg, i.v. or s.c. (Epinephrine injection**, 100 µg/ml; 1 in 10 000).
❏ **Etamiphylline camsylate, 20 mg/kg, 1 ml/7 kg (Millophylline**, Arnolds).
❏ **Methylene blue**, about **10 ml** of **2% aqueous solution i.v.** Repeat if necessary after 6 to 8 hours.

Kale

Haemolytic anaemia

See Chapter 17.

Goitre

See Chapter 9.

Ragwort

Goats demonstrate an apparent tolerance to ragwort but are susceptible if enough is consumed over a long period (a total plant intake in excess of 100% of body weight may be required for toxicity to occur).

Aetiology

❑ Pyrrolizidine alkaloids contained in the plant are hepatotoxic. Poisoning can occur from the fresh plant or hay or silage.

Clinical signs

❑ Depression, inappetence, emaciation.
❑ Incoordination.
❑ Jaundice, anaemia.
❑ Hepatic neurotoxicity, coma, death.

Postmortem findings

❑ Enlarged cirrhotic liver.
❑ Petechial haemorrhages in the digestive tract.
❑ Spongy degeneration of brain and spinal cord.

Treatment

❑ None.

Comfrey

Comfrey contains pyrrolizidine alkaloids and although goats have some resistance to these toxins, long-term consumption could lead to poisoning. The feeding of comfrey and the use of dietary supplements containing comfrey should be discouraged. Comfrey preparations used externally are not a cause for concern.

Plants affecting milk

Table 20.3 lists plants that are reported to affect milk, but of course many also have far more serious affects.

Table 20.3 Plant affecting milk. (From Cooper and Johnson, 1984)

Reduction in milk yield

Monkshood	Alder buckthorn	Buckthorn
Onion and garlic	Ash	Castor oil plant
Beet	Ivy	Sorrel
White bryony	Henbane	Water betony
Fat hen	St. John's wort	Potato, green
Cowbane	Laburnum	Yew
Ergot	Mercury	Clover
Meadow saffron	Poppy	Hemlock
Bracken	Hawthorn	Oak
Cypress	Buttercup	Hound's tongue
Radish	Bluebell	Rhododendron
Horsetail		

Plants that can taint milk

Fool's parsley	Sweet clover
Onion and garlic	Mint
Beet	Wood sorrel
Turnip	Pea
Shepherd's purse	Bracken
Compositae spp.	Oak
Hemlock	Buttercup
Cress	Radish
Horsetail	Potato, green
Ivy	Yew
Henbane	Laburnum
Birdsfoot trefoil	

Further reading

Baker, I. (1993) Poison, laburnum. *In Practice*, **15** (1), 20.

Boermans, H.J., Ruegg, P.L. and Leach, M. (1988) Ethylene glycol toxicosis in a Pygmy goat. *J. Am. Vet. Med Assoc.*, **193** (6), 694–6.

Clarke, E.G.C. (1975) *Poisoning in Veterinary Practice.* Association of the British Pharmaceutical Industry, London.

Cooper, M.R. and Johnson, A.W. (1984) *Poisonous Plants in Britain.* MAFF Ref. Book 161, HMSO, London.

Gunn, D. (1992) Poison, water dropwort. *In Practice*, **14** (5), 203.

Gunn, G.J. (1992) Poison, cyanobacteria (blue–green algae). *In Practice*, **14** (3), 132.

Jones, T.O. (1988) Nitrate/nitrite poisoning in cattle. *In Practice*, September 1988, 199–203.

Mayer, S. (1990) Ragwort poison. *In Practice*, May 1990, 112.

Mayer, S. (1991) Poison, acorns. *In Practice*, **13** (4), 167.

Mayer, S. (1991) Poison, rhododendron. *In Practice*, **13** (6), 232.

Mayer, S. (1991) Poison, brassicas. *In Practice*, **13** (5), 216–17.

Panter, K.E. and James, L.F. (1990) Natural plant toxins in milk: a review. *J. Animal Sci.*, **68**, 892–904.

Seawright, A.A. (1984) Goats and poisonous plants. *Proc. Univ. Sydney Post Grad. Comm. Vet. Sci.*, **73**, 544–7.

Spratling, R. (1980) Is it plant poisoning? *In Practice*, March 1980, 22–31.

21 Anaesthesia

Initial clinical examination

A routine clinical examination should be carried out in all animals to determine the degree of anaesthetic risk.

❏ General condition – fat cover, anaemia, etc., age.
❏ Auscultation of heart and lungs:
  ■ normal respiratory rate 15 to 20/minute;
  ■ normal pulse rate 70 to 95/minute.
❏ Accurate assessment of weight (*weigh* if necessary) – it is very easy to overdose if the estimation is inaccurate.

General anaesthesia

Preoperative considerations

> Endotracheal intubation with a cuffed tube is essential whenever general anaesthesia is induced in an adult goat.

Except for young kids, which are essentially monogastric, goats should be routinely starved for 12 to 24 hours preoperatively if elective surgery is being undertaken. Some authorities also recommend withholding water for a few hours. Longer periods of starvation may result in the rumen contents becoming more fluid, with a greater likelihood of regurgitation occurring, and may also predispose to the development of metabolic acidosis. Starvation means no food offered and no clean bedding, e.g. straw, either in the pen or in the vehicle used to bring a goat to the surgery.

Recumbency causes respiratory depression and hypoxaemia. The inspired gases should contain at least 30% oxygen (supply oxygen by mask if the goat is not intubated).

Sedatives

Premedication before general anaesthesia is usually *not* necessary and often undesirable because of the increased time required for recovery, but sedation is often used to reduce the required dose of induction agent or allow minor procedures to be carried out under regional analgesia.

❏ **Xylazine, 0.05 mg/kg, 0.1 ml/40 kg** slowly **i.v.** or **0.1 mg/kg, 0.2 ml/ 40 kg i.m. (Rompun**, Bayer; **Chanazine**, Chanelle; **Virbaxyl**, Virbac).

> The alpha-2 adrenoceptor stimulants xylazine, medetomidine and detomidine have sedative, muscle relaxant and analgesic properties in goats.
> The majority of anaesthetic deaths in goats are caused by xylazine overdose.

Minute doses are required in young animals and it is very easy to overdose, resulting, at least, in a very prolonged recovery. In kids, **0.025 mg/kg i.m.** is probably the maximum safe dose. The standard 2% solution can be diluted and administered via an insulin syringe to enable more accurate dosing. Angora goats are reported to require lower levels of the drug than dairy goats. Xylazine is probably contraindicated in late pregnancy.

Xylazine has also been combined in the same syringe with
  Butorphanol, 0.07–0.1 mg/kg i.v., 0.3–0.4 ml/40 kg (Torbugesic, Fort Dodge)
to provide additional analgesia for procedures such as dental work.

❏ **Medetomidine, 25–35 μg/kg, 1–1.5 ml/40 kg i.m. (Domitor**, Pfizer). Sedation is evident in 5 to 15 minutes.

The sedative effects of medetomidine can be reversed by an equal volume of
  Atipamezole, 125–175 μg/kg, 1–1.5 ml/40 kg, half **i.v.** and half **i.m. (Antisedan**, Pfizer).

❏ **Detomidine**, 20–40 μg/kg, **0.08–0.16 ml/40 kg i.v.** or **i.m. (Domosedan**, Pfizer).

Quicker, better and deeper sedation is achieved when the drug is administered intravenously. At 20 μg/kg, mild sedation is produced but the goat will remain standing with slight ataxia; 40 μg/ kg will produce deeper sedation with sternal recumbency and some analgesia for about 70 to 110 minutes, with complete recovery in about 200 minutes.

❏ **Acepromazine maleate, 0.05–0.1 mg/kg, 1–2 ml/40 kg** slowly **i.v. (ACP 2 mg/ml**, C-Vet).

Acepromazine is contraindicated in shocked animals because it produces a fall in blood pressure. Although it smooths induction and recovery with barbiturates, it also greatly increases the risk of regurgitation.

❏ **Diazepam, 0.25–0.5 mg/kg, 2–4 ml/40 kg** slowly **i.v. (Valium,** Roche).
Provides 30 minutes of sedation but no analgesia.

Overdosage of sedatives

Overdosage of sedatives can be treated with:
Doxapram hydrochloride, 0.5–1 mg/kg, 1–2 ml/40 kg i.v. (Dopram V, Fort Dodge).
Overdosage of xylazine and other alpha-2 adrenoceptor stimulants can be reversed by:
Atipamezole (Antisedan, Pfizer).
Atipamezole is specifically authorised to reverse medetomidine at 5 times the dose of medetomidine (i.e. the same volume of medetomidine previously administered). Resedation may rarely occur if atipamezole is used a short time after administration of the sedative because the effect of the atipamezole may subside before that of the sedative.

Antimuscarinic pre-anaesthetic medication

❏ **Atropine, 0.6–1 mg/kg, 1–1.5 ml/kg i.m. (Atropine sulphate,** C-Vet; **Atrocare,** Animalcare).
At this dose rate, atropine will reduce the flow of saliva but also render it more viscous, which may result in endotracheal tubes being blocked.
Most authorities do not recommend that atropine be given routinely as a premedication, although recognising its use in situations where handling viscera may cause bradycardia and possibly cardiac arrest because of vagal inhibition.

Positioning of goat during general anaesthesia

❏ Head down – allowing saliva to drain from the mouth.
❏ Neck placed over a sandbag.
❏ Hindquarters lowered – decreases pressure on diaphragm, reduces risk of regurgitation.

Injectable anaesthetic agents

Barbiturates

❏ **Pentobarbital sodium, 10–15 mg/kg, 40–60 ml/40 kg i.v. (Sagatal,** Merial).

❏ **Thiopental sodium,** 10–15 mg/kg, 8–12 ml/40 kg **i.v.** (**Intraval Sodium 5 g,** Merial; **Thiovet 5 g,** C-Vet).
❏ **Methohexital sodium,** 4 mg/kg, 6.5 ml/40 kg (**Brietal,** Animalcare) as 2.5% solution.

In general, the barbiturate drugs produce a marked respiratory depression, with delayed recovery if additional amounts are given to maintain anaesthesia. Regurgitation is particularly likely if thiopentone is used. Their use as sole anaesthetic agents is thus limited, but they are very useful induction agents before intubation and maintenance with gaseous anaesthesia.

Pentobarbital sodium is metabolised between three and four times faster in small ruminants than in dogs. Any commercial preparation containing propylene glycol should be avoided as haemolysis of red blood cells may be produced.

The short-acting barbiturates give a rapid, smooth induction. Giving half the calculated amount rapidly followed by the remainder over a 2-minute period may reduce the period of apnoea which occurs following rapid injection of the whole amount. Premedication with acepromazine or diazepam will reduce the barbiturate dose.

Alphaxalone/alphadolone

❏ **Alphaxalone/alphadolone** 3 mg/kg, 10 ml/40 kg slowly **i.v.** (**Saffan,** Schering-Plough).

Note: the dosage is the sum of both drugs, i.e. alphadolone 3 mg/ ml + alphaxalone 9 mg/ml = 12 mg/ml total.

❏ Anaesthesia can be maintained with infusions of **2–2.5 mg/kg/ minute i.v.**

Saffan provides a reliable smooth induction agent in the goat, with rapid recovery, minimal respiratory depression and less fetal depression than barbiturates, although a transient fall in blood pressure and heart rate occurs. Small goats, such as Angoras, require about 10 ml and larger dairy breeds up to 20 ml to produce a sufficient depth of anaesthesia for intubation. Kids presented for disbudding require between 1 and 2 ml intravenously. Laryngospasm and laryngeal oedema have been recorded in goats.

Propofol

❏ **Propofol,** 3–5 mg/kg, 12–20 ml/40 kg slowly **i.v.** (**Rapinovet,** Schering-Plough).

Propofal can be used to provide short duration anaesthesia with the advantage of rapid recovery or for induction followed by intubation. Kids presented for disbudding require between 1 and 2 ml intravenously.

Ketamine

❏ **Ketamine, 10–15 mg/kg, 4–6 ml/40 kg** slowly **i.v.** (**Ketaset**, Fort Dodge; **Vetalar**, Pharmacia & Upjohn).

When ketamine is used on its own, there is inadequate muscle relaxation for abdominal procedures and excessive trembling. Better results are obtained by using ketamine in combination with diazepam or an alpha-2 adrenoceptor stimulant like xylazine, medetomidine or detomidine.

Diazepam and ketamine

❏ **Diazepam, 0.25–0.5 mg/kg, 2–4 ml/40 kg** slowly **i.v.** (**Valium**, Roche), wait 2–3 minutes, then
Ketamine, 4 mg/kg, 1.6 ml/40 kg i.v. (**Ketaset**, Fort Dodge; **Vetalar**, Pharmacia & Upjohn).

The lower level of diazepam is used in larger animals. This combination provides adequate time for intubation and maintenance on gaseous anaesthesia.

Xylazine and ketamine

❏ **Xylazine, 0.1 mg/kg, 0.2 ml/40 kg i.m.** (**Rompun**, Bayer; **Chanazine**, Chanelle; **Virbaxyl**, Virbac), followed by
Ketamine, 10 mg/kg, 4 ml/40 kg i.m. or **5 mg/kg, 2 ml/40 kg i.v.** (**Ketaset**, Fort Dodge; **Vetalar**, Pharmacia & Upjohn).

Lower doses of xylazine, **0.025 mg/kg**, should be used in kids. Anaesthesia may be prolonged by an incremental intramuscular dose of ketamine at **2.5–5 mg/kg** or by use of gaseous anaesthetics such as halothane. The combination gives 15 to 20 minutes anaesthesia with good analgesia, and intubation is not essential, although advisable for abdominal surgery in case of regurgitation or passive reflux.

A total intravenous technique using *xylazine, ketamine* and *guaifenesin* has also been used: 200 mg ketamine is combined with 2 mg xylazine and 100 ml 5% guaifenesin (5 g/100 ml). This solution is administered intravenously at 2 ml/kg to give 30 minutes of surgical anaesthesia; then according to the patient's response. Total surgical time should not exceed 60 minutes. The solution should be given through a jugular catheter as it is very irritating to tissues.

> Most alpha-2 adrenoceptor stimulants have been used in goats, either alone or combined with ketamine.

Medetomidine and ketamine

❏ **Medetomidine, 25–35** μg/kg, **1–1.5 ml/40 kg** (**Domitor**, Pfizer), mixed in same syringe with
Ketamine, 1–1.5 mg/kg, 0.4–0.6 ml/40 kg i.m. (**Ketaset**, Fort Dodge; **Vetalar**, Pharmacia & Upjohn).

Adult animals require higher doses than young animals. Induction of anaesthesia takes 5 to 10 minutes and the combination provides 30 to 40 minutes of anaesthesia.

The sedative effects of medetomidine can be reversed by
Atipamezole, 125–175 μg/kg, **1–1.5 ml/40 kg,** half **i.v.** and half **i.m.** (**Antisedan**, Pfizer).

> Atipamezole can be used to reverse all alpha-2 adrenoceptor stimulants.

Etorphine hydrochloride/acepromazine maleate

❏ Etorphine hydrochloride/acepromazine maleate, **0.01 ml/kg i.v.** or **i.m.** (**Large Animal Immobilon/Revivon**, C-Vet).

Large Animal Immobilon produces a reversible neuroleptanalgesia in goats as in other species and has been used for minor surgical procedures, but there is reportedly a high mortality and morbidity rate. Relapse due to recycling may occur, particularly if the intramuscular route of administration is used, and can be countered by a further injection of Revivon.

The goat needs to be well restrained to avoid undue risk to the anaesthetist or assistant from an accidental self-injection of the drug and the *relevant safety precautions should be carefully followed at all times.*

Tiletamine–zolazepam

❏ **Tiletamine–zolazepam, 5.5 mg/kg i.v.** (**Telazol**, Fort Dodge), not available in the UK.

Note: the dosage is the sum of both drugs, i.e. tiletamine 50 mg/ ml + zolazepam 50 mg/ml = 100 mg/ml total.

It provides adequate anaesthesia for about 1 hour and anaesthesia can be extended by incremental doses at **0.5–1.0 mg/kg** as needed.

Gaseous anaesthetic agents

Halothane

❏ Induction of anaesthesia – gradual increase to 4%.
❏ Maintenance of anaesthesia 2%.

Halothane (**Halothane RM**, Merial; **Fluothane**, Schering-Plough) and oxygen is the most commonly used gaseous anaesthetic, providing excellent safe anaesthesia, either via mask for induction and maintenance of kids for disbudding, or for maintenance of older goats via endotracheal tube following induction by injection.

An oxygen flow of 11 ml/kg/minute is adequate.

Halothane hepatotoxicity has been reported (see Chapter 11).

Methoxyflurane

Methoxyflurane (**Metofane**, C. Vet) will provide adequate anaesthesia in goats, with a smooth recovery, but induction takes longer than with halothane and recovery is slower. Methoxyflurane is generally used for maintenance following induction with an injectable agent.

Isoflurane

❏ Induction of anaesthesia 2 to 5%.
❏ Maintenance of anaesthesia 0.25 to 5%.

Faster recovery occurs after maintenance with isoflurane (**Isoflo**, Schering-Plough; **Isoflurane RM**, Merial) as compared with halothane, but isoflurane is much more expensive.

Nitrous oxide

Nitrous oxide can be used during the induction of anaesthesia but should then be discontinued because it accumulates in the rumen and can potentiate ruminal tympany. When used for induction, nitrous oxide should be 50% of the total gas flow.

Intubation

Intubation of goats can be performed with or without a long-bladed laryngoscope. Endotracheal tubes about sizes 8 to 9 are generally suitable for adult goats. Comparatively, goats have a much smaller laryngeal opening than a dog and need relatively small tubes. An adequate depth of anaesthesia is essential for intubation. If a laryngoscope is not available, a technique of threading the tube through the larynx is relatively easy with experience. The goat is placed in lateral or dorsal recumbency and the tube inserted until the top touches the larynx; the larynx is then manipulated from the outside over the tube. A distinct click is usually felt as the tube passes into the laryngeal cartilages. The use of a wire stiffener in the tube may make the intubation easier.

Goats especially kids are prone to *laryngospasm* generally following regurgitation at the time of intubation. Spraying the cords with lignocaine will reduce the hazard. In an emergency, a tracheotomy may be necessary.

Hazards of general anaesthesia

Regurgitation

Genereal anaesthesia (or deep sedation) can lead to passive regurgitation and aspiration of rumen contents. The risk of regurgitation can be minimised by:

- ❑ Preoperative starvation.
- ❑ Correct positioning of the goat on the operating table. The thorax and neck should be raised if possible by tilting the table to lower the hindquarters, while the head is tilted downwards to allow free drainage of saliva.
- ❑ If problems arise during intubation, a cuffed tube in the oesophagus will help to protect the airway from regurgitation.
- ❑ If regurgitation occurs, the pharynx should be drained, the trachea sucked out and atropine administered if there is a danger of bronchospasm.

Salivation

Like all ruminants, goats salivate copiously during anaesthesia and it is important that the saliva is allowed to drain freely from the mouth and not pool in the pharynx. Except for very short procedures the goat should be intubated with a cuffed inflated endotracheal tube.

Hypovolaemia and acidosis can occur through loss of alkaline saliva during long periods of anaesthesia (more than 2 to 3 hours). Therefore, during long periods of anaesthesia, the saliva should be collected and replaced on a volume for volume basis with **lactated Ringer's solution**

(**Hartmann's solution**) and **sodium bicarbonate, 1 mmol/kg/hour** (4.2% bicarbonate contains 0.5 mmol/ml = 2 ml/kg/hour).

Ruminal tympany

Ruminal tympany becomes progressively more important with the length of the operation as continuous gas production puts pressure on the diaphragm, interfering with respiration and leading to hypoxia. In elective surgery, preoperative starvation will reduce the risk of tympany, or in non-elective surgery, rumen contents can be emptied by stomach tube, the contents kept at 37°C and then returned to the rumen postoperatively.

Removal of rumen contents by stomach tube may be possible if tympany occurs or the distension may be relieved by trocarisation using a 14- or 16-gauge needle.

Cardiovascular and respiratory embarrassment

During lateral and, particularly, dorsal recumbency the large mass of the rumen puts pressure on the diaphragm and great vessels, leading to decreased tidal volume and inadequate ventilation, with increased areas of lung tissue not ventilated and consequently respiratory acidosis and hypoxaemia. All anaesthetic procedures, particularly those requiring dorsal recumbency, should be kept as short as possible.

Hypoxaemia can be prevented by the provision of at least 30% inspired oxygen and respiratory acidosis prevented by the use of intermittent positive pressure ventilation.

Depth of anaesthesia

No single reflex is reliable enough to be used on its own to assess the depth of anaesthesia. The assessment must be based on a combination of:

❏ Response to surgery – the anaesthetist should monitor the heart rate, pulse, respiratory rate, colour of mucous membranes, gingival perfusion time (normally 1 to 2 seconds) and muscle relaxation.
❏ Experience with the drug being used.
❏ Examination of a number of reflexes.

(1) *Jaw tension:* this decreases with an increasing depth of anaesthesia, but some tone persists even in deep anaesthesia. As the anaesthetic level lightens, swallowing or chewing movements can be elicited.

(2) *Eye rotation:* unlike cattle, eye rotation is *not* a useful method of assessing the depth of anaesthesia.

(3) *Pupils:* during surgical anaesthesia, the eye is normally *central* and the pupil moderately *constricted.* During both light and deep anaesthesia, the pupil is *dilated.*

(4) *Palpebral reflex:* this usually (but *not* always) disappears as surgical anaesthesia is obtained.

(5) *Limb withdrawal reflexes:* these are reduced during light anaesthesia with barbiturates or halothane and are generally absent under deep anaesthesia. However, they may persist if ketamine is used. Generally, they are not as good an indicator of the depth of anaesthesia as in dogs and cats.

(6) *Corneal reflex:* this persists through all levels of anaesthesia.

Local anaesthetics

Paravertebral anaesthesia

Use: flank laparotomy for caesarian section or other abdominal surgery.
Technique: Figure 21.1a shows the area served by each of the nerves T13, L1, L2 and L3. The nerves run caudally at an angle. The sites for injection can be palpated – 'walk' the needle over the anterior edge of the transverse process of the vertebra caudal to the nerve being blocked and inject approximately 2 cm from the midline, i.e. halfway between midline and the tip of the transverse process. The transverse process is 4 to 5 cm deep. Use **5 ml** of **1** or **2% lignocaine plus adrenaline**. Inject 2 ml into skin and muscle above the intertransverse ligament and 3 ml below the ligament.

Caudal epidural anaesthesia

Use: desensitises the perineal area, tail and vagina; useful for perineal surgery and some obstetrical conditions (see Figure 21.1b).
Technique: the area over the tailhead is clipped and surgically prepared. The first intercoccygeal space or sacrococcygeal space (preferred) is identified by digital palpation as the tail is moved gently up and down. In dairy goats, an 18- or 19-g × 35-mm needle is inserted vertically and cranially at an angle of 15 degrees. The correct position of the needle is determined by failure to strike bone and lack of resistance to injection of the anaesthetic solution.

Inject **2–4 ml** of **2% lignocaine** solution, depending on the size of animal, or **2 ml** of **2% lignocaine** (0.5 mg/kg) + **0.25 ml xylocaine (0.07 mg/kg)** (**Rompun**, Bayer); these can be mixed in the same syringe.

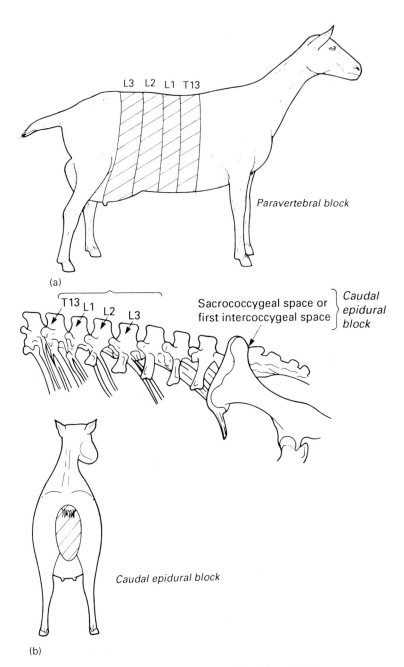

(a)

(b)

Figure 21.1 (*a*) Paravertebral block. (*b*) Caudal epidural block.

Injection of a combination of xylazine and lignocaine provides adequate analgesia to permit replacement of rectal, vaginal or uterine prolapses after 5 to 10 minutes, although loss of tail tone and perineal sensation occurs within 2 minutes. Overdosage with lignocaine/xylazine may cause pelvic limb paresis, which can persist for 36 hours or more.

Local infiltration

> Total dose of lignocaine by local infiltration should be < 10 mg/kg.

Goats, particularly kids, are sensitive to the toxic effects of lignocaine, which include drowsiness and respiratory depression. **Convulsions occur at about 6 mg/kg i.v. or 10 mg/kg i.m.** Care must be taken not to exceed recommended doses, e.g. 30 ml of 2% solution in 45- to 70-kg goats and 40–50 ml in larger animals.

❑ Infiltration analgesia is useful for suturing wounds and as a line block for laparotomy where the anaesthetic is infiltrated along the line of the incision.
❑ *Inverted L block* – local anaesthetic is injected as an inverted L into the skin and full thickness of the body wall, so as to block the nerves entering the operation site, creating an area of analgesia. The horizontal arm of the L is ventral to the transverse processes of the lumbar vertebrae and the vertical arm is posterior to the last rib (Figure 21.2a). This technique avoids oedema of tissues, with subsequent delayed wound healing in the area of the incision.

Intravenous regional analgesia

Intravenous regional analgesia (IVRA) is a technique for obtaining analgesia of the lower limb using **5 ml of 2% lignocaine** (without adrenaline) injected via a 23-g needle into a superficial vein such as the medial radial vein in the fore leg and the lateral saphenous vein in the hind leg. The injection should be directed distally, with pressure on the injection site to avoid a haematoma. A tourniquet is applied above the carpus or hock to localise the effect of the lignocaine and prevent its leakage into the circulation. A roll of bandage below the tourniquet on the lateral surface of the hock allows better occlusion of the blood vessels.

The onset of analgesia is about 5 to 10 minutes after injection and

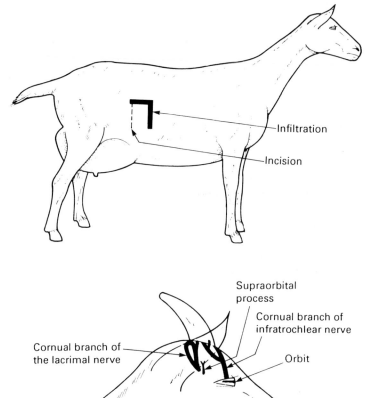

(a)

(b)

Figure 21.2 (*a*) Inverted L block. (*b*) Local anaesthesia for dehorning.

persists for as long as the tourniquet is left in place. The tourniquet should not be removed for at least 20 minutes and should not be left in place for more than 2 hours.

Dehorning

Inject **2–3 ml of 2% lignocaine** at each of the following sites (see Figure 21.2):

❏ Cornual branch of the lacrimal nerve is blocked as in the calf using the supraorbital process as a landmark.
❏ Cornual branch of the infratrochlear nerve is blocked dorsomedial to the eye close to the orbit.
❏ In kids, use a maximum of 1 ml of 0.5 or 1% lignocaine on each side. General anaesthesia is safer and easier for routine disbudding (see Chapter 22).

Note: under most conditions, general anaesthesia is to be preferred to local anaesthesia for dehorbing. For technique, see Chapter 22.

Further reading

Gray, P.R. and McDonell, W.M. (1986) Anaesthesia in goats and sheep. Part I. Local analgesia. *Comp. Cont. Ed. Pract. Vet.*, **8** (1), S33–9.

Gray, P.R. and McDonell, W.M. (1986) Anaesthesia in goats and sheep. Part II. General anaesthesia. *Comp. Cont. Ed. Pract. Vet.*, **8** (3), S127–35.

Taylor, P. (1980) Goat anaesthesia. *Goat Vet. Soc. J.*, **1**, 4–11.

Taylor, P.M. (1991) Anaesthesia in sheep and goats. *In Practice*, **13** (1), 31–6.

22   Disbudding and Dehorning

Disbudding and dehorning of goats can only be performed by a veterinary surgeon and the patient must be anaesthetised (Veterinary Surgeons Act 1966 as amended 1982).

Anatomy

❏   The horn bud in the kid is proportionately much larger than in the calf.
❏   Two nerves supply the horn:
  (1)   cornual branch of the lacrimal nerve;
  (2)   cornual branch of the infratrochlear nerve.

See Figure 21.2.

Disbudding of kids

Age

Kids should preferably be disbudded between 2 and 7 days of age, particularly males where horn growth is rapid.

Selection of anaesthetic agent for disbudding kids

> Kids are the youngest animals most veterinary surgeons ever anaesthetise.

See also Chapter 21. Of all the domestic species, only kids are routinely anaesthetised so soon after parturition. Because they are alert and active and relatively large when compared to, say, an adult cat, it is easy for the veterinary surgeon to forget that they are dealing with a neonatal animal.

Like all neonates, kids are very sensitive to lignocaine – analgesic doses are very close to toxic doses – and overdosage will result in lethargy, unwillingness to feed and even death. The toxic dose of lignocaine is about 10 mg/kg, i.e. 2 ml of 2% lignocaine for a 4-kg kid. Similarly, only *minute* doses of xylazine are required – the ruminant dose is much less than that routinely used in the dog and cat and it is preferable to dilute the standard 2% solution.

At the surgery, induction and maintenance with halothane or iso-flurane in oxygen by mask is simple, quick and safe and recovery is very rapid. On the farm, **Saffan** (Schering-Plough), 2–6 mg/kg is easy to administer, induction smooth and recovery quiet and relatively rapid. Depending on the size of the kid, 1 or 2 ml of Saffan is injected into the cephalic or jugular vein.

Equipment

Calf disbudding irons are quite adequate for disbudding small kids, provided they reach a satisfactory temperature. In this respect gas irons are probably better than electric irons. Dehorning irons, heated in a gas blow torch to 600°C, are also suitable. A technique for disbudding kids using a tubular cutting edge has been described (Boyd, 1987).

Note: halothane/oxygen mixtures will support combustion of hair, resulting in a rather singed kid – the anaesthetic mask should therefore be removed before a gas iron is applied.

Procedure

Clip the hair from around the horn bud. With larger buds clip off the tip of the buds with scissors or bone forceps if necessary. Apply the iron to the bud with an even action to ensure the whole bud tissue is destroyed – it is important to use a hot iron for the minimum time necessary to remove the bud. Excessive pressure or exposure may result in cortical necrosis, cerebral oedema and a brain-damaged kid or even fracture of the skull. The whole bud is best removed, rather than just burnt around, as this reduces the risk of infection.

Where the disbudding iron has a recessed head or the iron is not very hot, scraping the burnt out area with a scalpel blade and then briefly reapplying the iron ensures the tissue is destroyed. If the cauterised area is not large enough, a further ring of tissue can be removed with a scalpel blade or, even better, with an electric cautery knife. Several superficial vessels, especially the superficial temporal artery on the lateral side of the horn, may require recauterising.

Finally, the cauterised areas are sprayed with tetracycline spray, and broad spectrum antibiotics and tetanus antitoxin given.

Large buds are best removed with embryotomy wire as described in dehorning. Where kids are presented at about 3 or 4 weeks, it is extremely difficult to remove successfully all horn tissue with a calf disbudding iron – in these cases it may be best to wait for a few more weeks until the horn can be removed with wire.

Descenting of kids

Burning a semi-circular area caudomedially behind the horn buds will also remove the scent glands from the area, reducing to some extent buck odour. However, the presence of musk cells in other parts of the body and the habit of spraying urine means that even 'descented' males will still smell during the breeding season.

Dehorning

> Removal of very large horns is probably contraindicated and should be undertaken with trepidation!

Horned goats, particularly when running with hornless animals, are often dominant within the herd. Dehorning can thus have profound psychological implications for the goat, involving loss of status, reduced milk yield or impaired fertility. Possible complications from surgery include sinusitis, myiasis and tetanus. After surgery, breathing can be seen to occur through the frontal sinuses and haemorrhage may occur down the nostrils. For these reasons the whole procedure should be carefully discussed with the owner and the timing of surgery arranged accordingly – surgery is best carried out in a dry, non-pregnant goat during the autumn, winter or early spring.

Removal of the horns exposes the openings into the frontal sinuses which extend into the hollow base of the horn. It is important that the openings are kept as clean as possible after surgery by treating regularly with antibiotic powders or sprays, feeding hay from the floor rather than a rack, and housing the goat in clean surroundings. The head is likely to remain tender for a month or more. Bandaging of the head is sometimes recommended or the holes can be covered in Stockholm tar.

Anaesthesia

With general anaesthesia, intubation should be considered but is not usually necessary if the operation is performed quickly on a starved animal.

Surgical technique

❏ If the horns are relatively small, as for instance in a large kid or yearling animal, there is no need to suture the skin over the exposed area of the frontal sinuses, provided the area can be kept clean postsurgically, as the hole will seal naturally within a few days and the skin will grown back over the area fairly quickly.

The area around both horns is clipped and routinely prepared for surgery and the skin incised in a ring about 1 cm from the base of the horn. The horns are removed in turn with embryotomy wire, working from the back of the horn forward and leaving the wire as low as possible to avoid leaving scurs. Any haemorrhage should be controlled by cautery.

❏ In mature animals, particularly males, the exposed area of the frontal sinuses should be closed by suturing the skin across the wound.

The area around both horns is clipped and prepared for surgery and the skin incised about 1 cm from the base of the horns. The skin incision starts on the cranial aspect of the horn, encircles the horn and is then directed caudally towards the ear. It is important to leave plenty of skin to make closure easier, using the loose skin around the ears. The edges of the skin are undermined using sharp dissection with scissors and the horns removed as above. After horn removal, the skin is undermined for an additional 2 to 3 cm to permit closure.

The surgical site is flushed with sterile saline and the skin closed with interrupted horizontal mattress sutures, using a non-absorbable material. The wound is dressed and the head bandaged until suture removal after 10 to 14 days, with the bandage changed after 4 days. Antibiotics should be given for 5 to 7 days, together with tetanus antitoxin. A non-steroidal anti-inflammatory drug, carprofen or flunixin, should be given daily for 2 or 3 days.

Descenting of adult goats

Descenting of polled, horned or disbudded adult males can be carried out under general anaesthesia.

A triangular skin flap is made, with the base of the triangle approaching the caudal aspect of the head and the apex 3 to 4 cm in front of a line between the horns or polls (Figure 22.1). The skin flap is separated from the underlying tissue and folded caudally to its base. The large scent glands, which generally lie within the borders of the triangle, are exposed, grasped with forceps and removed with scissors

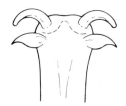

Figure 22.1   Incision line for scent gland removal.

or a scalpel blade, taking care to remove all glandular tissue. The skin flap is replaced with simple interrupted sutures. Antibiotic cover and tetanus antitoxin should be given.

Further reading

Anon (1984) Disbudding. *Goat Vet. Soc. J.*, **5** (2), 32–3.

Boyd, J. (1987) Disbudding of goat kids. *Goat Vet. Soc. J.*, **8** (2), 77–8.

Buttle, H.L. *et al.* (1986) Disbudding and dehorning of goats. *In Practice*, March 1986, 63–5.

Johnson, E.H. and Steward, T. (1984) Cosmetic descenting of adult goats. *Agri. Practice*, **5** (9), 16.

Mobini, S. (1991) Cosmetic dehorning of adult goats. *Small Ruminant Res.*, **5**, 187–91.

Taylor, P. (1983) Goat anaesthesia. *Goat Vet. Soc. J.*, **1**, 4–11.

Turner, A.S. and McIlwraith, C.W. (1982) Dehorning the mature goat. In: *Techniques in Large Animal Surgery*. Lea and Febiger, Philadelphia, 317–19.

23　Surgical Techniques

Castration

Goats are commonly castrated if:

❏　they are to be kept for meat for longer than 4 months;
❏　they are to be retained as wethers for fibre production;
❏　they are to be kept as pets;
❏　they are to be used as pack animals or harness goats.

Castration renders the animal infertile and prevents the development of male odour and unpleasant secondary sexual behaviour, such as spraying urine. Uncastrated kids show better growth rate, efficiency of feed utilisation and carcass yield than castrated kids, but, in older kids, the meat is likely to be darker and more strongly flavoured. Early castration may lead to a greater risk of urolithiasis, because the urethra remains relatively small. It may be better to delay castration in animals which are to be kept for work or as pets, but an uncastrated male should never be sold as a pet, without full discussion with the new owner and arrangements for castration having been made. There is a difference in the law regarding the castration of lambs and kids – kids over 2 months of age must be castrated by a veterinary surgeon using anaesthesia, whereas lambs up to 3 months of age can be castrated surgically by a lay person without anaesthesia (see Table 23.1).

Table 23.1　Castration of kids.

Age of animal	Technique	Person who may perform castration	Anaesthetic required
First week of life	Rubber ring or burdizzo	Any Any	No No
<2 Months	Surgical	Any	No
>2 Months	Surgical	Veterinary surgeon	Yes

Rubber rings

Very young kids can be castrated with elastrator rings placed round the neck of the scrotum using a special applicator. The ring constricts the blood flow to and from the testes and scrotum, which wither and drop off in about 2 to 6 weeks. It is essential to confirm that both testicles are fully trapped within the scrotal sac beneath the ring, or an induced inguinal cryptorchid may be produced. Conversely, placing the ring too high can trap the urethra – ensure that the teats are proximal to the ring.

There is a risk of infection around the ring and also of tetanus. Kids castrated by rings show behavioural evidence of acute pain for at least 3 hours. There is evidence in lambs that a combined technique of rubber ring and bloodless castrator, or Burdizzo emasculator (see below), causes less acute pain. The Burdizzo emasculator is applied for 10 seconds, just distal to the rubber ring, across the full width of the scrotum.

Emasculator (Burdizzo)

Each spermatic cord is crushed in turn using the emasculator, depriving the testicle of its blood supply and causing the testicle to atrophy and become non-functional after several weeks, whilst leaving the scrotum intact. By staggering the placing of the emasculator on the two cords, the skin in the middle of the scrotum is left undamaged, retaining sufficient blood supply to retain scrotal viability.

Each cord is generally crushed twice, with the second crush below the first, although a single application for 6 to 10 seconds of a correctly functioning emasculator should be effective. The scrotum should be carefully palpated before application of the emasculator to check both testicles are descended and that there is no scrotal hernia.

This technique is less painful than using a rubber ring, at least in the first few hours after castration.

Surgical (open) castration

Kids

The scrotum is cleaned and scrubbed with **chlorhexidine (Hibiscrub**, Schering-Plough) or **povidone–iodine (Pevidine**, C-Vet; **Vetasept**, Animalcare), the bottom of the scrotum pulled downwards and the distal third removed with a scalpel blade. In very young kids, each testicle is grasped individually, the testicle and spermatic cord with intact tunica freed from the fascia by traction and blunt dissection and the cremaster muscle and tunica then ruptured by continuing controlled traction. Traction to the spermatic vessels produces rupture in the inguinal area as the testicle is removed. Ligation of the spermatic vessels is unnecessary in newborn kids, but is recommended in kids over a few days of age. Kids mature rapidly and are sexually mature by 3 months of age. Older kids, even Pygmies, have relatively large testicles.

Adults

An emasculator with catgut ligation can be used on adult animals. The ventral third of the scrotum is removed with a scalpel, as in kids, or an incision just shorter than the length of the testicle is made in the ventral scrotum. Each testicle is then individually exposed and the fascia bluntly separated from the spermatic cord. The vascular and non-vascular portions of the spermatic cord are identified. The non-vascular portion is crushed for about 10 seconds just proximal to the epididymis, then the vascular portion is crushed to remove the testicle, leaving the emasculator in place for at least 1 minute. A catgut suture is placed around the cord, 1 cm proximal to the emasculator blade. Before releasing the emasculator, an artery forcep is placed on the edge of the cord and a check made for haemorrhage before the cord is released.

Open castration should not be carried out in warm weather when fly strike may be a problem. Prophylaxis against tetanus should always be given. After castration, the goat should be placed in a clean, dust-free environment and exercise encouraged.

Anaesthesia

Anaesthesia is desirable in all animals, although only legally required in kids over 2 months. Kids can be conveniently castrated at the same time as they are anaesthetised for disbudding. In other animals general anaesthesia (see Chapter 21) or local infiltration with lignocaine and adrenalin can be used. Because goats are sensitive to the toxic effects of lignocaine, care should be taken not to exceed recommended doses – toxic effects occur at 10 mg/kg intramuscularly, i.e. 5 ml of 2% lignocaine in a 10-kg kid.

Surgical treatment of obstructive urolithiasis

> It is not possible to catheterise male goats as far as the bladder so surgical intervention is always necessary in cases of obstructive urolithiasis.

Treatment of urolithiasis presents major problems for the veterinary surgeon, because of the need to make rapid decisions so that the discomfort of the animal can be relieved, the problematical outcome of many of the techniques used and the high recurrence rate in many animals. It is essential that the owner is fully involved in the discussion concerning the possible options for treatment and is aware of the costs and long-term prognosis before surgery is undertaken. Stud males present particular problems, as surgery must not impair fertility, and in harness goats the backward direction of urination following a urethrostomy can present major difficulties for the owner. Many owners may opt for euthanasia. Figure 23.1 attempts to provide a rational framework for surgery. How far each goat is taken down the surgical pathway will depend on the value of the goat, its future use and owner preference.

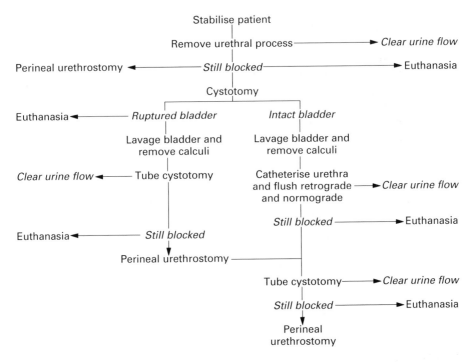

Figure 23.1   Obstructive urolithiasis.

Animals with obstructive urolithiasis are usually uraemic, with BUN levels often <40 mmol/l, and with elevated serum creatinine levels. Electrolyte abnormalities include hyponatraemia, hypochloraemia and hyperkalaemia and most animals show an elevated white cell count due to a neutrophilia. Intravenous fluid therapy should be given pre-operatively and for as long as necessary postoperatively to correct electrolyte imbalances. After successful removal of the obstruction, BUN levels fall rapidly to below 20 mmol/l within 24 hours and below 10 mmol/l within 48 hours.

Antibiotic cover should be given to present ascending infection – use broad-spectrum antibiotics or procaine penicillin, which is excreted unchanged by the kidney and is effective against *Corynebacterium renale*. Temporary pain relief is achieved by use of caudal epidural anaesthesia (see Chapter 21).

Surgical removal of the urethral process

The urethral process is a common site for blockage with urinary calculi. Gritty or sandy material can occasionally be milked out without resorting to surgery, particularly in kids and if the animal is sedated. If this is unsuccessful, amputation of the process may alleviate the blockage. If only the urethral process is blocked, urine will flow within 5 minutes. Placing an Angora goat on its rump and flexing its back may be sufficient to exteriorise the penis, which can be held with a swab or cotton wool. Alternatively, the animal can be laid on its back and front and hind legs tied together. In larger dairy goats, exteriorisation of the penis is often more difficult (occasionally very difficult) and is easier under sedation. With the glans penis held manually, the urethral process is removed with a pair of scissors. Removal of the process does not affect the future fertility of stud males.

Urethrotomy

If the blockage is in the distal portion of the urethra, a low urethrotomy, with or without urethral closure, may relieve the obstruction, at least temporarily. Although plain or contrast radiography or ultrasound studies may help to locate calculi and determine the numbers of calculi present, in many cases it is difficult to establish the precise location of the calculi and several calculi may be present at different sites, so that the urethra may subsequently become obstructed again as additional calculi travel down the urethra. Postsurgical fibrosis and chronic stenosis commonly occur and result in even smaller calculi causing reobstruction. Urethrotomy should thus be considered an emergency procedure to relieve the pressure on the goat and the surgeon, giving time to consider the options for the long-term surgical solution of the problem.

Anaesthesia: caudal epidural or general anaesthesia.

The surgical site is clipped and routinely prepared for surgery. A skin incision is made directly over the penis at the site of the obstruction and the penis located by blunt dissection of the underlying subcutaneous adipose tissue and elastic tissue surrounding the penis. A small incision is made in the ventral surface of the penis, directly over the calculus (calculi) and the calculus (calculi) removed.

A catheter is passed proximal and distally up the urethra as far as possible to ensure urethral patency. The urethral wall may be sutured with an absorbable material, using simple interrupted or continuous sutures, but urine often seeps through the incision and it is preferable to leave both urethra and skin to heal by secondary intention.

Broad-spectrum antibiotics should be given before and for several days after surgery. Amputation of the urethral process should be carried out at the same time as the urethrotomy to prevent the possibility of a smaller calculus causing obstruction later.

Cystotomy

Anaesthesia: general anaesthesia.

The goat is placed in dorsal recumbency and the abdomen clipped and routinely prepared for surgery. A 10- to 15-cm paramedian incision is made midway between the scrotum and the distal prepuce, 3 cm to the left or right of midline. The penis and prepuce are reflected and the abdomen opened through the linea alba. The bladder is exteriorised and packed off from the abdomen with moist swabs.

If the bladder is ruptured, a tube cystotomy should be considered (see below). If the bladder is intact, two stay sutures are placed on the ventral aspect of the bladder and a cystotomy performed, with a full thickness incision at the apex of the bladder. Urine is aspirated, any calculi removed and the bladder lavaged with sterile isotonic saline. Careful removal of all possible calculi will reduce the risk of further obstruction later. Calculi are flushed from the urethra with sterile saline (1) retrograde by means of a urinary catheter (8 to 10 fg) passed through the neck of the bladder into the urethra and (2) normograde by means of a urinary catheter inserted into the distal opening of the urethra (easier if the urethral process has been amputated). Care should be taken not to exert excessive pressure on the urethra during flushing as *overenthusiastic flushing can lead to rupture of the urethra.*

> Flushing of the urethra after catheterisation from the bladder is often unsuccessful in relieving obstruction and may cause urethral rupture if done too enthusiastically.

If the urethral obstruction is cleared by flushing, the bladder is closed with 2-metric synthetic absorbable suture, using a continuous inversion suture (Lembert or Cushing), or simple continuous suture followed by a continuous Lembert suture. The linea alba is closed with 3-metric synthetic absorbable suture in a simple interrupted pattern, the subcutaneous tissue closed in a simple continuous pattern and the skin sutured with non-absorbable material.

If the urethral blockage cannot be cleared, the surgical options are (1) a perineal urethrostomy or (2) a tube cystotomy.

Perineal urethrostomy

Perineal urethrostomy is a salvage procedure, unsuitable for breeding males. Even with good surgical technique, the long-term prognosis is poor, with less than 20% of animals surviving more than a year without stricture or recurrent obstruction.

Anaesthesia: caudal epidural or general anaesthesia.

The skin from anus to scrotal neck is routinely prepared for surgery and a midline skin incision is made from the dorsal aspect of ischium distally for about 10 cm – a relatively high site encourages urine to be expelled caudally, reducing urine scald of the hind legs which is often a major long-term problem postoperatively.

The penis is exposed by blunt dissection of the subcutaneous tissues and then incised longitudinally in the midline, separating the bulbo-urethral and ischiocavernosus muscles, so that the urethra, surrounded by the corpus cavernosum urethrae, is exposed. Adequate mobilisation of the urethra is important to ensure that the urethral mucosa and skin are well apposed and the sutures not under tension. Apart from urine scald, the most common complication of perineal urethrostomy is stricture formation.

A 1- to 2-cm incision is made in the urethra, releasing a flow of urine if the urethra is patent distal to the incision and the urethral mucosa, and a small amount of underlying fibrous tissue sutured to the skin with 2- or 3-metric polyglycolic acid (Dexon, Dains and Geck) attached to a swaged-on needle. The initial sutures are placed dorsally and ventrally, then the lateral sutures. An indwelling urinary catheter (8 to 10 fg) is placed in the bladder, sutured to the skin using a tape tab and left in situ for 3 days.

Broad-spectrum antibiotics should be given before surgery and continued for 3 days after catheter removal.

Tube cystotomy

Tube cystotomy is the treatment of choice for relief of obstructive urolithiasis in valuable animals and in animals where a ruptured bladder is suspected. It is expensive, involving a long period of hospitalisation or careful nursing at home and must be combined with dietary changes to prevent a recurrence of the problem.

The insertion of an indwelling Foley catheter into the urinary bladder temporarily relieves the obstruction, providing immediate relief to the animal by diverting urine flow from the blocked urethra. This gives time for the obstruction of the urethra to be resolved by eliminating urethral spasm associated with urethral pressure, allowing time for the urethritis to subside and the urinary calculi to dissolve. Dissolution of the calculi can be helped by altering the urinary pH by dietary change (see Chapter 14) and by dosing with ammonium chloride and ascorbic acid.

Anaesthesia: general anaesthesia.

A cystotomy is performed as described above. If the bladder is ruptured, the bladder wall is repaired with a 2-metric synthetic absorbable suture, using a continuous inversion suture (Lembert or Cushing), or a simple continuous suture, followed by a continuous Lembert suture. The bladder is thoroughly lavaged with isotonic saline and any residual calculi removed. Any calculi in the peritoneal cavity are harmless. As many calculi as possible are removed from the urethra by retrograde and normograde flushing.

An 8- to 20-fg silicone-treated latex Foley catheter ('Folec', SIMS Portex, distributed by Arnolds Veterinary Products) is placed through a small incision lateral to the paramedian incision and tunnelled subcutaneously a short distance before entering the abdominal cavity. The end of the catheter is passed through a stab incision into the bladder, where it is secured by two purse-string sutures. The balloon of the catheter is inflated with saline and traction applied to the distal portion of the catheter to draw the bladder closer to the body wall, although in most cases it does not come into direct contact with the wall. The abdominal incision is closed and the catheter sutured to the skin.

Broad-spectrum antibiotics should be given before surgery until 3 to 5 days after the catheter is removed, and urethral inflammation reduced by giving

> **Flunixin meglumine, 1.1 mg/kg, 1 ml/45 kg i.v. (Finadyne Solution,** Schering Plough; **Flunixin**, Norbrook; **Binixin**, Bayer) every 12 hours

until the urethral obstruction is resolved. The catheter is left open for 3 to 4 days after surgery and then intermittently closed to determine if the urethra is patent. If the animal shows signs of discomfort such as straining or crying, the catheter is again opened and the process repeated the following day. When urine starts to drip from the urethra, the catheter is closed for longer periods, until a steady stream of urine is produced. Once urination has been normal for 24 hours, the catheter can be removed. The time to dribbling of urine varies between 1 day and 3 weeks and the time to a steady stream of urine between 4 days and 5 weeks.

Dissolution of the calculi can be encouraged by:

- ❑ dosing the animal with **10 g ammonium chloride**, dissolved in 40 ml water, by mouth daily to acidify the urine;
- ❑ **ammonium chloride** fed at **40 mg/kg** daily in feed, but this is not very palatable and will need disguising in molassed food;
- ❑ dosing with **3 mg/kg ascorbic acid**, orally or s.c. daily;
- ❑ infusing the bladder daily with **200 ml Walpole's Buffer Solution** (Arnolds) through the Foley catheter;
- ❑ Urine pH should be monitored daily wherever possible (goats will often urinate when a stranger enters the pen). The urine pH should be stabilised at 5.5 to 6.0.

Tube cystotomy may not be successful in a small number of animals. In these animals, a urethrostomy should be carried out or euthanasia considered.

Caesarian section

Indications: dystocia, pregnancy toxaemia, as an aid to disease control (e.g. CAE).

A caesarian section in the goat can be successfully carried out using a variety of surgical approaches – flank, ventral abdominal midline, ventral abdominal paramedian – and with the goat in lateral or dorsal recumbency or standing. It is important that the surgeon adopts an approach with which he/she is comfortable and this may depend on whether the surgeon's experience is based largely on small or large animals. The most common surgical approaches are either a left flank or a ventral midline laparotomy.

In general, goats are less amenable than sheep to being restrained and restraint in lateral recumbency is much easier than in dorsal recumbency. A flank approach can be undertaken with minimal restraint under local anaesthesia, whereas a midline laparotomy will usually require general anaesthesia (but see Table 23.2).

Left flank laparotomy

Anaesthesia: local infiltration or inverted L block or paravertebral regional anaesthesia.

The goat is placed in right lateral recumbency and the surgical site in the mid-left paralumbar fossa routinely prepared for surgery. Most surgeons use a muscle incisional approach, although a grid or muscle-

Table 23.2   The pros and cons of left flank and ventral midline laparotomy.

Left flank laparotomy	
Pros:	local anaesthesia; less risk of wound breakdown; goat conscious so readily mothers kids.
Cons:	difficult to exteriorise and isolate uterus to prevent contamination of the abdominal cavity when kids are dead and putrefied.
Ventral midline laparotomy	
Pros:	easier access to gravid uterus; easier to prevent abdominal contamination.
Cons:	general anaesthesia; greater risk of wound breakdown in active animal or from interference by suckling kids.

splitting approach can be used if preferred. The skin, internal and external abdominal oblique muscles, transversus abdominis muscle and peritoneum are incised and the uterus exposed. The abdominal muscles are fairly thin and easily incised. Muscle layers should be carefully identified to avoid penetrating the abdominal contents. The peritoneum should be incised by puncturing it and enlarging the incision with scissors. The exposed horn of the uterus is packed off with swabs. The usual site for incision into the uterus is over the greater curvature of one horn, which will usually allow all the fetuses to be removed from one site and avoids major blood vessels, so reducing haemorrhage. The incision into the uterine muscle should be large enough to permit delivery of the kids without causing tearing of the uterus. It may be possible to deliver a kid from the other horn through the same incision, but often a second incision is necessary in the other horn.

If the umbilical cord does not break during delivery, it is clamped with two pairs of forceps and broken between them. Ligation is not usually necessary but should be considered if haemorrhage is excessive. The placental membranes are removed from the uterus if they come away easily. Closely attached membranes are left in situ. Intrauterine antibiotics are of limited value and should not be used routinely.

The uterine incision is closed using an inverting suture, such as Lembert or Cushing, with 3-metric catgut or synthetic absorbable material swaged on an atraumatic needle. Any tears in the uterine horn should be carefully sutured. Entry of uterine fluid into the abdominal cavity does not present a problem, unless there is intrauterine infection associated with an emphysematous kid. In cases of grossly infected fluids, removal should be attempted by swabs, lavage and aspiration. In all cases, the uterus should be swabbed to remove excessive blood and fetal fluids before returning it to the abdominal cavity, as this will help prevent adhesions during healing.

The transversus abdominis muscle and peritoneum are closed using a 3.5- or 4-metric absorbable suture material in a simple continuous or interrupted pattern, followed in turn by the internal and external abdominal oblique muscles and the subcutaneous truncus muscle and fascia. The skin is closed with a non-absorbable suture, using simple interrupted or a horizontal mattress suture pattern.

Ventral midline laparotomy

Anaesthesia: general anaesthesia.

The goat is placed in dorsal recumbency and the surgical site, from the umbilicus to just in front of the udder, routinely prepared for surgery. The incision is made through the skin, subcutaneous tissues and linea alba. The greater omentum is pushed cranially and the gravid uterine horn exteriorised. The surgical procedure is then as for the flank incision. The peritoneum and linea alba are closed with a continuous mattress eversion suture of 5-metric absorbable synthetic material such as polyglycolic acid (Dexon, Dains and Geck). Bury this layer with a continuous simple layer of absorbable suture material and then suture the skin and subcutis with interrupted mattress sutures of 4- or 5-metric monofilament nylon. Leave the ends long so the sutures are easier to find for suture removal.

Following caesarian section

If surgical sterility is doubtful or in cases of uterine infection, broad-spectrum antibiotics should be given parenterally for 3 to 5 days and tetanus antitoxin should be given routinely if the goat is not vaccinated.

Perioperative pain relief is very important and will greatly speed recovery:

Carprofen, 1.4 mg/kg, 1 ml/35 kg i.v. (Zenecarp Solution, C-Vet)

Flunixin meglumine, 2 mg/kg, 2 ml/45 kg i.v. (Finadyne Solution,
Schering-Plough; **Flunixin,** Norbrook; **Binixin,** Bayer)

If necessary, milk letdown can be encouraged by administering **Oxytocin:**

Hyposton (G) (Pharmacia & Upjohn) **20–50 U, 2–5 ml i.m.** or **s.c.**

Oxytocin-S (G) (Intervet) **2–10 U, 0.2–1 ml i.m.** or **s.c.** or **0.5–2 U,**
0.05–0.25 ml, diluted 1 in 10 with water for injection slowly **i.v.**

There are no figures available for postoperative fertility following caesarian section, but levels appear to be close to those following normal parturition.

Care of kids following caesarian section

> Have assistance available to deal with the kids.

Live kids should be dried thoroughly with towels and placed in a warm environment with their mother as soon as she is sufficiently recovered to respond to them. A live kid will usually produce a positive response even from a very weak dam and may be the deciding factor in a goat which is deciding whether to live or die! As soon as the kid is delivered, ensure the respiratory tract is cleared of mucus. Towelling will help stimulate respirations or respiration can be stimulated by

> **Doxapram hydrochloride, 5–10 mg, 0.25–0.5 ml, sublingually** (**Dopram V**, Fort Dodge).

Where necessary the umbilical cord should be shortened and then treated with strong tincture of iodine or antibiotic spray.

Exploratory laparotomy to examine the uterus and ovaries

Anaesthesia: general

The goat is placed in dorsal recumbency and a midline incision is made through the skin, subcutaneous tissues and linea alba. The incision starts as close to the pelvis brim as possible (and may need to extend on to the udder septum) and extends cranially for about 5 or 6 cm. Tilting the table cranially makes finding the uterus easier (but increases pressure on the diaphragm from the abdominal contents and may compromise respiration!).

The uterine horns and ovaries of a non-pregnant animal can be completely exteriorised through the incision by inserting a finger into the abdominal cavity, hooking it round the uterus and applying gentle traction. The uterus should be handled gently to avoid unnecessary trauma which might lead to adhesions forming. Talc on gloves has also been implicated to causing adhesions.

Mastectomy

> As with all surgery, prior knowledge of the anatomy of the area is recommended – watch for those large blood vessels!

Mastectomy is a straightforward procedure but major surgery so far as the animal is concerned, and intravenous fluid therapy is indicated during surgery.

Indications: chronic mastitis or gangrenous mastitis.

Anaesthesia: general.

The goat is placed in dorsal recumbency, if a bilateral mastectomy is being carried out, or lateral recumbency, with the hind leg pulled caudally, for a unilateral mastectomy. The site is routinely clipped and prepared for surgery. The weight of the udder can be supported by attaching Allis tissue forceps to the teats and suspending the udder above the table from a hook or drip stand.

An elliptical incision is made around the base of the udder, *leaving as much skin as possible* to facilitate closure. The gland is separated from the skin and underlying tissue by blunt dissection. In the case of unilateral mastectomy, the gland is separated medially from the medial suspensory ligament. The mammary lymph glands, which lie caudal and dorsal to each gland, should be removed at the same time as the gland.

Several major blood vessels will require ligating during the dissection. These include the external pudendal artery (which should be *double ligated*), the external pudendal vein, the subcutaneous abdominal vein and the perineal vein. As much dead space as possible is reduced by means of several rows of absorbable simple continuous subcutaneous sutures and drains should be used if necessary. The skin is closed with simple interrupted sutures using 3-metric non-absorbable material.

Further reading

General

Noordsy, J.L. (1994) *Food Animal Surgery*, 3rd edn. Veterinary Learning Systems Co., Inc., Trenton, New Jersey.

Mastectomy

Kerr, H.J. and Wallace, C.E. (1978) Mastectomy in a goat. *Vet Med., Small Animal Clin.*, **73** (9), 1177–81.

Obstructive urolithiasis

Haven, M.L., *et al.* (1993) Surgical management of urolithiasis in small ruminants. *Cornell Vet.*, **83**, 47–55.

Rakestraw, P.C., *et al.* (1995) Tube cystotomy for treatment of obstructive urolithiasis in small ruminants. *Vet. Surgery*, **24**, 498–505.

Stone, W.C., *et al.* (1997) Prepubic urethrostomy for relief of urethral obstruction in a sheep and a goat. *J. Am. Vet. Med. Assoc.*, **210** (7), 939–41.

Reproductive system

Noakes, D.E. (1985) Surgical answers to reproductive problems in the female goat. *Goat Vet. Soc. J.*, **6** (2), 61–3.

Appendix 1
The Normal Goat

Unlike most other domestic ruminants, goats are *browsers* rather than grazers, preferentially ranging over a large area, often consuming as many as 25 different plant species. Many of the 'weed' species consumed by goats have a higher mineral and protein content than grasses, because of their greater root depth. In extensive grazing systems, goats will reject any plants contaminated with the scent of their own species' urine or faeces, thus limiting parasite infestation. However, this means that, conversely, goats have not evolved with the ability to develop an acquired immunity to gastrointestinal parasites and remain susceptible throughout their lives in intensive grazing systems. In confinement, goats remain extremely fussy eaters, often to the despair of their owners. Goats can distinguish between bitter, salt, sweet and sour tastes and will reject apparently similar batches of food because of a small variation in flavour. Goats have a higher tolerance for bitter-tasting feeds than most ruminants, presumably because browsings – bark, leaves, shrubs etc. – have a more bitter taste than grasses.

Kids are *hiders*, like deer, rather than followers, like lambs or calves, remaining concealed in one spot whilst their mothers graze and freezing at the sound of danger, so that predators will hopefully pass them by. Groups of kids will actively huddle together and seek out shelter in the form of a kid box or packing case.

Goats have a well defined social *hierarchy*, which is enhanced by crowding or limited feeding space. Once a dominance order is established, it may remain stable for several years, but any new goats introduced to the herd will have to fight to establish their own level. To prevent excessive conflict, goats should be kept as much as possible in permanent groups, without overcrowding and with adequate trough and rack space.

Physiological values

Temperature $\quad$ 38.6–40.6°C (102–104°F) (average 39.3°C)
Respiration – adults $\quad$ 15–30/minute
$\qquad$ – kids $\qquad$ 20–40/minute

Heart rate	70–95/minute
Rumination	1–1.5/minute

Weight

Adult dairy doe	55–105 kg
buck	75–120 kg
Adult Angora doe	35–55 kg
buck	50–70 kg
Adult Pygmy doe	22–27 kg
buck	28–32 kg

Weight can be estimated by measurement of the heart girth (see Table A1.1). For best results, the goat should stand square with its head erect and the tape should fit snugly around the circumference of the goat, just behind the front legs. A tape is more accurate with dairy goats than

Table A1.1   Goat weight table.

Girth (cm)	Dairy goats Weight (kg)	Pygmy does Weight (kg)	Pygmy males Weight (kg)
30	2.75		
35	4		
40	6		
45	9		
50	12	9	9
52.5	14	10.4	10.4
55	16	12.2	12.2
57.5	18	14	14.5
60	21	16	17
62.5	23	17.6	19
65	25	19.2	21.4
67.5	28	21	23.4
70	30	23.2	24.8
72.5	34	26.4	28
75	36	28.6	30
77.5	40	31	33.2
80	43	33.6	35.6
82.5	47	35.6	38
85	51	37.4	40.4
90	60		
95	69		
100	78		
105	88		

Table A1.2 Age to weight relationship (dairy goat).

Age (months)	Weight (kg)
Birth	4
1	11.5
2	18
3	25
4	29.5
5	34
6	38.5
7	42
8	45.5
9	50
10	52
11	54.5
12	59
18	70
24	77
30	81.5
36	93

Table A1.3 Age to weight relationship (Pygmy goats).

Age (months)	Weight (kg)	
	Male	Female
Birth	1.55	1.4
1	4.8	4.3
2	8.3	6.8
3	11.8	9.1
4	13.2	11.1
5	14.5	12.8
6	15.5	14.7
8	19	17.2
10	21	19.5
12	22.7	22.2
24	29	25
36	32	28

with Pygmies. Age is related to weight by a normal growth curve (see Tables A1.2 and A1.3). Estimating the weight of immature Pygmy goats is not easy. Table A1.3 gives very approximate weights that can be expected at different ages. Females are considered mature at 24 months, males at 30 months.

Haematology

Red blood cell parameters

Test	Range (VLA)[2]	Units
RBCC	10–18	$\times 10^{12}/l$
Hb	8–15	g/dl
PCV	0.24–0.39	l/l
MCH	7–9	pg
MCHC	31–42	g/dl
MCV	16–34	fl
Platelets	3–6	$10^5/ul$

White blood cell parameters

Test	Range (VLA)[2]	Units	%
WBCC	6–14	$\times 10^{12}/l$	
Neutrophil (mature)	1.2–7.2	$\times 10^{12}/l$	30–48
Neutrophil (band)	Rare		Rare
Lymphocyte	2–9	$\times 10^{12}/l$	45–70
Monocyte	0–0.5	$\times 10^{12}/l$	0–4
Eosinophil	0.05–0.5	$\times 10^{12}/l$	1–8
Basophil	0–0.1	$\times 10^{12}/l$	0–1

Urinalysis

Specific gravity	1.015–1.050
pH	7–8
Colour	Yellow
Turbidity	Clear
Volume	10–40 ml/kg body weight/day

Cerebrospinal fluid

Specific gravity	1.005
Colour	Colourless
Total protein	0–0.39 g/l
Glucose	3.0–4.0 mmol/l
White blood cells	0–4 cells/µl

Biochemistry

Test	Range (Vettest 8008)[1]	(VLA)[2]	Units
ALB	28–38	29–43	g/l
ALKP	75–228	0–300	U/l
ALT	23–44		U/l
Amylase	1–30		U/l
AST	122–321	0–300	U/l
BHB	0–1.2	0–1.2	mmol/l
BUN	3.6–7.5	4–8.6	mmol/l
Calcium	2.05–2.45	2.3–2.9	mmol/l
Chloride		98–110	mmol/l
Cholesterol	1.63–2.79	1.0–3.0	mmol/l
CK	28–130	0–100	U/l
Copper		9–25	µmol/l
Creatinine	53–124	54–123	µmol/l
GGT	60–101	0–30	U/l
GLDH		0–10	U/l
Globulin	36–40	23–46	g/l
Glucose	3.0–5.2	2.4–4.0	mmol/l
GSH-Px		>60	U/ml RBCs
Haptoglobulin		<0.1	g/l
LDH	811–1250	0–400	U/l
Magnesium		0.8–1.3	mmol/l
Pepsinogen		0–1	U/l
Phosphate	1.35–2.45	1–2.4	mmol/l
Potassium		3.4–6.1	mmol/l
Sodium		135–156	mmol/l
T4		43–90	nmol/l
Total bilirubin	0.9–6.0	0–7	µmol/l
Total protein	64–78	62–79	g/l
Triglycerides	0.11–0.33		mmol/l
Vitamin B_{12}		>221	pmol/l

Values for enzymes are shown for assays carried out at 37°C. All values shown are for serum with the exception of phosphate and glucose (oxalate fluoride plasma) and copper (whole blood). Variations may occur within ranges according to breed, age and sex, etc.

Individual laboratories will have their own reference ranges and should be consulted before attempting to interpret haematological or biochemical results.

Reference ranges are based on published and unpublished data supplied by:

[1] Idexx Laboratories Ltd., Chalfont St. Peter, Buckinghamshire, UK. (Vettest 8008 is an automated biochemistry analysis in use in many practice laboratories.)
[2] Veterinary Laboratories Agency, New Haw, Weybridge, Surrey, UK.

Reproductive data

Breeding season (northern hemisphere): September to March
Oestrus cycle (days)   : 21 (18–21)
Oestrus duration (hours)   : 32–96
Ovulation after start of oestrus (hours) : 36–48
Age at puberty (months) male   : 4–5
                       female : 4–5
Gestation period (days)   : 150 (145–154)
Semen volume (ml)   : 0.5–1.5
    concentration ($\times 10/$ml)   : 1500–5000
    total sperm ($\times 10$)   : 750–7500
    good motility (%)   : 70–90
    normal morphology (%)   : 75–95

Appendix 2
Drug Dosages

Under The Medicines (Restrictions on the Administration of Veterinary Medicinal Products) Regulations 1994, a veterinary surgeon, or someone acting under his or her direction, may only administer a product to a food-producing animal if it contains substances found in a product authorised for use in food-producing animals. Because there are so few drugs licensed for goats in the UK (ten at the last count by the Goat Veterinary Society), it will generally be necessary to use drugs licensed for use in other species of farm animal. Manufacturers should be consulted about suitable drug doses for goats. Drug metabolism shows species variation, with the result that dose rates and excretion times for goats cannot be simply extrapolated from sheep and cattle data. For instance, the half-life of some drugs, including many anthelmintics, that are eliminated mainly by hepatic metabolism is, in goats, about half that for sheep. Furthermore, there are species differences between breeds of goats. Pygmy goats are reported to metabolise sulphonamides, chloramphenicol and probably other drugs that are metabolised by hepatic microsomal enzymes faster than other breeds.

All drugs, which are not specifically licensed for goats, carry a mandatory *7-day withholding time for milk* and *28-day withholding time for meat*.

Drug doses mentioned in this book have been gleaned from the world literature. Wherever possible, drugs are matched with licensed products currently available in the UK, but these change monthly, and not all drugs quoted have a current licence for food-producing animals in the UK. It is the reader's responsibility to ensure that he/she is legally entitled to use any drug mentioned.

The Veterinary Medicines Directorate has stated that

'at present [they] cannot envisage that the Ministry would wish to take action against veterinary surgeons prescribing and using anaesthetics and analgesics which are necessary for the health and welfare of animals in circumstances where no suitable authorised product exists and where the imposition of the withdrawal period set down in the Regulations would protect consumers.'

Drugs discussed below and in the text marked G are licensed for use in goats in the UK.

Administration of drugs

Intramuscular injections

> Lameness, sometimes permanent, is a common sequel to intramuscular injections.

Because the goat has relatively small muscle masses in the hind leg, particularly the gluteal region, temporary lameness is common after injections of irritant substances such as tetracyclines and fluoro-quinolones. More permanent lameness may result from damage to the sciatic nerve if the gluteal muscle mass is used, or to the peroneal nerve if the injection is in the caudal thigh region.

An alternative site for intramuscular injections is the cleido-occipitalis muscle in the mid neck region, but induced pain in this region may result in the goat being unwilling to feed. A preferable site in the neck is the triangular area bordered by the vertebral column ventrally, the nuchal ligament dorsally and the shoulder caudally. The triceps muscle mass and the longissimus muscles of the back in the lumbar region can also be used.

The volume of drug administered at one site should never be more than 5 ml, using a needle of 18 g or less and 25 to 38 mm (1 to 1.5 inches) in length in adult goats. Smaller amounts and shorter needles should be used in kids.

It is always safer to use the subcutaneous route rather than give intramuscular injections and this route should be adopted wherever possible.

Subcutaneous injections

Subcutaneous injections are normally given in the chest wall just behind the elbow or in the loose skin of the neck just in front of the shoulders.

Intravenous injections

Intravenous injections are generally given via the external jugular vein:

❏ Animal is held standing, with head restrained by hand on the nose.
❏ Clip hair over jugular furrow at approximately mid point of neck.

❏ Clean site with surgical spirit or iodophor.
❏ Apply external pressure with fingers or tourniquet on the jugular groove in the lower part of the jugular furrow to dilate the external jugular vein.
❏ A needle 18 g × 38 mm (1.5 inches) is suitable for adult goats, 20 g × 25 mm (1 inch) for smaller animals; puncture the vein; blood should flow through the needle.
❏ Infuse drug slowly.

Oral medication

Oral medication can be given relatively easily by means of syringes, drenching guns or boluses, if the goat is properly restrained. Back the animal into a corner with one side against a wall; then either straddle the animal or stand against the shoulder in a larger animal. The head should be held normally in a horizontal position, and not tilted, to reduce the chance of inducing aspiration pneumonia. Holding the lower jaw with one hand, the syringe or drenching gun is slipped into the corner of the mouth at the commissure of the lips, so that the tip is just over the base of the tongue.

Goats are generally tolerant of the passage of a stomach tube but tend to bite through it unless a suitable gag is available. Any of the varieties of sheep gag are suitable or use a block of wood with a hole drilled through it.

Closure of the reticular groove

The absorption of many drugs from the rumen is problematical. Closure of the reticular groove, allowing orally administered drugs to pass straight to the abomasum, can be achieved by:

❏ oral administration of **5 ml** of a solution of **copper sulphate** (a tablespoonful in 1 l of water);
❏ injection of **0.25 U/kg lysine–vasopressin i.v.** also results in groove closure;
❏ in cattle, oral administration of 60 ml sodium bicarbonate 10%.

Sedatives and anaesthetics

Sedatives

❏ **Acepromazine maleate, 0.05–0.1 mg/kg, 1–2 ml/40 kg** slowly **i.v.** (**ACP 2 mg/ml**, C-Vet).
❏ **Detomidine, 20–40 µg/kg, 0.08–0.16 ml/40 kg i.v.** or **i.m.** (**Domosedan**, Pfizer).

❏ Diazepam, 0.25–0.5 mg/kg, 2–4 ml/40 kg, slowly **i.v.** (**Valium**, Roche).

❏ **Medetomidine, 25–35 μg/kg, 1–1.5 ml/40 kg i.m. (Domitor**, Pfizer).

❏ **Xylazine, 0.05 mg/kg, 0.1 ml/40 kg** slowly **i.v.** or **0.1 mg/kg, 0.2 ml/ 40 kg i.m.(Rompun**, Bayer; **Chanazine**, Chanelle; **Virbaxyl**, Virbac).

Overdosage of sedatives can be treated by:

❏ **Doxapram hydrochloride, 0.5–1 mg/kg, 1–2 ml/40 kg i.v.** (**Dopram V**, Fort Dodge).

Overdosage of xylazine and other alpha-2 adrenoceptor stimulants can be reversed by:

❏ **Atipamezole, 125–175 μg/kg, 1–1.5 ml/40 kg**, half **i.v.** and half **i.m.** (**Antisedan**, Pfizer).

Injectable anaesthetics

❏ **Alphaxolone/alphadolone, 3 mg/kg, 10 ml/40 kg** slowly **i.v.** (**Saffan**, Schering-Plough).

❏ **Etorphine hydrochloride/acepromazine maleate, 0.01 ml/kg i.v.** or **i.m.** (**Large Animal Immobilon/Revivon**, C-Vet).

❏ **Ketamine, 10–15 mg/kg, 4–6 ml/40 kg** slowly **i.v.** (**Ketaset**, Fort Dodge; **Vetalar**, Pharmacia & Upjohn) (for ketamine combined with other drugs see Chapter 21).

❏ **Methohexital sodium, 4 mg/kg, 6.5 ml/40 kg** (**Brietal**, Animalcare) as 2.5% solution.

❏ **Pentobarbital sodium, 10–15 mg/kg, 40–60 ml/40 kg i.v.** (**Sagatal**, Merial).

❏ **Propofol, 3–4 mg/kg, 12–16 ml/40 kg** slowly **i.v.** (**Rapinovet**, Schering-Plough).

❏ **Thiopental sodium, 10–15 mg/kg, 8–12 ml/40 kg i.v.** (**Intraval Sodium 5 g**, Merial; **Thiovet 5 g**, C-Vet).

❏ **Tiletamine–zolazepam, 5.5 mg/kg i.v.** (**Telazol**, Fort Dodge); not available in the UK.

Analgesics and anti-inflammatory drugs

Opioid analgesics

❏ **Butorphanol, 0.07–0.1 mg/kg, 0.3–0.4 ml/40 kg i.v.** (**Torbugesic**, Fort Dodge).

Non-steroidal anti-inflammatory drugs

❏ **Aspirin, 50–100 mg/kg po** every 12 hours (aspirin is poorly absorbed from the rumen so relatively high doses are needed).

❏ **Carprofen, 1.4 mg/kg, 1 ml/35 kg s.c. or i.v. (Zenecarp Solution,** Pfizer) every 36 to 48 hours.

❏ **Carprofen, 1.4 mg/kg, 0.5 sachet/75 kg orally (Zenecarp Granules,** Pfizer) once daily.

❏ **Flunixin meglumine, 2 mg/kg, 2 ml/45 kg i.v. or i.m. (Finadyne Solution,** Schering-Plough; **Flunixin,** Norbrook; **Binixin,** Bayer; **Meflosyl 5%,** Fort Dodge; **Resprixin,** Intervet) daily for up to 5 days.

❏ **Flunixin meglumine, 2 mg/kg, 100 kg horse calibration/50 kg orally (Finadyne Paste,** Schering-Plough) daily for up to 5 days
                          0.5 sachet/50 kg orally (Finadyne Granules, Schering-Plough) daily for up to 5 days.

❏ **Ketoprofen, 3 mg/kg, 1 ml/33 kg i.v. or i.m. (Ketofen,** Merial) daily for up to 3 days.

❏ **Meloxicam, 0.5 mg/kg, 1 ml/10 kg i.v. or s.c. (Metacam 5 mg Solution,** Boehringer Ingelheim) every 36 to 48 hours.

❏ **Phenylbutazone, 4 mg/kg, 1 ml/50 kg i.v. or 10 mg/kg orally.**

Note: under present legislation, phenylbutazone is banned from use in food-producing animals in the EU.

Corticosteroids

❏ **Betamethasone, 0.04–0.08 mg/kg, 1 ml/30 kg [Betsolan** (G), **Betsolan Soluble** (G), Schering-Plough].

❏ **Dexamethasone, 0.1 mg/kg, 1 ml/20 kg i.v. (Azium,** Schering-Plough; **Colvasone,** Norbrook; **Dexadreson,** Intervet).

❏ **Methylprednisolone, 10–30 mg/kg i.v. (Solu-medrone,** Pharmacia & Upjohn) every 4 to 6 hours for 24 to 48 hours.

Other anti-inflammatory drugs

The following have all been used empirically in non-lactating pet goats with dose rates extrapolated from those for other species as there are no published results of clinical trials in goats.

❏ **Pentosan polysulphate sodium, 3 mg/kg s.c. (Cartrophen Vet,** Arthropharm) weekly for 4 weeks, then a single injection every 4 to 6 months. Do not use concurrently with steroids or non-steroidal anti-inflammatory drugs, including aspirin and phenylbutazone.

❏ **Polysulphated glycosaminoglycan, 125 mg, 1.25 ml i.m. (Adequan,** Janssen) for a 50- to 80-kg doe (large animals may need increased amount), weekly for 4 weeks, then a single injection every 4 to 6 months.

❏ **Sodium hyaluronate, 20 mg, 2 ml i.v. (Hyonate,** Bayer).

Anthelmintics

Dose rates for sheep cannot be directly extrapolated to goats. Higher dose rates are often required in goats.

Benzamidazoles

Dose at **1.5–2 times sheep dose rate**.

- ❏ Albendazole, febental, fenbendazole, oxfendazole, **7.5 mg/kg orally**.
- ❏ Mebendazole, **22.5 mg/kg orally**.
- ❏ Netobimin, **11.25 mg/kg orally**.

Levamisole

Dose at **1.5 times sheep dose rate**, i.e. **12 mg/kg orally** (do not exceed this rate as levamisole is toxic in goats at dose rates approaching 20 mg/kg; do not use injectable preparations).

Avermectins

Use sheep dose rate, i.e. 200 µg/kg, 10 mg/50 kg, 1 ml/50 kg s.c. The only anthelmintics licensed for use in goats in the UK are the avermectin

- ❏ **Ivermectin, 200 µg/kg, 2.5 ml/10 kg orally** (**Oramec Drench**, Merial)

and the probenzimidazole

- ❏ **Thiophanate, 9 kg/tonne feed** as single dose or **2.8 kg/tonne feed** daily for 5 days (**Nemafax 14**, Merial).

Drugs for flukes (trematodes)

Chronic fascioliasis

- ❏ **Oxyclozanide, 15 mg/kg orally** (**Zanil**, Schering-Plough).
- ❏ **Albendazole, 7.5 mg/kg orally** (**Valbazan**, Pfizer); also effective against intestinal worms and tapeworms.
- ❏ **Triclabendazole, 10 mg/kg orally** (**Fasinex**, Novartis).
- ❏ **Netobimin, 20 mg/kg orally** (**Hapadex**, Schering-Plough).
- ❏ **Closantel, 10 mg/kg orally** (**Flukiver**, Janssen).
- ❏ **Nitroxynil, 10 mg/kg s.c.** (**Trodax**, Merial).

Acute and subacute fascioliasis

❏ **Triclabendazole, 10 mg/kg orally** (**Fasinex**, Novartis), active against all stages of fluke from 2 days old to adult fluke.
❏ **Closantel, 10 mg/kg orally** (**Flukiver**, Janssen), moderately effective in fluke from 3 to 4 weeks old and highly effective against adult fluke.
❏ **Nitroxynil, 10 mg/kg s.c.** (**Trodax**, Merial), moderately effective in fluke from 8 to 9 weeks old and highly effective against mature fluke.

Drugs for tapeworms (cestodes)

❏ **Albendazole, 10 mg/kg; febental, 7.5 mg/kg; fenbendazole, 15 mg/ kg;** and **oxfendazole, 10 mg/kg** are effective against *Moniezia* spp. at higher doses than required for nematode control.
❏ **Praziquantel, 5 mg/kg, 1 ml/10 kg s.c.** or **1 tablet/10 kg orally** (**Droncit**, Bayer) is effective, but not licensed for food-producing animals in the UK. Some goats are irritated by the injection.

Antibiotics

There are no antibiotic preparations presently licensed specifically for goats in the UK. In general, it is safe to extrapolate from recommendations for sheep or cattle, but it cannot always be assumed that the pharmokinetics of a particular drug will be the same in the goat as in other species, e.g. oxytetracycline is more rapidly excreted in the goat than in cattle. Because mandatory 7-day withholding times are required for milk, the use of depot preparations, e.g. ampicillin, amoxycillin, oxytetracycline and penicillin, may permit a shorter total withholding time than when daily injections are given.

Do not use tilmicosin (Micotil, Elanco) in goats, as injection has been fatal.

Anticonvulsants

❏ **Diazepam, 0.25–0.5 mg/kg, 2–4 ml/40 kg i.v.** to effect (**Valium**, Roche).
❏ **Phenobarbitone, 0.04 ml/kg i.v.** to effect (**Sagatal**, Merial), then **0.22 ml/kg i.v.** every 8 to 12 hours as required.

Coccidiosis

Treatment

- ❏ **Sulphadimidine 200 mg/kg, 6 ml/10 kg** initial dose, then **100 mg/ kg, 3 ml/10 kg s.c.** or **i.v.** (preferred) (**Bimadine 33 1/3**, Bimeda; **Intradine**, Norbrook; **Sulfoxine 333**, Vetoquinol; **Vesadin**, Merial) daily for up to 5 days total.
- ❏ **Sulphadimidine, 200 mg/kg** initial dose, then **100 mg/kg orally** (**Bimadine Oral Powder**, Bimeda) daily for 5 days total.

Note: sulphadimidine injectable solutions can be given orally in milk or water as an alternative to powder.

- ❏ **Sulphamethoxypyridazine, 20 mg/kg, 1 ml/12.5 kg s.c.** (**Bimalong**, Bimeda; **Midicel**, Pharmacia & Upjohn; **Sulfapyrine LA**, Vetoquinol) daily for 3 days,
- ❏ **Decoquinate, 100 g/tonne feed** or **1 mg/kg** (**Deccox, Deccox prescription**, Merial) for 28 days,
- ❏ **Diclazuril 1 mg/kg, 1 ml/2.5 kg orally** (**Vecoxan**, Janssen) as a single dose.
- ❏ **Amprolium, 5–10 mg/kg orally** daily for 3 to 5 days and
- ❏ **Toltrazuril, 20 mg/kg orally** (**Baycox**, Bayer) once every 3 to 4 weeks
  have been used successfully to control coccidiosis in kids but are only licensed for use in poultry in the UK.

Prophylaxis

In feed

- ❏ **Decoquinate, 100 g/tonne feed** or **1 mg/kg** (**Deccox, Deccox prescription**, Merial) for 28 days to kids.
- ❏ **Decoquinate, 50 g/tonne feed** or **0.5 mg/kg** (**Deccox, Deccox prescription**, Merial) for 28 days to does.
- ❏ **Monesin** is now classified as a growth promoter in the UK and cannot be used in the control of coccidiosis in goats. Similarly, other growth promoters such as **lasalocid** and **salinomycin** are also prohibited.

In milk

- ❏ **Sulphadimidine, 200 mg/kg** initially, then **100 mg/kg** for a further 2 to 4 days every 3 weeks. Sulphadimidine will reduce the level of environmental contamination of oocysts as 3 weeks is close to the prepatent period for many goat *Eimeria*. Sulphadimidine can be given as oral powder or the injectable solution can be added to milk.

❏ **Toltrazuril, 20 mg/kg (Baycox**, Bayer) every 3 to 4 weeks (only licensed for poultry in the UK).

Orally

❏ **Diclazuril, 1 mg/kg, 1 ml/2.5 kg orally (Vecoxon**, Janssen) at about 4 to 6 weeks of age. Under conditions of high infection pressure a second treatment can be given about 3 weeks after the first dosing.

Drugs acting on the digestive tract

To reduce intestinal motility

❏ **Loperamide hydrochloride, 100–200** μg/kg, **0.5–1 ml/kg orally (Immodium Syrup**, Janssen-Cilag) every 8 or 12 hours or **1–2 capsules/20 kg orally (Immodium Capsules**, Janssen-Cilag); dissolve contents in small amount of water every 8 to 12 hours.

Spasmolytics

❏ **Metamizole, hyoscine butylbromide, 0.5–5 ml i.v. (Buscopan Compositum**, Boehringer Ingelheim).

To restore abomasal tone and promote emptying

❏ **Metaclopramide, 0.5–1 mg/kg, 0.5–1 ml/5 kg i.v. (Emequell**, Pfizer).

To stimulate appetite

❏ **Chlorpromazine, 0.5 mg/kg i.v.**
❏ **Diazepam, 0.04 mg/kg i.v.**

Positive effect on feeding lasts approximately 30 minutes.

External parasites

Amidines

❏ **Amitraz 0.025% solution**, by **spray** or **wash (Taktic**, Hoechst Roussel), dilute 1 volume in 250 volumes of water, or (**Aludex**, Hoechst Roussel), dilute 1 volume in 200 volumes of water.

Pyrethrins and synthetic pyrethroids

❏ **Cypermethrin 1.25% solution, 'pour-on' 0.25 ml/kg** (maximum 20 ml) (**Crovect**, Crown; **Provinec**, C-Vet; **Vector**, Young's).
❏ **Deltamethrin 1%**, by **'spot-on'** (**Spot On**, Schering-Plough).
❏ **Permethrin 4%, 'pour-on'** (**Ridect**, Pfizer; **Ryposect**, C-Vet; **Swift**, Young's).
❏ **Pyrethrins**
There are also many preparations containing permethrin marketed for use in dogs and cats as shampoos and powders and containing pyrethrins and piperonyl butoxide marketed as dog and cat sprays and powders which can be used on pet and Pygmy goats.

Avermectins and milbemycin

❏ **Abamectin, 10 mg/50 kg, 1 ml/50 kg s.c.** (**Enzec**, Janssen).
❏ **Doramectin, 10 mg/50 kg, 1 ml/50 kg s.c.** (**Dectomax**, Pfizer).
❏ **Ivermectin, 10 mg/50 kg, 1 ml/50 kg s.c.** (**Ivomec**, **Panomec**, Merial).
❏ **Moxidectin, 10 mg/50 kg, 1 ml/50 kg s.c.** (**Cydectin 1%**, Fort Dodge).
Doramectin, Ivermectin and **Moxidectin** are also available as cattle 'pour-on' applications at **500 m/kg, 1 ml/10 kg**.
❏ **Eprinomectin, 500 m/kg, 1 ml/10 kg** [**Eprinex**, Merial].

Fipronil

Fipronil (Frontline Spray, Merial) is suitable for Pygmy goats or individual pet goats as it is expensive! It is not licensed for use in food-producing animals in the UK.

Phosmet

❏ **Phosmet 0.09% solution** (**Vet-Kem Sponge-On**, Sanoffi), dilute 30 ml with 3.8 l water.
❏ **Phosmet 20 mg/kg, 200 mg/ml, 'pour-on'** (**Dermol Plus**, Crown; **Poron 20**, Young's).

Dips

Fibre goats can be dipped using products approved for sheep. The body should be immersed for at least 30 seconds, until the coat is completely saturated. The head should be immersed once or twice, allowing the animal to breathe between immersions. Products available include **amitraz** (**Taktic**, Hoechst Roussel), **pyrethroids – cypermethrin** (**Crovect**, Crown; **Provinec**, C-Vet) and **flumethrin** (**Bayticol Scab and Tick Dip**, Bayer).

Fertility

Prostaglandins

- ❏ **Dinaprost, 2 ml i.m.** or **s.c.** (**Lutalyse**, Pharmacia & Upjohn).
- ❏ **Clorprostenol, 0.5 ml i.m.** or **s.c.** (**Estrumate**, Schering-Plough).

Oxytocin

- ❏ **Oxytocin, 2–10 U, 0.2–1 ml i.m.** or **s.c.** (**Oxytocin-S**, Intervet) (G) or **0.5–2 U, 0.05–0.25 ml, diluted 1 in 10 with water** for injection slowly **i.v.**
- ❏ **Pituitary extract (posterior lobe), 20–50 U, 2–5 ml i.m.** or **s.c.** (**Hyposton**, Pharmacia & Upjohn) (G) or **2–10 U, 0.2–1 ml i.m.** (preferred) or **s.c.** (**Pituitary Extract (Synthetic)**, Animalcare) (G).

Chorionic gonadotrophin

- ❏ **Chorulon** (Intervet), **500 U, i.m.** (at time of service) or **1000 U, i.m.** (cystic ovaries).

Gonadotrophin releasing hormones

- ❏ **Gonadorellin** (**Fertagyl**, Intervet), **2.5 ml i.m.** (at time of service or to prevent luteolysis) or **5 ml i.m.** (cystic ovaries).
- ❏ **Buserelin** (**Receptal**, Hoechst) **2.5 ml i.m., s.c.** or **i.v.** (at time of service or to prevent luteolysis) or **5 ml i.m., s.c.** or **i.v.** (cystic ovaries).

Serum gonadotrophin

- ❏ **Folligon** (Intervet), **Fostim** (Pharmacia & Upjohn) (G) **s.c.** or **i.m.**, dose depends on time of year, weight of goat and milk yield (see Chapter 1).

Myometrial relaxants

- ❏ **Clenbutarol hydrochloride, 0.8 μg/kg, 1.25 ml/50 kg**, slowly **i.v.** or **i.m.** (**Planipart, Ventipulmin**, Boehringer Ingelheim).

❏ **Vetrabutine hydrochloride, 2 mg/kg, 1 ml/50 kg i.m.** (Monzaldon, Boehringer Ingelheim).

Fungal treatments

Topical fungicides

❏ **Copper naphthenate (Kopertox,** Crown).
❏ **Eniliconazole (Imaverol,** Janssen), 0.2% solution, by **wash** or **spray**, every 3 days for 3 or 4 applications.
❏ **Natamycin (Mycophyt,** Intervet), 0.01% solution locally, repeat after 4 or 5 days and again after 14 days if required.

Oral preparations

❏ **Griseofulvin, 7.5 mg/kg orally** for 7 days.

Note: under present EU legislation, griseofulvin cannot be used in food-producing animals as no official residue limits have been set.

Respiratory disease

❏ **Clenbuterol, 0.8 mcg/kg, 1.25 ml/50 kg** slowly **i.v.** or **i.m.** (**Ventipulmin**, Boehringer Ingelheim) or **2.5 g/50 kg orally** (**Ventipulmin Granules**, Boehringer Ingelheim) in feed twice daily.

Appendix 3
Diagnostic Reference Charts

3.1 Weak kids: principal causes

❏ **Prematurity**
❏ **Low birth weight**
❏ **Birth injury**
❏ **Malnutrition**

   (1) **Intrauterine malnutrition**
     Maternal malnutrition
     underfeeding of doe
     multiple fetuses
     pregnancy toxaemia
     lameness
     Trace element deficiency
     copper deficiency [enzootic
      ataxia]
     iodine deficiency [goitre]
     selenium deficiency [white
      muscle disease]
     Congenital infection
     chlamydia
     salmonella
     toxoplasmosis
     neosporosis
     listeriosis
     Q-fever
     border disease
     sarcocystis

   (2) **Postnatal malnutrition**
     inability to suckle
     mismothering
     agalactia
     poor udder conformation
     teat abnormalities

❏ **Congenital defects**

   (1) **Genetic**
     atresia ani
     arthrogryposis (contracted
      tendons)
     microphthalmia
     hydrocephalus
     cerebellar hypoplasia
     beta mannosidosis

   (2) **Developmental abnormalities**
     hyper/hypoflexion of limbs
     ventricular septal defect
     hydronephrosis
     cleft palate
     spinal abnormalities

❏ **Postnatal infection**
   Escherichia coli
   Clostridia spp.
   Pasteurella spp.
   Staphylococcus aureus
   Streptococcus spp.
   Corynebacterium spp.
   Tick pyaemia

❏ **Floppy kid syndrome**

❏ **Exposure**
   Primary hypothermia
   Secondary hypothermia

3.2 Chronic weight loss: principal causes

❑ **Primary nutritional deficiency**
starvation
  neglect
  inexperience
trace element deficiency
  cobalt
  copper
  vitamin E/selenium

❑ **Inability to utilize available foodstuffs**
dentition
mouth lesions
facial paralysis
lameness
blindness
bullying

❑ **Unwillingness to utilize available foodstuffs**
male goats at the start of the
  breeding season
unpalatable feed – spoilage,
  mould etc
change in feed

❑ **Inability to increase feed intake to match production demands**
peak lactation
periparturient toxaemia
  (pregnancy toxaemia,
  postparturient toxaemia,
  ketosis, acetonaemia)

❑ **Interference with absorption of nutrients/loss of nutrients**
gastrointestinal parasitism
Johne's disease
  (paratuberculosis)

liver disease
  chronic fascioliasis
  abscess
  tumour
  ragwort poisoning
  visceral cysticercosis
  hydatid disease
diabetes mellitus

❑ **Interference with rumen/ intestinal mobility**
chronic rumen impaction
ascites – chronic fascioliasis
ruminoreticular ulceration
adhesions following surgery
tumour – carcinomas
cestode infection
left-sided displacement of the
  abomasum

❑ **Presence of chronic diseases**
pneumonia
  pasteurella
  CAE
  lungworm infection
  viruses
  mycoplasma
  caseous lymphadenitis
peritonitis
enteritis
mastitis
metritis
tuberculosis

❑ **Pruritic conditions**
lice
sarcoptic mange
scrapie

3.3 Nervous diseases: principal causes

Neonatal kids
congenital infections
hypoglycaemia
birth trauma
enzootic ataxia (swayback)

Kids up to one month
spinal abscess
trauma
congenital vertebral lesions
tick pyaemia
bacterial meningitis
focal symmetrical encephalomalacia
   (enterotoxaemia)
tetanus
disbudding meningoencephalitis
louping ill

2–7 months
trauma
delayed swayback
spinal abscess
coccidiosis
CAE (viral leucoencephalitis)

7 months–adult
❏ **Infectious disease**
   listeriosis
   scrapie
   louping
   tetanus
   CAE
   pseudorabies (Aujesky's disease)
   rabies

❏ **Metabolic disease**
   cerebrocortical necrosis
      (CCN, polioencephalomalacia)
   hypocalcaemia (milk fever)
   hypomagnesaemia (grass tetany)
   transit tetany
   periparturient toxaemia

❏ **Space-occupying lesions of the
    brain**
   cerebral abscess
   coenuriasis (gid)
   pituitary abscess syndrome
   oestrus ovis
   tumour

❏ **Space-occupying lesions of the
    spinal cord**
   spinal meningitis
   spinal abscess
   vertebral osteomyelitis
   tumour
   coenuriasis
   cerebrospinal nematodiasis

❏ **Trauma**

   Vestibular disease
   otitis media/interna
   ear mite infection

❏ **Hepatic encephalopathy**

   Poisonings
   lead
   plant
   organophosphates
   rafoxanide
   urea

❏ **Epilepsy**

3.4   Diarrhoea: principal causes

❏ **Birth–4 weeks**
nutritional
enterotoxigenic *E.coli*
Salmonella spp.
Clostridium perfringens type C
Clostridium perfringens type B
Campylobacter jejuni
rotavirus
coronavirus
cryptosporidium
Strongyloides papillosus

❏ **4 weeks–12 weeks**
parasitic gastroenteritis
coccidiosis
Clostridium perfringens type D
salmonella
giardiasis
yersiniosis
nutritional factors
Campylobacter jejuni
toxic agents

❏ **Over 12 weeks**
parasitic gastroenteritis
coccidiosis
Cl. perfringens type D
salmonella
nutritional factors
toxic agents
liver disease
copper deficiency
(Johne's disease)

Further Reading

Anatomy

Garrett, P.D. (1988) *Guide to Ruminal Anatomy Based on the Dissection of the Goat.* Iowa State University Press, Iowa.

Owen, N.L. (1977) *The Illustrated Standard of the Dairy Goat.* Dairy Goat Publishing Corporation, Lake Mills, Wisconsin.

Haematology and biochemistry

Davies, D.M. and Sims, B.J. (1985) Welsh and Marches Goat Society survey to determine normal blood biochemistry and haematology in domestic goats. *Goat Vet. Soc. J.,* **6** (1), 38–42.

Mews, A. and Mowlem, A. (1981) Normal haematological and biochemical values in the goat. *Goat. Vet. Soc. J.,* **2** (1), 30–31.

Management

Gall, C. (ed.) (1981) *Goat Production.* Academic Press, London.

Guss, S.B. (1977) *Management and Diseases of Dairy Goats.* Dairy Goat Publishing Corporation, Lake Mills, Wisconsin.

Mackenzie, D. (revised and ed. by R. Goodwin) (1993) *Goat Husbandry,* 5th edn. Faber and Faber, London.

Mowlem, A. (1992) *Goat Farming,* 2nd edn. Farming Press Books, Ipswich.

Peacock, C. (1996) *Improving Goat Production in the Tropics.* Oxfam/Farm-Africa, Oxford.

Medicine and surgery

Baxendell, S.A. (1988) *The Diagnosis of the Diseases of Goats.* Vade Mecum. Series No. 19. Univ. Sydney Post Grad. Found. Vet. Sci., Sydney, Australia.

Dunn, P. (1994) *The Goatkeeper's Veterinary Book,* 3rd edn. Farming Press Books, Ipswich.

Goat Veterinary Society Journals (ed. by R. Goodwin). Available from J. Matthews, The Limes, Chalk Street, Rettendon Common, Chelmsford, Essex CM3 8DA.

Goats (1984) No. 73. Proc. Univ. Sydney Post Grad. Found. Vet. Sci., Sydney, Australia.

Goat Health and Production No. 134 (1990) Proc. Univ. Sydney Post Grad. Found. Vet. Sci., Sydney, Australia.

Howe, P.A. (1984) *Diseases of Goats.* Vade Mecum No. 5. Proc. Univ. Sydney Post Grad. Found. Vet. Sci., Sydney, Australia.

Linklater, K.A. and Smith, M.C. (1993) *Color Atlas of the Diseases and Disorders of the Sheep and Goat.* Mosby-Wolfe, London.

Lloyd, S. (1982) Goat medicine and surgery. *Br. Vet. J.*, **138**, 70–85.

Smith, M.C. (ed.) (1983) Sheep and goat medicine. *Vet. Clin. North Am.: Large Animal Practice*, **5** (3), November 1983.

Smith, M.C. (ed.) (1990) Advances in sheep and goat medicine. *Vet. Clin. North Am.: Large Animal Practice*, **6** (3), November 1990.

Smith, M.C. and Sherman, D.M. (1994) *Goat Medicine.* Lea & Febiger, Philadelphia.

Nutrition

AFRC Technical Committee on Responses to Nutrients (1998) *The Nutrition of Goats.* Report No. 10. CAB International, Wallingford.

British Goat Society (1997) *Feeding Goats, a Modern Guide to Healthy Nutrition.* British Goat Society, Bovey Tracey.

National Research Council (1981) *Nutrient Requirements of Goats. Nutrient Requirements of Domestic Animals*, No. 15. National Academy Press, Washington, DC.

Orskov, B. (1987) *The Feeding of Ruminants, Principles and Practice.* Chalcombe Publications, Canterbury.

Reproduction

Artificial Breeding in Sheep and Goats (1987) No. 96. Proc. Univ. Sydney Post Grad. Found. Vet. Sci., Sydney, Australia.

Embryo Transfer/Goats and Sheep (1989) No. 127. Proc. Univ. Sydney Post Grad. Found. Vet. Sci., Sydney, Australia.

Evans, G. and Maxwell, W.M.C. (1987) *Salamon's Artificial Insemination of Sheep and Goats.* Butterworths, London.

Index